Malaria Frontline

Malaria Frontline

AUSTRALIAN ARMY RESEARCH
DURING WORLD WAR II

Tony Sweeney

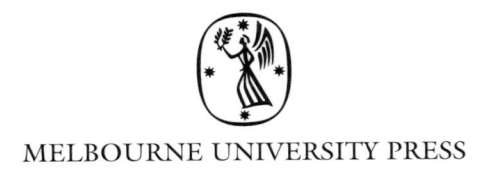

MELBOURNE UNIVERSITY PRESS

MELBOURNE UNIVERSITY PRESS
(an imprint of Melbourne University Publishing)
PO Box 1167, Carlton, Victoria 3053, Australia
mup-info@unimelb.edu.au
www.mup.com.au

First published 2003
Text © A. W. Sweeney 2003
Design and typography © Melbourne University Publishing 2003

This book is copyright. Apart from any use permitted under the *Copyright Act 1968* and subsequent amendments, no part may be reproduced, stored in a retrieval system or transmitted by any means or process whatsoever without the prior written permission of the publishers.

Designed by Alice Graphics
Typeset in Malaysia by Syarikat Seng Teik Sdn. Bhd.
Printed in Australia by Openbook Print

National Library of Australia Cataloguing-in-Publication entry

Sweeney, Tony, 1941– .
Malaria frontline: Australian Army malaria research during World War II.
Bibliography.
Includes index.
ISBN 0 522 85033 2.

1. Australia. Army. Land Headquarters Medical Research Unit. 2. Malaria—Research—Australia. 3. World War, 1939–1945—Health aspects—Australia. 4. World War, 1939–1945—Medical care—Australia. I. Title.

940.547594

Publication of this work was assisted by a generous contribution from the Commonwealth Department of Veterans' Affairs.

*To Katie,
for putting up with me*

Foreword

THE PURPOSE OF THIS BOOK is to place on record, in the public domain, an account of the major research into malaria carried out by the Australian Army during World War II and its unique contribution to the success of the Allied Forces in the Pacific Area. The research work carried out, its results and application are described in detail. The book encompasses its background, relationship to malaria research being carried out in the United States of America and the United Kingdom at the time, and its dependence upon the large number of volunteers who experienced malaria during the clinical trials.

In 1977 I presented a brief account of this research work as an example of successful problem solving in a lecture given at the McMaster Medical School, Hamilton, Ontario. I said it was successful because 'the right man was in the right place at the right time'. That man was Neil Hamilton Fairley, who was in the Australian Army directing a research unit at Cairns when a malaria epidemic occurred in the Australian armed forces operating in the South West Pacific Area during World War II. The malaria epidemic was controlled so the problem was solved, and during the process significant additions were made to the scientific knowledge of malaria infections in humans. A remarkable feature of the malaria research unit was the speed with which it was established and began carrying out multidisciplinary research involving entomology, parasitology, haematology, biochemistry, drug estimations and, above all, drug trials on volunteers—all within a few months of conception. Such a multidisciplinary approach is taken for granted now, but in those days was very rare indeed, particularly in war time. In *Malaria Frontline*, Tony Sweeney tells the whole story.

I was in charge of the Cairns unit for a little over two years, after taking over from Major Roderick R. Andrew, and the experience was unforgettable. I took over a wonderful research team of pathologists, entomologists, clinicians, nurses, support staff and volunteers. It was a unique experience to be committed full-time to the solution of a single broad but specific problem with the support of the most senior people in the armed forces who ensured that we could obtain what we needed. As is described in the book, some enormous obstacles had to be overcome before the highly complicated studies needed could be carried out—for example, the breeding of large numbers of mosquitoes of the appropriate type and their infection with malaria at the required times. More important still, there was a steady stream of volunteers coming to the unit to take part in the clinical trials—they quickly saw what malaria attacks could be like, and then experienced them. They regarded their role as of major importance in helping their friends and colleagues deal with the malaria that they faced in action—their spirit was admirable.

Neil Fairley visited the unit regularly for detailed discussion, writing, and planning of new programs based on his wide-ranging visits in the South West Pacific area, the United States and the United Kingdom, and from time to time he brought senior officers of the Allied Forces with him to show them how the unit worked. He regularly made a point of having personal meetings (which were greatly appreciated) with the heads of the various sections of the unit. Among the specific outcomes of these visits was the development of plans for studying new drugs that had been shown to be safe for administration to humans before they were sent to us to be tested in the volunteers. He also took the opportunity to brief us on results of studies, albeit limited, being carried out overseas. There was no current relevant journal in the unit, and of course no detailed data on malaria research were published at the time.

A. W. Sweeney, MSc Agr PhD, Lieutenant Colonel (retired), entomologist, was in command of the Army Malaria Research Unit at Ingleburn, New South Wales, and is unusually well qualified to have undertaken the huge task of research, collation of material and authorship of this book. He has put the whole story together into a readable and informative narrative based on 'hard data', and has not avoided contentious issues. His major contribution to medical history is to place the unique Australian malaria research effort in perspective in relation to the control of malaria in the Allied Forces during World War II and to the research being carried out simultaneously in the United States and United Kingdom. The Cairns unit was the only such centre using mosquito-transmitted New Guinea strains of malaria parasites in healthy Army volunteers living in a tropical environment. It was also the only place where potential protective and therapeutic antimalarial drugs could be tested under 'field conditions' and within an appropriate time scale—answers could be obtained in a matter of a few weeks rather than six or more months as in the United States. This unique capacity was recognised at the time, and was the basis for requests to test 'new' drugs from both the United States and the United Kingdom.

Readers will probably ask the question 'Could you do these studies now?' This was the first question put to me in Hamilton in 1977 on the occasion of my lecture there: The answer I gave then was 'no', and I would still say it is no unless major and critical changes in the research program were made, which could well have made it less effective.

Hepatitis B was not prevalent in the Australian Army and the definitive studies on its transmission were not done until 1944.[1] Hepatitis C was unknown and apparently absent from the Australian Army as was HIV infection. All members of the unit, particularly the volunteers, were imbued with the imperative of winning the war and avoiding an invasion of Australia. For that reason it was critical to have available enough fit subjects in whom the usefulness of chemoprophylactic drugs could be studied. In the absence of the immediate threat of the war with Japan, I doubt whether the motive would be there. In addition to that motive for working extraordinarily long hours, days, and weeks, there had to be a leader, and an opportunity to establish a unit with excellent personnel and appropriate facilities without major financial restrictions. Perhaps terrorist attacks such as the recent ones on New York and Washington might provide a milieu in which another such unit could function —this time to deal with the issues of bio-terrorism.

C. R. B. Blackburn
Professor Emeritus

Contents

Foreword, by C. R. B. Blackburn — vii
Acknowledgements — xvii
Conversions — xxi

Prologue   Escape from Rabaul — 1
1   War and Malaria — 10
2   Critical Shortages of Antimalarial Supplies — 18
3   Our Worst Enemy — 27
4   Anti Sweat — 36
5   Priority Neill — 43
6   Neil Desperandum — 53
7   Atebrin — 62
8   The Atherton Conference — 77
9   Subinoculation — 86
10   Setbacks and Dilemmas in the US Program — 94
11   Captured from the Enemy — 104
12   'SB' — 115
13   The Birth of Chloroquine — 128
14   The Problem of Vivax — 137
15   Reorientation of the US Program — 147
16   The Answer to the Maiden's Prayer — 156
17   The Possibility of an 'X' Factor — 167
18   Paludrine — 191
19   Mode of Action — 203
20   Tolerance and Immunity — 214

21	Guinea Pigs	223
22	The Military Value of the Cairns Research	239
23	A Glorious Gamble in Science	250
24	Press Reports	258
Epilogue	The Rise of Drug Resistance	264
Appendix 1	Nominal Roll of Volunteers	272
Appendix 2	Nominal Roll of Donors	294
Appendix 3	Nominal Roll of Staff	302
Appendix 4	Summary of Findings from Repatriation Medical Authority Workshop, July 1999	305
Glossary		309
Abbreviations		314
Notes		317
Bibliography		340
Index		348

Illustrations

Plates

Neil Hamilton Fairley, World War I   *following* 74
Australian Academy of Science

Brigadier Neil Hamilton Fairley, Director of Medicine Australian Army Medical Corps, World War II
Australian Academy of Science

Australian infantry on patrol in the Milne Bay area
Australian War Memorial negative number 013335

Lieutenant Colonel Ted Ford
Ms D. Ford

Buildings and tents of the Malaria Experimental Group at 5 Australian Camp Hospital, Cairns
Mrs. R. Adams

Major Richard Andrew
The late Professor R. R. Andrew

Major Jo Mackerras (oil painting by Nora Heysen)
Australian War Memorial accession number 24395

Lieutenant Colonel Ruthven Blackburn (oil painting by Nora Heysen)
Australian War Memorial accession number 24376

Collecting mosquito larvae in a swamp near Cairns for malaria experiments   *following* 106
Australian Academy of Science

Field-collected mosquito larvae in rearing dishes being fed with Farex baby food
Australian Academy of Science

Lieutenant Tom Lemerle collecting mosquito pupae from larval rearing dishes (oil painting by Nora Heysen)
Australian War Memorial accession number 24374

Private Patricia Johnson sorting mosquito cages used for feeding female mosquitoes on carriers and volunteers for experimental transmission of malaria
Australian Academy of Science

xiv *Illustrations*

Staff Sergeant Jack McNamara removing adult mosquitoes from a cage
Australian War Memorial accession number F07251 (still from movie film)

Gunner Gilbert Seaton (sketch by Nora Heysen)
Australian War Memorial accession number 24269

Volunteer (Corporal James Clune) receiving a regulated number of bites from infected mosquitoes
Australian Academy of Science

The subinoculation technique: transmission of malaria by direct blood transfusion from infected donor to recipient volunteer
Australian War Memorial accession number F07251 (still from movie film)

Major Jo Mackerras and entomology staff examining mosquito salivary glands under the compound microscope *following* 138
Australian Academy of Science

Entomology staff LHQ Medical Research Unit with guinea pigs used for mosquito feeding
Australian Academy of Science

Pathology staff, LHQ Medical Research Unit
Australian Academy of Science

Routine blood collection from malaria-infected volunteers
Australian Academy of Science

Private Harry Harper staining blood slides taken from volunteers before examination under the microscope
Australian Academy of Science

War artist Nora Heysen sketching Lieutenant Max Swan
The late T. A. Akhurst

Lieutenant Max Swan examining blood slides under the microscope (sketch by Nora Heysen)
Australian War Memorial accession number 24304

Headquarters staff, LHQ Medical Research Unit *following* 170
Australian Academy of Science

Nursing staff, LHQ Medical Research Unit
Australian Academy of Science

Lieutenant Colonel Ruthven Blackburn, Major Jo Mackerras, Brigadier Neil Hamilton Fairley
Emeritus Professor C. R. Blackburn

American malaria scientists attached to US 42 General Hospital, Brisbane
Professor W. Trager

Lieutenant Ken Pope taking a blood sample from volunteer Sergeant L. T. Goble for atebrin estimation (sketch by Nora Heysen)
Australian War Memorial accession number 24300

Participants, 'Prevention of Disease in Tropical Warfare' conference, Atherton, Queensland, June 1944
Australian Academy of Science

Lieutenant Colonel Ian Mackerras and Major John Tonge
Mrs R. Adams

Major Jo Mackerras and Warrant Officer Bill Winterbottom *following* 234
Australian Academy of Science

Staff of LHQ Medical Research Unit, Christmas 1944
Australian Academy of Science

'The little yellow atebrin tablet issued by an officer was taken with a great deal of ceremony'
John Sands Pty Ltd

Lieutenant J. J. Garrick placing atebrin tablets in the mouths of his men during the daily 'atebrin parade'
Australian War Memorial negative number 094177

Private J. P. Merity heeding the anti-malaria sign to roll down sleeves after 1830 hours
Australian War Memorial negative number 089678

Brigadier Neil Hamilton Fairley, Brigadier J. A. Sinton VC and Lieutenant Colonel Ruthven Blackburn, June 1945
Emeritus Professor C. R. Blackburn

Captain Robert Black and the mobile laboratory in which he grew malaria parasites in test tubes
Australian Academy of Science

'Los Medicos' (ink sketch by Gunner Donald Friend)
National Library of Australia MS 5959/16/64

Soldiers who have volunteered for malaria research lining up for inspection in a mosquito-proof ward *following* 266
Australian Academy of Science

Drug parade
Australian Academy of Science

AAMWS Nursing orderly (Private Hazel Lugge) sponging a volunteer (Private Ken Glover) suffering an attack of malaria (oil painting by Nora Heysen)
Australian War Memorial accession number 24375

Volunteers pausing by a waterfall during a march up the railroad track from Cairns to the Atherton Tablelands
E. E. Viant

Volunteers in the library at LHQ Medical Research Unit
Australian Academy of Science

Volunteers boarding a truck to spend a day at the beach
Australian Academy of Science

Professor Sir Neil Hamilton Fairley (oil painting by William Dargie)
Hans Hamilton Fairley

Figures

1	Map showing track followed by Major Palmer and others from Rabaul	5
2	The malaria cycle	13
3	South West Pacific theatre of operations, 1942–45	29
4	Plan of experiments at Cairns for mosquito-transmitted malaria	45
5	Plan of experiments at Rocky Creek, Atherton Tablelands, for blood-induced malaria	46
6	LHQ Medical Research Unit, Cairns, floor plan	68
7	'This was our longest and dearest campaign' *Salt*, vol 9, no 1, 11 September 1944, pp. 10–14	84
8	Experiment to investigate the length of time that sporozoites remain in the bloodstream	89
9	The timing of experiments on SN-6911 and SN-7618 at Cairns and Atlanta	145
10	Area of operations during the Aitape–Wewak campaign	168
11	Monthly malaria incidence among troops of 6th Australian Division in the Aitape–Wewak area during 1945	173
12	Sites of action of antimalarial drugs in mosquitoes and humans determined by experiments at Cairns	208
13	Effects of paludrine on the mosquito stages of *Plasmodium falciparum*	209
14	Clinical experiments on naturally acquired immunity to vivax malaria	217
15	Clinical experiments on the development of immunity to vivax malaria	220
16	Commander-in-Chief's card signed by General Blamey, awarded to Ted Viant E. E. Viant	235
17	Monthly incidence of malaria in Australian troops on overseas operations, December 1943 to September 1945	240

Tables

1	Chronology of first series of Cairns experiments with sulphonamide drugs, and sulphonamides combined with atebrin	57
2	Cairns experiments with M.4888, first series	165
3	Experiment AW-1: first documented evidence of drug-resistant malaria	181

Acknowledgements

My interest in malaria and the problems it caused during World War II began in 1963. At that time debris from the military campaigns was evident throughout the New Guinea islands, particularly in Rabaul, the main town in the region, where I was based as entomologist for the malaria control program. Bomb craters from American air raids on this major Japanese base still provided prolific breeding sites for *Anopheles* malaria vectors 20 years after the war. This was the location of the Australian Army's first encounters with two enemies in the South West Pacific: the armed forces of Japan, and malaria. For the war to be won both foes had to be defeated. The scientific articles of Brigadier Sir Neil Hamilton Fairley's research team from the Land Headquarters Medical Research Unit at Cairns, which were published in medical journals after the war, formed a significant part of my introduction to the job. These documented the scientific basis of the fight against malaria that underpinned the successful outcomes of the military campaigns.

In early 1970 I returned to Australia and joined the Army to take up an appointment at 1 Malaria Research Laboratory (later the Army Malaria Research Unit). This laboratory was formed to continue the pioneering work at Cairns in order to face the renewed malaria threat to our forces during the Vietnam War. I studied the published record again, and came to appreciate the magnitude of the Australian Army's wartime contribution to the malaria problem. The research group at Cairns undertook the largest single series of clinical trials of human malaria that has ever been undertaken. In less than three years they discovered more about the drug control of malaria than had been found out in the previous 50 years—and more than would be discovered in the next 20. How had this extraordinary achievement been accomplished?

Scientific papers describe the outcomes of research in a logical sequence: introduction, materials and methods, results, and discussion. This is the tried and proven method of reporting to the scientific community what has been accomplished in a particular study in relation to pre-existing knowledge. However, such publications do not provide a complete account of all the milestones that led to a particular discovery. Research projects rarely proceed as originally planned. Avenues of investigation that initially appear promising often lead to dead ends or unexpected detours, which could not have been foreseen at the outset. Negative or inconclusive results are often omitted or mentioned briefly, so that it is not possible to understand the chronological sequence of significant intermediate steps (positive, negative, or uncertain) that happened along the way. Such information is crucial to an historical appreciation of how a particular scientific undertaking was carried out. This deficiency is apparent in the publications that emanated from the Land Headquarters Medical Research Unit. There is a useful summary in the official history by Allan S. Walker, but the full story has not previously been published.

Fortunately, the extensive correspondence, reports, and data-sheets in the Fairley Papers at the Basser Library, Australian Academy of Sciences, provided the raw material from which I was able to understand the circumstances that led to the formation of the research group, and to appreciate how the remarkable experimental program was planned and executed. I am very grateful to the Basser Librarian, Rosanne Walker. For more than a decade she has helped me through the archival labyrinth.

I was extremely fortunate to obtain the wholehearted encouragement of Emeritus Professor Ruthven Blackburn when I started the background research to this account in 1990. As Commanding Officer of the unit from February 1944 until the last experiments were completed in April 1946, his contribution to the success of the enterprise was second only to that of Fairley himself. His progress reports and correspondence form a substantial component of the documentary record. With Ruthven's unfailing guidance I have attempted to trace the sequential development of experiments, and to see how the interim results were viewed by the research team as the work progressed. He has been my mentor and staunchest supporter over the last 12 years, not only by enabling me to comprehend the true significance of cryptic archival references, but also by assisting with clinical interpretation of the results. Furthermore, he carefully scrutinised each draft of every chapter and provided a wealth of constructive comments that have substantially improved the quality of this book.

Before his death in 1995 Emeritus Professor Rod Andrew provided very useful background information about the early days at 5 Australian Camp Hospital during his tenure as Officer in Command of the Malaria Experimental Group. I am indebted to the late Dr Max Swan, the first laboratory technician appointed to the experimental group and the longest serving member of the unit. Soon after I contacted him in 1991 I received in the mail two audiotapes on which he had recorded his memories at Cairns. His candid comments on life in the unit acted as a catalyst that spurred me on to complete this book. Max's tapes are now lodged with the Fairley Papers. My thanks are due to Mrs Rosemary Adams (née Gore). As senior clerk in the orderly room her reminiscences on the administration of the unit and on various personalities of the group were most helpful. I wish to acknowledge the following members of the unit who also assisted my enquiries: the late Tom Akhurst, Dr Don Colless, Hazel Crow (née Lugge), Joyce Goodwin (née Bullock), George Merritt, and Dr John Tonge.

I owe much to Ted Viant. The personal story of his wartime experiences, which he wrote for his family, contains a lucid and balanced account of his service as a volunteer at Cairns during 1944. During many conversations with Ted over the last decade I have gained an appreciation of what it was like to be an experimental subject at the Land Headquarters Medical Research Unit. Moreover, he has made a very substantial contribution to this book by compiling, at his own expense, the first computerised list of the participants in the Australian wartime malaria experiments. This formed the draft database from which the nominal rolls of volunteers and donors, attached as appendices to this book, were derived. I am grateful to Ken Glover and Ray Whiteley, who provided lively reminiscences of their experiences as volunteers during the last series of long-term experiments at Cairns during 1945.

The medical historian Brendan O'Keefe provided generous assistance during the course of my research. He helped me access relevant material in the Australian War Memorial and Australian Archives in Canberra. I am particularly grateful for his find of some notebooks and other original records from the Cairns unit, now lodged in the Fairley Papers, which clarified the chronology of experiments undertaken in 1945. Chris Shanahan, of Defence Sydney, is a tireless worker who has helped considerably by tracking down obscure references in journals, books and newspaper articles. Professor Frank Fenner provided most useful background information on the malaria problem from the viewpoint of a wartime malariologist in New Guinea. Dr S. J. Goulston gave me an account of his time in London during 1944–45 when he accompanied Fairley during visits and meetings with British medical scientists. Thanks are also due to Brenda Heagney, Librarian of the History of Medicine Library, Royal Australasian College of Physicians in Sydney, who facilitated my search of the papers of Sir Edward Ford.

I set out to write this book from a global rather than a parochial perspective. I wished to portray the impact of the wartime research at Cairns on the continuing world fight against malaria. In order to do this I needed to understand the genesis and development of the massive wartime efforts in the USA, as well as the smaller but equally important program in Britain, devoted to the search for new antimalarial drugs. Professor William Trager, of Rockefeller University, New York, was of great assistance by providing recollections of his wartime experiences as a US Army malaria scientist in Australia and New Guinea. Professor Robert Joy, of the Uniformed Services University of the Health Sciences in Maryland, alerted me to the work of Dr Mary Ellen Condon-Rall of the US

Army Center of Military History in Washington, DC. She generously provided some very relevant material, including an indexed list of the wartime reports of the Board for the Co-ordination of Malarial Studies and guided me to the archives section of the National Academy of Sciences in Washington. This repository has all the reports and minutes of the US Board meetings, as well as many wartime British reports, and some documents pertaining to the research at Cairns that are not in the Fairley Papers. I wish to thank Janice Goldbloom, of the Archives Section, NAS, for her assistance during my visits to Washington in 1993 and 1994.

However, there were still some gaps in the story, particularly to do with Fairley's visit to Java during his return from the Middle East and his many duty tours to Cairns and New Guinea, as well to two extended visits to the USA and Britain in 1942 and 1944–45. I am most grateful to Dr James Hamilton Fairley of Caversham, Reading, UK, who answered my queries and generously provided copies of his father's diary entries. He later deposited the original diaries and other important documents and photographs in the Fairley Papers. This new information provided an additional window through which to view Fairley's contribution to the malaria problem, as well as to throw new light on how the problem was dealt with by Australia, the USA and Britain at key stages during the war.

Dr Keith Horsley, Medical Services Advisor, Department of Veterans' Affairs, Canberra, has been of great help during the last three years. He strongly advocated that the Department of Veterans' Affairs should support the publication of this book, and, with the capable assistance of Fiona Tuckwell, he paved the way for this to happen. I am grateful to Bob Connolly, Department of Veterans' Affairs, Brisbane, and Alistair Kerr, Central Army Records Office, Melbourne, for their help in finalising the nominal rolls in the appendices.

The staff of Melbourne University Press have been most helpful. I owe a particular debt to Bernadette Hince whose keen editorial eye found many inconsistencies in the text. Finally, I would like to thank my wife Kay for her patience, support and understanding.

Tony Sweeney

Conversions

1 tonne/1000 kilograms	= .98 tons
1 kilogram	= 2.2 pounds
1 gram/1 000 000μg	= 0.035 ounces
1 litre	= 1.76 pints
1 ml	= 0.03 fluid ounces
1 km	= 0.62 miles
1 metre	= 3.28 feet
100°C	= 212°F
37°C	= 98.6°F

Plasmodium falciparum and *P. vivax* are common in many tropical areas of the world where they pose serious threats to public health. Nowadays, the diseases caused by them are termed falciparum malaria and vivax malaria, but until the end of World War II they were commonly called malignant tertian (MT) malaria and benign tertian (BT) malaria, respectively.

Prologue
Escape from Rabaul

BEFORE THE 1994 volcanic eruption Rabaul was one of the most picturesque ports of the South Pacific. Situated within five degrees of the equator on the north-eastern extremity of New Britain, a banana-shaped island 480 km in length, it epitomised the best of the tropics. The town lies within the rim of an ancient volcanic crater that forms a steeply sloping irregular ridge surrounding the bay. The perennially green vegetation contrasts with the black sand beaches and the tranquil blue water of Simpson Harbour—one of the most secure and commodious natural anchorages in the Pacific. This lush tropical environment is complemented by the elegant symmetry of the three volcanic peaks—the Mother, North Daughter and South Daughter—overlooking the town. Formerly the capital of German New Guinea, it became part of the Mandated Territory of New Guinea under Australian control after World War I. But it was not a good place for an Australian to be in January 1942.

Following the attack on Pearl Harbor on 7 December 1941 the Japanese advanced rapidly into Malaysia and the Philippines. Their powerful naval and land forces were in a position to expand, at will, into the islands of the South Pacific and threaten the mainland of Australia. Allied forces in the area at this time were few and isolated. The Rabaul garrison of approximately 1400 troops comprised the 2/22 Battalion of the 23rd Brigade, AIF, under Lieutenant Colonel H. H. Carr, together with a militia detachment of the New Guinea Volunteer Rifles, a coastal defence battery, two obsolete anti-aircraft guns, an anti-tank battery and support troops. Their role was to protect the airfield and seaplane anchorage that constituted a link in the chain of forward bases to the north of Australia. There were plans to increase these units to the equivalent of a brigade group and a new commander, Colonel J. J. Scanlan, arrived in October 1941 to prepare for this expansion. However, events moved too rapidly for this scheme to be implemented. The Australian military authorities accepted that the existing garrison was not sufficient to withstand a large-scale Japanese assault, but they felt that the island should not be given up without a fight. The problem with this approach was that the force was too small to mount any kind of effective defence against a determined land attack supported by strong naval and air units.[1]

The coastal defence battery was sited at Praed Point on the northern approach to the harbour at the foot of the South Daughter. The anti-aircraft guns, on a ridge adjacent to the North Daughter, had good all-round visibility to cover both northern and southern approaches to the harbour. The town and Lakunai airfield were on a strip of flat land on the north side of Simpson Harbour between the base of the North Daughter and the Mother. There are numerous gently sloping beaches in the vicinity, both inside and outside the harbour, which could provide suitable landing points for a seaborne invasion. The Australian troops were too few in number to cover all possible approaches, and the bulk of them were initially deployed adjacent to the town and airfield. If they made a stand in these positions against a superior force, they would run the risk of being quickly overrun. The vulnerable situation of the force was apparent to some of the officers and men. There were suggestions that a portion of the two year's supply of rations, together with ammunition and other essential supplies, should be hidden in the mountains to the west where they could be retrieved in the event of a withdrawal. This proposal was not seriously considered as there were no contingency plans for retreat into the jungle. In fact, all such ideas were actively discouraged by Colonel Scanlan, who issued an order on New Year's Day 1942 that the men should fight to the last, with the injunction 'there shall be no thought of withdrawal'.

Four Hudson bombers and 10 Wirraway fighters were sent to provide air support to the force in December 1941. During the same month individual Japanese planes began to fly over the area at a great height. The first air raid, by 22 bombers flying at high altitude, was on 4 January 1942. This caused little damage, as did several other high-level raids made in the following two weeks, but the worst was yet to come. On 20 January the garrison was attacked by more than 100 aircraft. The obsolete Wirraways were no match for the superior Zero fighters: three were quickly shot down; while another three were damaged but managed to crash land. The enemy bombers and fighters then made unopposed low-level passes over the harbour, strafing ships, troop concentrations and installations. At the end of the raid only one Hudson and two Wirraways remained unscathed, and they were moved to Vunakanau, the second airfield in the area, approximately 16 km south of the town.

There were no air raids on the following day but a group of enemy cruisers were reported off the west coast of New Ireland steaming towards Rabaul, and Scanlan ordered Carr to move from the exposed positions around the harbour to avoid being destroyed by naval gunfire. The remaining aircraft were flown to Lae and the airfields were prepared for demolition. Early on 22 January dive bombers destroyed the battery at Praed Point, and Scanlan ordered that the town be evacuated. The troops were redeployed on the south side of the bay and at Vunakanau in order to prevent the possibility of part of the force being isolated and cut off if the enemy landed within the harbour. Unfortunately, the men had originally been told that the move was to be considered 'as an exercise only', so most left behind important equipment, including emergency rations, mosquito nets and their personal supplies of the antimalarial drug quinine. This was to have serious consequences for the health and survival of those who avoided capture.

The first enemy landings in the harbour occurred around 1 a.m. on 23 January. Enemy troops landed from barges in front of the Australian positions around 2.30 a.m., where they were held back until just before dawn with small arms and mortar fire. When the sun came up, more than 30 enemy ships were in the harbour, some still discharging troops into landing barges while others began to fire on the Australian positions. The men around Vunakanau came under constant dive bombing and strafing attacks. Later in the morning the entire Australian defensive positions became completely untenable as the enemy advanced in great strength with air and naval gunfire support. Amidst considerable confusion, the various platoons and companies disengaged and fell back to the south-west, some by road in trucks and others on foot through the bush. Scanlan ordered Carr to withdraw, saying that 'it is now every man for himself'. The latter took this to mean to withdraw in small parties, but these orders were somewhat academic as there was no effective command and control of the overall situation. Most of the men were already isolated in groups of various sizes and were acting independently, either on their own initiative, or under their subunit commanders.

Medical support for the garrison consisted of a detachment of 2/10 Australian Field Ambulance under the command of Major E. C. (Ted) Palmer, comprising two officers and 22 other ranks together with six nursing sisters. There was also a regimental medical officer (RMO) of the 2/22 Battalion and a part-time RMO (civilian practitioner) of the New Guinea Volunteer Rifles. Major Palmer's detachment did not receive the order to evacuate the town until the afternoon of 22 January, when they were instructed to proceed to Vunapope Mission Hospital at Kokopo, 32 km around the coast on the southern side of the bay. On the morning of 23 January he decided to leave all of the patients in the care of the four civilian doctors and the army nurses at the mission hospital.

He then led Medical Corps personnel to join the force in the Vunakanau area. Palmer later wrote:

> I had considered that the greatest probability was that those of us who were alive would be prisoners of war in a short time and had been more concerned with taking equipment for coping with possible wounded. I filled my pack exclusively with medical equipment and distributed the rest amongst . . . the detachment.[2]

The administration in Rabaul had a reserve of two million quinine tablets and had reluctantly handed over 15 000 to Palmer. He gave 5000 to the RMO of 2/22 Battalion and took the remainder with him, together with another 3000–4000 tablets obtained from missions and other sources.

By late afternoon the Australians had been forced from their positions around Vunakanau and had fallen back along the main native tracks into the jungle of the Gazelle Peninsula leading away from Rabaul. The force followed two main lines of withdrawal. One group, which included Battalion Headquarters and the two RMOs, went towards the north coast across the Keravat River, while another group, including Palmer and his medical detachment, headed off across the Warangoi River towards the south coast. There were no vehicular roads at all outside the Rabaul–Kokopo area, which was not to say that the rest of New Britain was a trackless expanse of jungle. Coconut plantations, usually occupied by European managers, were scattered along the bays and inlets of both north and south coasts. There were also a number of mission stations at irregular intervals. The usual method of transport between plantations and missions was by canoe, sailing vessel or motor pinnace. The island was rather thinly inhabited with the local population in villages and hamlets on the coast and scattered throughout the inland mountains. There was a network of rough bush paths linking villages, plantations and mission outstations, though the normal practice was for those paths across mountainous regions to go straight up and down precipitous ridges. Swift-flowing streams and rivers posed a serious hindrance, particularly after heavy rain. A spine of high mountains runs along the length of New Britain so that crossing from the north coast to the south coast was a major difficulty.

Nevertheless, orderly withdrawal along the length of the island was not an impossible task for a force that was well equipped, well supplied, and trained to move through the jungle. It was, however, a perilous undertaking for the troops of the Rabaul garrison who had never patrolled outside the town area. This situation was exacerbated by the fact that none of them had made provision for a long trek through the bush. The first obstacle after leaving the town was the Bainings Range, which extends across the Gazelle Peninsula from coast to coast about 30 km from Rabaul. Many of the peaks are over 1500 metres and the track traversing the range crosses numbers of ridges and valleys 300–500 metres deep without regard for grade. On the third day of walking amongst this inhospitable terrain, through thick jungle, over tracks wet and slippery with intermittent rain, approximately 300 men of the force arrived at Lamingi Catholic Mission in the Central Bainings area (see Fig. 1). They were fed by the missionary, Father Maierhofer, and were able to sleep for a night under shelter

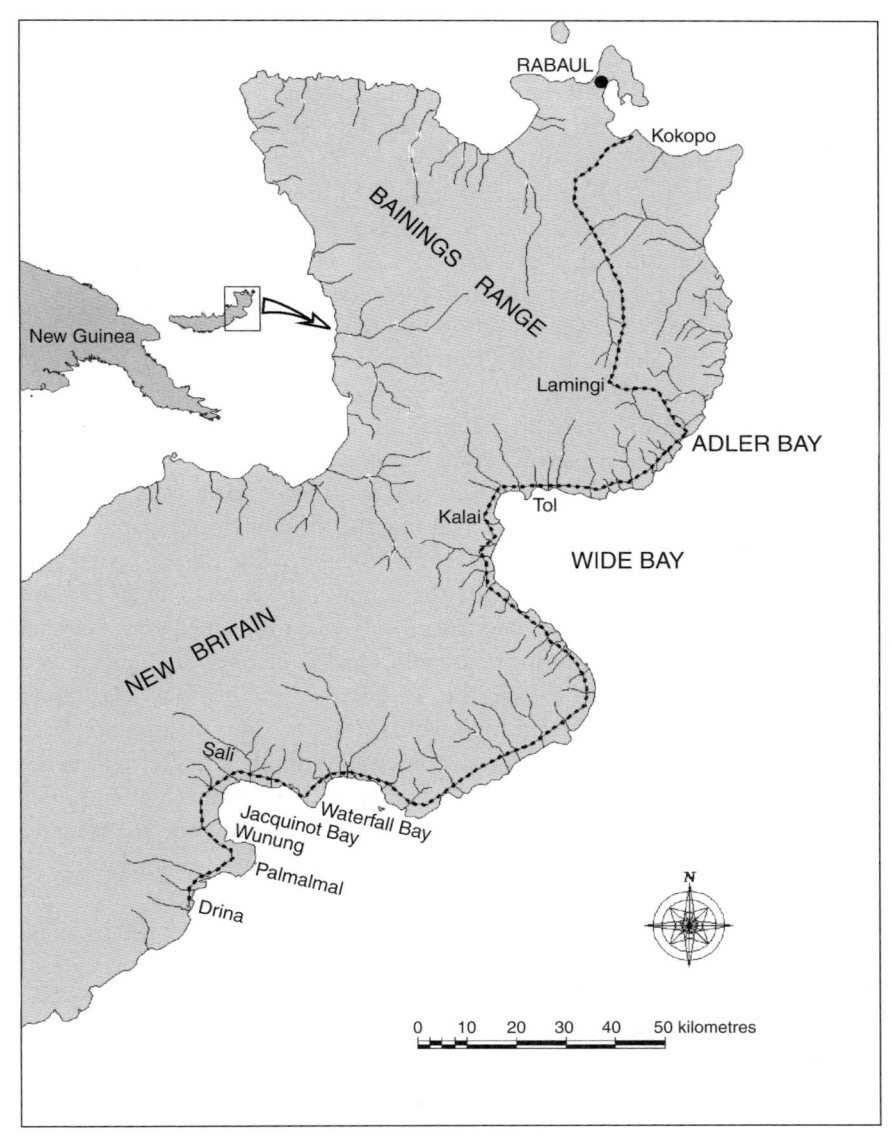

Fig. 1 Map showing track followed by Major Palmer and survivors of 2/22 Battalion from Rabaul along the south coast of New Britain, January–April 1942

before heading down the range to the south coast. Palmer's detachment provided treatment for minor injuries of all troops passing through and then divided into two parties—the larger medical group moving on, and a smaller group remaining for an extra day to tend to any stragglers who might come through.

After a further three days travelling over very rough country on ill-defined tracks they reached Adler Bay, about halfway along the south coast of the Gazelle Peninsula. The general idea at this stage was to follow the coast southwest to Wide Bay as there were several plantations and a mission where it was hoped that food would be plentiful. By this time small parties of men were spread out over 30–50 km of coast. Major W. T. Owen, of 2/22 Battalion, decided to muster the troops together at Kalai Mission on the southern side of Wide Bay, so he pushed ahead with a small group including Palmer. Most of the troops were very exhausted, as even the track down the coast was very hilly and difficult, and many had abandoned their rifles coming across the mountains.

On 3 February, while the move towards Kalai was in progress, six landing barges of Japanese landed at Tol Plantation in the central part of Wide Bay. About 20 men surrendered on the beach as soon as the Japanese landed, and many others apparently made little attempt to escape. Many of those coming behind walked into enemy patrols before they could be warned of their presence in the area. Those who surrendered on the beach were taken back to Rabaul but the remainder (about 140) were tied together in groups and marched into the jungle where they were either bayoneted or shot. The forward party and some other groups managed to elude the enemy patrols and Palmer did not learn of the massacre until two days afterwards when four men with bayonet wounds were brought to him for treatment. One, a member of Palmer's own unit—2/10 Field Ambulance—said that 14 others of the medical detachment had been killed. The Japanese left for Rabaul on the day after the massacre with the captured officers and men who surrendered on the beach after telling the local villagers that they would return in a week. The prospect of summary execution indicated to the survivors that capture was clearly not an attractive option, so they were reconciled to moving further down the coast in search of food, even though most felt that there was little prospect of rescue.

The first case of malaria occurred on 6 February, shortly after the Japanese left Tol. This man was promptly treated by Palmer with a five-day course of 20 quinine tablets.[3] Palmer collected all the quinine he could from the troops and, with what he carried himself, his inventory then amounted to around 3000 tablets.

On 10 February he started down the coast with a party of 25 men including the wounded. After 10 days they arrived at Waterfall Bay where there was a sawmill that was supposed to have a radio transmitter. The radio was smashed, and the party found that all five plantations they passed on the way had been looted. In every house they found an empty quinine bottle. About half a dozen of Palmer's group developed malaria and were treated with quinine as they moved further down the coast to Jacquinot Bay. On arriving at Sali village on the north side of the bay they came across a number of troops held up by sickness. They were told that three men had died the previous day from what Palmer believed was malaria. Two others were critically ill with the disease—one comatose, and the other delirious. Both died the next day. Lieutenant D. M. (David) Selby, Officer Commanding the anti-aircraft detachment at Rabaul, travelled with the medical party on this part of the trek. He later published a vivid account of his experiences:

> I saw for the first time the pathetic coma vigil which almost invariably precedes death from malaria . . . They lay in a state of coma, their faces yellow, lips parted, noses waxen and pinched and their eyes wide open and staring, staring into space, as though looking for those Catalinas which would never come.[4]

The group at Sali had small quantities of quinine with them, but had not used it as they thought that the sick men were suffering from scrub typhus. About a quarter of the remainder had malaria, and Palmer gave each of them 20 tablets of quinine to carry out their treatment.

Palmer's party reached Wunung plantation on 23 February; here they met the main body of men under Major Owen, and learned that the Japanese had occupied Gasmata, about 100 km further down the south coast, where there was an airstrip. They decided to stay near Jacquinot Bay, as there was a reasonable amount of local food in the area, and because continued movement along the coast towards Gasmata might lead to capture. About 100 troops had already arrived and others were still on their way, so Palmer and his assistants remained with the sick at Wunung while the main body went on to Drina plantation, 20 km further on, where there was also a fair amount of food. Considerable assistance was provided by Father T. Harris, an Australian missionary at Mal Mal mission, but the problem of malaria increased despite the rest and better conditions. Palmer later wrote:

> On the night of our arrival . . . there were two men apparently moribund. One was practically unconscious, unable to speak and with incontinence of urine and faeces. With a great deal of difficulty he was induced to put out his tongue and a quinine bisulphate tablet put on it, water poured into his mouth from a water bottle, and he was finally forced to swallow it by forcibly opening and closing his mouth. Now the process was repeated with a second tablet. The other man was persuaded with difficulty to swallow tablets (2). Next morning the comatose man was quite sensible, said he felt fairly well and ate some food. The other man was somewhat improved. Both subsequently recovered.[5]

The main party at Drina was in a similar state: two died of malaria on the track, another two died on the night of their arrival, and several others were critically ill. Palmer sent a quantity of quinine there, along with written instructions for its use, with one of the officers. The drug was to be given only to men with temperatures of 39°C or over, at a dose of four tablets daily for four days, and a written record of their course was to be kept. During the following fortnight Palmer visited Drina for a few days each week. Forty to fifty men were treated according to his instructions but none died.

By this time the supply of quinine had diminished considerably and, with no prospect of replenishing it, Palmer decided that it would be impossible to continue treatment indefinitely on the same dosage schedule. He reserved the meagre amount of the drug remaining for cases where he thought the patient would die without it, and then gave it only in small amounts to tide the man over his crisis. Another man died during the next week, at which time there was always about a third of the men with fever, some lasting for days on end. Three other men died during March. The immediate cause of two of these deaths was dysentery, but Palmer thought that concurrent malaria was a major factor and that they might have been saved if he had enough quinine to give them. Over the same period he managed to save the lives of two other men with cerebral malaria. Lieutenant Selby described the devotion with which Palmer cared for the sick and wounded. On the way down the coast he invariably refused to touch his evening meal until he had ministered to every one of his patients. Selby said that he 'positively bullied [one man] into living, forcing him to eat and to swallow his quinine . . . until finally [he] did not dare to die'.[6]

By the end of March the physical condition of most troops in the Jacquinot Bay area was very bad. It was difficult to find sufficient men to do simple routine chores such as carrying water and cooking. To dig a grave required almost all the fit men available. In a report dated 28 March Palmer noted that everyone had malaria, with 90 per cent suffering two or more recurrences, and at least 15 per cent being so debilitated that they would not remain alive for more than a few weeks.

On 5 April 1942 the launch *Mascot*, with an officer and two signallers on board, arrived in Jacquinot Bay. Their instructions were to find survivors of the Rabaul garrison and to transmit the details to Port Moresby by radio so that a rescue could be organised. The yacht *Laurabada* was promptly dispatched to New Britain, and the men were ordered to gather at Palmalmal plantation, the designated evacuation point. This was only 16 km from Drina, but they were in such poor condition that this movement took over 12 hours. Tragically, two men died of malaria soon after their arrival at Palmalmal, even though rescue was close at hand. Both were deeply unconscious and Palmer was not able to save them with intravenous or oral medication. A total of 136 men (soldiers with a few civilians) were evacuated on the *Laurabada* to Port Moresby; one man died of dysentery and was buried at sea. All of the survivors were in a greatly debilitated condition and required convalescence for many months in Australia before they were fit for further military operations.

In a report to Colonel Neil Hamilton Fairley, the Australian Army Director of Medicine, Palmer wrote:

> I am unable to assess the importance of vitamin deficiencies in producing the marked physical and in some cases mental deterioration in most of the men. It is possible that lack of vitamins played some part but in view of the well marked difference between those who had little or no malaria and the rest of the troops I feel that malaria was by far the most important factor.[7]

He noted that 33 of the troops who escaped to the south coast of New Britain were definitely known to have died from causes other than enemy action. Three drowned, but, in all of the other recorded cases, death was due to malaria, even though the immediate cause was dysentery in some of them. He observed that 'Deaths would have occurred at a greatly increased rate but for our timely rescue . . . Men without anti-malarial precautions or quinine will begin to die in about a month in hyper malarious areas'.[8]

Major Ted Palmer was clearly one of the unsung heroes of the Australian Army Medical Corps. His report concludes:

> To travel through uninterrupted jungle in pouring rain, along unknown tracks and across an apparently interminable series of steep hills and swiftly flowing streams, with the silence of the jungle broken only by the roar of the rain on the trees, can be the most depressing of experiences.[9]

His meticulously documented clinical observations graphically highlighted the overwhelming importance of malaria as the major health problem confronting military operations in the islands of the South West Pacific.

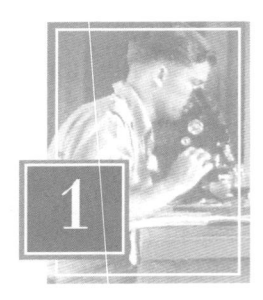

War and Malaria

EXPERIENCES IN MACEDONIA and Palestine during World War I demonstrated dramatically what malaria could do to a modern army. Opposing forces were bogged down in trench warfare in northern Macedonia from 1915 until the end of the war in a protracted campaign in which both sides were ravaged by malaria. The British were initially fortunate in arriving at the end of the year after the malaria season was over but, during the next three summers, it severely limited their capacity for offensive action. Official records cite that out of an average strength of 200 000 there were 162 000 hospitalised malaria casualties during the campaign, compared with 28 000 battle casualties.[1] In the autumn of 1916 the French could put no more than 20 000 men in the line out of a total force of at least six times that number. The official British history of the campaign quotes a senior medical officer, Major General W. H. S. Nickerson:

> In any attack or even in a strategical move, the great question . . . was 'how many fit men can I raise for the prosecution of the operation and . . . how many are likely to fall out with malaria'. Many of our failures would have had a very different end had they been entrusted to fit troops . . . To have brought the campaign to a speedy end, a huge army would have been needed. The bigger the army the quicker it went down with malaria, and we couldn't have had hospitals enough to house half a million men.[2]

The First AIF encountered malaria in September 1915 at Gallipoli, but there were few cases as mosquitoes were rare. The situation was entirely different during the closing stages of the war in Palestine in 1918, when the disease incapacitated almost half of the Desert Mounted Corps. The Jordan Valley was recognised as being highly malarious during the warmer months of the year, and specific steps were taken to minimise the exposure of British and ANZAC troops at the outset of the campaign. Systematic attempts were made to drain the mosquito-breeding swamps and the valley was held lightly by cavalry, predominantly ANZAC Light Horse troops, with the different formations rotated regularly to reduce the chances of infection. In spite of these measures, there were significant numbers of cases throughout the summer of 1918, though the disease was not an overwhelming problem. During the last two weeks of September the force made a rapid advance through the north of the valley to capture Damascus. However, in less than a week the victorious troops were struck by a major epidemic of severe illness. The British 4th Cavalry Division was immobilised with barely enough fit men to feed their horses, and the ANZAC Mounted Division fared little better.

> At Damascus the medical situation had become in the course of a few days about as bad as it was possible to be; accommodation, equipment and medical personnel were hopelessly inadequate for the inrush of cases . . . It was impossible to send all the seriously ill to these hospitals . . . for practically all the sick were serious cases.[3]

Battle casualties during this last campaign of the war in the Middle East were surprisingly light, with less than 200 killed and about 450 wounded. But the sickness casualties amounted to 11 300 (41% of the Corps).[4]

The exact nature of the disease outbreak was not immediately evident. Damascus was experiencing an epidemic of pneumonic influenza, and other diseases—including dysentery, typhus, and cholera—were suspected. The situation was clarified after a malaria diagnostic station was set up in the second week of October: 'All supposed cholera and cerebral cases and a large proportion of those of dysentery, were found malarial'.[5] Most troops diagnosed with influenza were also found to have malaria. The official history of the Australian Army Medical Services concluded that 'simultaneously with an outbreak of pneumonic influenza, a huge rise took place at this moment in the incidence of malignant malaria'.[6] There were 6437 cases of malaria diagnosed by blood examination for the seven weeks of the final offensive (22 per cent of the force), but this was considered to be much less than the true number of cases. For the whole campaign in Sinai and Palestine there were 865 recorded deaths from malaria, with 101 from the AIF. It is sobering to consider what might have happened if the final assault on Damascus had been held up for a week. It is likely that the result may have been a disastrous defeat rather than a decisive victory. The historian C. E. W. Bean recorded that 'for the Light Horse, despite full measures against malaria, this was the hardest service of the war'.[7]

Malaria has always been an intractable problem for humans. Physicians of the ancient world noted the peculiar intensity of its fever (alternating with chills) that recurs at regular intervals. Hippocrates characterised these 'intermittent fevers' according to the days of their recurrence: tertian—every third day; quartan—every fourth day; and quotidian—daily. Later Greek and Roman observers associated the disease with swamps and marshes. They believed that the fever was caused by stagnant waters, and advocated drainage for its control in places like Rome. The name itself is derived from the supposed association with bad air—'mala aria'.

It was not until the latter half of the nineteenth century, after the development of the achromatic compound microscope, that the disease was shown to be caused by small living organisms that grow within human red blood cells. During this time medical scientists were able to augment clinical observations of malaria patients with microscopic examination of their blood to unravel the complex development cycle of the malaria parasite (see Fig. 2). Captain Ronald Ross, a British army medical officer working in India, discovered that malaria of birds was transmitted by mosquitoes. This breakthrough paved the way for other workers to confirm that *Anopheles* mosquitoes are responsible for transmitting human malaria. The microscopic appearance of the various blood and mosquito stages was described in the scientific literature by 1900, and we now know that there are four separate species of human malaria parasites. The most virulent species, *Plasmodium falciparum*, is often fatal to non-immune humans who are not treated with antimalarial drugs. A second species, *P. vivax*, is rarely lethal, but it may relapse for several years to cause subsequent episodes of fever after the initial attack is controlled. Another less common species, *P. malariae*, is the agent of quartan malaria. The fourth species, *P. ovale*, which was not described until 1922, is quite rare.

The first effective treatment for malaria was discovered in the seventeenth century, more than 150 years before the nature of the disease was understood. During the early part of the seventeenth century reports from South America described a certain kind of bark, called Peruvian bark or quina quina bark, which was reputed to cure fevers. The Jesuits tried it on shivers due to intermittent fevers, and confirmed that it worked. It was then introduced into Europe as a fever remedy (febrifuge), but the results were sometimes erratic as the active component was not known and the bark of other trees was sometimes used instead. The tree was described scientifically by Charles de la Condamine, a French astronomer who led an expedition to South America in 1735, and it was named *Cinchona* by the Swedish botanist Linnaeus.

The value of cinchona bark against malaria fevers was first noted in England by T. Sydenham in 1666. The Italian physician F. Torti differentiated the fevers it cured from those it didn't in 1712. His observations clearly pointed to its activity against the intermittent fevers of malaria, and he emphasised that these were distinct from other fevers that did not respond to cinchona. The active ingredient, quinine, was chemically assayed in 1830, and thereafter the value of the bark was related directly to the quinine content. Large-scale cultivation of cinchona trees started in India in the 1860s, but the most successful com-

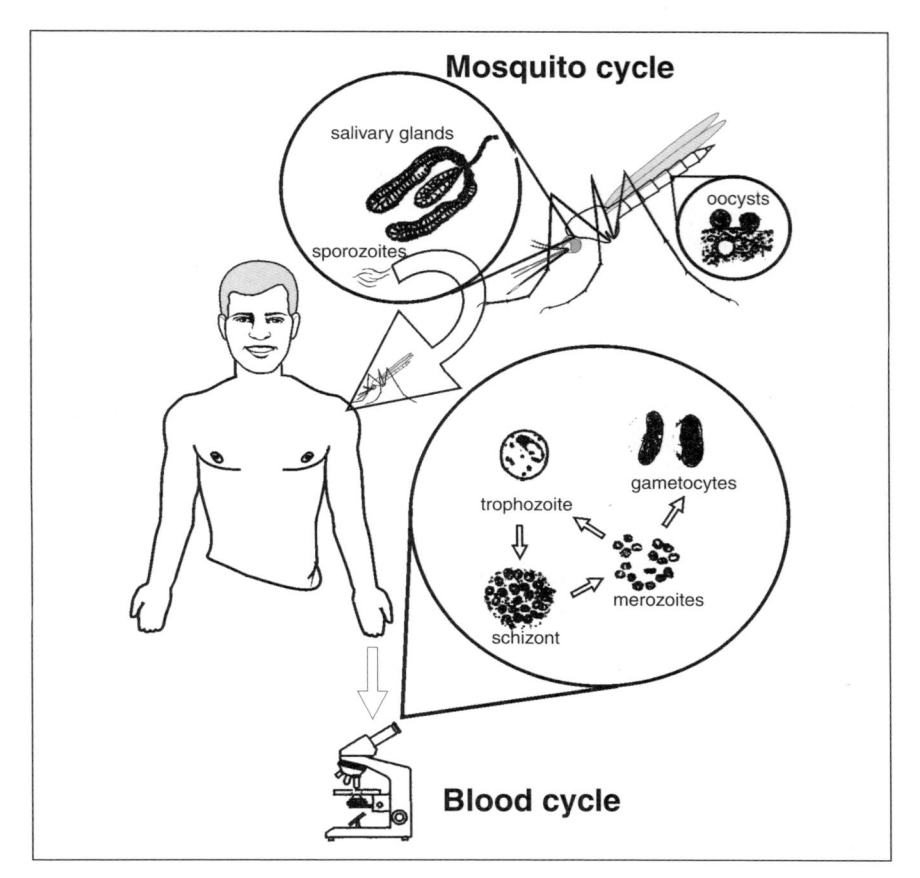

Fig. 2 The malaria cycle

The blood cycle in humans: The onset of fever is associated with rupture of infected red blood cells (erythrocytes) when parasites (merozoites) are released and invade other erythrocytes for another cycle of growth and multiplication. The early stages (trophozoites) develop within infected erythrocytes to form mature stages (schizonts) before rupture to release another batch of merozoites. Some of the parasites undergo successive cycles within erythrocytes, whereas others develop into stages, called gametocytes, which persist within the blood for several days or weeks.

The mosquito cycle: When the gametocytes are ingested in a meal of blood by a susceptible female mosquito they start a cycle of development in the mosquito entirely different from that in humans. The gametocytes undergo sexual fusion in the mosquito gut to form ookinetes, which penetrate the gut wall and become enclosed in cysts on its interior surface. These cysts develop into translucent bodies (oocysts), which later rupture to release sporozoites—small, thread-like stages that migrate to the salivary glands. The mosquito cycle takes about two weeks, and is completed when the soprozoites are injected into a new human host during a subsequent blood meal.

mercial enterprise was that of the Dutch in Java using seed derived from the 'best' trees obtained in Bolivia by the Englishman Charles Ledger. From the mid-nineteenth century quinine became widely available as a specific remedy against malaria. Five grains (325 mg) of quinine daily was widely used by Europeans living in malarious areas to suppress the symptoms of the disease.

Quinine was the only effective malaria drug during World War I. The first systematic attempts to develop synthetic drugs as alternatives to quinine were carried out at the Bayer-Meister-Lucius Research Laboratories at Elberfeld, Germany, in the early 1920s. Here, the chemists W. Schulemann, F. Schonhofer and A. Wingler synthesised chemicals related to quinine and cinchona alkaloids. They modified the chemical arrangement and structure of the components to make a whole range of new compounds, whose activity was tested in an experimental system developed by Wilhelm Roehl in canaries infected with the avian malaria parasite, *Plasmodium relictum*. The birds were given test substances, and their blood was examined daily for appearance of parasites. The results were compared with that of untreated 'control' birds that were infected but not treated with the drug. Roehl noted a delay in appearance of parasites in birds treated with a compound named plasmoquine (also called pamaquine), which was selected for trials in 1925 on the basis of its favourable toxicological and chemotherapeutic properties.[8] In the following year the German scientist F. Sioli showed that plasmoquine was active against human malaria, and subsequent observations by Roehl showed that it destroyed the gametocytes of falciparum malaria. Quinine does not have this effect as it only affects the schizogonic stages. Studies by J. A. Sinton and his co-workers in India suggested that it also reduced the relapse rate of vivax malaria.[9] This first synthetic antimalarial drug came into limited use during the 1930s, particularly in combination with quinine, to prevent vivax relapses. Unfortunately, its toxicity in humans is high and it can only be taken in relatively low doses.

Roehl died in 1929, but his position was filled by Walter Kikuth who collaborated with the chemists F. Mietzsch and H. Mauss to continue the work at Elberfeld.[10] Their efforts culminated in a second drug called atebrin (also known as quinacrine or mepacrine), a yellow powder with a bitter taste, originally called erion or plasmoquin E by the Germans. In 1932 W. Kikuth and Sioli noted its activity against schizonts of avian malaria and found that it was not a gametocide like plasmoquine. Later tests showed that this drug had good activity against blood stages of vivax and falciparum malaria in humans. Yellowing of skin can occur, but atebrin is less toxic than plasmoquine and it persists within the body much longer than quinine.

In the 1930s the Malaria Commission of the Health Organization of the League of Nations sponsored a series of controlled field experiments on the curative and prophylactic treatment of malaria to compare the activity of the new synthetic drugs, atebrin and plasmoquine, with quinine. They hoped to use such drugs for the eradication of the disease. However, the results of trials in Algeria, Italy, Malaya, Romania and the Soviet Union indicated that, even though such treatment 'may greatly diminish morbidity, yet it cannot suppress the parasites in all the carriers'.[11] While acknowledging that the new synthetic drugs represented 'a notable scientific advance' the Malaria Commission concluded that quinine 'still ranks first in current practice'.[12] Plasmoquine was too toxic for general use, and atebrin was considered to be of secondary importance to quinine. This view was supported by the widespread belief that long-term use of atebrin might not be safe, as the associated skin yellowing could indicate that the drug caused jaundice and damaged the liver.

The combatant forces on both sides entered World War II as ill-prepared for the fight against malaria as their predecessors of the Great War. But the Australian Army was particularly fortunate to have Neil Hamilton Fairley, a supremely competent scientist and physician, who addressed the wartime problem of malaria and led a uniquely Australian research effort that was to have far-reaching consequences for its control.

Fairley was born in Inglewood, Victoria, in 1891. He graduated in medicine with first-class honours from the University of Melbourne in 1915, and was commissioned in the AIF with the rank of Captain. He served as pathologist in 14th Australian General Hospital in Egypt, where he made a distinguished clinical and research contribution to a range of tropical diseases: schistosomiasis, malaria, dysentery and typhus. By the end of the war he had been promoted to Lieutenant Colonel, was awarded an OBE, and was Mentioned in Dispatches. He returned to Australia after the war as research assistant to Charles Kellaway, Director of the Walter and Eliza Hall Institute, Melbourne, where he worked on diagnostic tests for hydatid disease.

He departed for India in 1922 to take up a new Chair in Clinical Tropical Medicine in Bombay. On arrival, he discovered that the government had decided not to form a School of Tropical Medicine and that his services were not required. After protracted negotiations he was offered a research appointment at the Bombay Bacteriological Laboratory where he worked on schistosomiasis and guinea worm disease. While working on tropical sprue he developed the condition himself.

Fairley returned to the Hall Institute in 1926 where he worked with Kellaway on snake venoms. In 1928 he went to England and became established as a Harley Street consultant in tropical medicine with a teaching appointment at the London School of Hygiene and Tropical Medicine. Fairley's interest in malaria continued during visits to Macedonia where he investigated blackwater fever that was prevalent in highly malarious areas. This research led to his discovery of methaemalbumin (a previously unknown blood pigment) for which he was elected to the Royal Society in 1942. By this time he was at the pinnacle of his career, with an internationally acclaimed reputation as a medical researcher and as a physician in tropical medicine.

Fairley enlisted in the Second AIF in 1939 in England, and went to the Middle East in August 1940 as consultant physician to the Australian forces with the rank of colonel. He also became a consultant in tropical diseases to British forces in the Middle East. His dual appointments fostered a close liaison between Australian and British medical services in this theatre. Fairley collaborated closely with Colonel J. S. K. Boyd of the Royal Army Medical Corps to confirm the efficacy of sulphaguanidine against bacillary dysentery, which was a severe medical threat to the campaign. The adage that the lessons of history have to be relearned by each generation is certainly valid in the case of malaria, as the Macedonian debacle of 1916–18 was almost repeated in 1941.

Plans were made to send British and Australian troops to Macedonia to counter the threat of a German invasion of Greece. In his war diary Fairley wrote 'From remotest times war and malaria have been loyal allies'.[13] This comment was based on first-hand experience, as he had seen the effects of the devastating epidemic of malaria among troops of the Light Horse at Damascus in 1918, and had performed autopsies of some men who had died of cerebral malaria. He was also familiar with the malaria situation in Macedonia from his work there in the 1930s. He and Boyd prepared a 'memorandum of the danger of malaria in south east Europe and Asia Minor',[14] which summarised the incidence of the disease in the region, related the situation that occurred in Macedonia during World War I, and reviewed the health risks of undertaking military operations in this area during the present conflict. It pointed out that 'the heavy morbidity from malaria in Macedonia in the last war ... occurred despite an intensive anti-mosquito campaign directed by eminent malariologists', and that there had been no significant improvements in methods of controlling mosquitoes or in protecting troops from mosquito bites. Fairley and Boyd wrote that there was no drug known to them that could prevent a susceptible person exposed to the bite of an infected mosquito from developing malaria. Drugs such as atebrin and quinine would reduce fever and help keep the army on its feet, but they may be of little direct benefit in preventing a malaria epidemic. They concluded that 'there can be no reasonable doubt that, given the same circumstances, the melancholy history of the British Army in Macedonia during the last war would re-enact itself'.

The memorandum was passed up to the Commander-in-Chief General Archibald Wavell. His initial response was very unfavourable: 'I have read these very pessimistic reports but refuse to accept the attitude shown in them that nothing can be done, which seems to me typical of a very non-medical and non-military spirit'.[15] He admitted that there was an undoubted risk of malaria if the army had to campaign in the Balkans, but asked if the authors of the report were aware of the considerable drainage works implemented in Macedonia since the last war. Colonel R. G. Shaw, replying on behalf of the Director of Medical Services, suggested that the Commander-in-Chief might like to discuss this matter directly with Colonels Fairley and Boyd. Shaw added: 'I feel sure that they would indicate that their attitude is not that nothing can be done, but rather that much has already been done with indifferent results'.[16] Following an interview with Fairley and Boyd next day Wavell wrote 'I . . . withdraw any suggestion that their attitude was defeatist or unhelpful. It is obviously a very serious problem. I had been given to understand that the canalisation and drainage done since the war had probably halved the incidence of malaria, but [this] is not so, apparently'.[17]

As a result of these representations the force was committed to Greece instead of Macedonia. This was probably the first time that disease considerations had ever played a major role in planning of a campaign. The campaign in Greece was a failure, but this was not due to malaria. In fact, the disease did not pose a major threat during operations in the Middle East, though the Second AIF first became acquainted with it at this time. In the summer of 1941, 1400 cases were reported in I Australian Corps in Syria. After their return to Australia, in March 1942, many men of the 7th Division suffered relapses of vivax malaria.

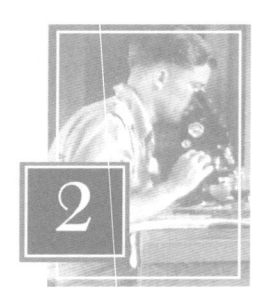

Critical Shortages of Antimalarial Supplies

THE TRIBULATIONS OF the survivors from the garrison at Rabaul foreshadowed the prospect that malaria would be on a vastly different scale in the South West Pacific to that experienced by the AIF in the Middle East—the mountainous tropical islands on Australia's northern doorstep are among the most highly malarious in the world. An additional vital concern was that more than 90 per cent of the world supply of quinine was produced in Indonesia, which was directly in the line of the Japanese advance.

These issues were immediately apparent to Colonel Fairley when hostilities broke out with Japan. He was sent on a mission to Java from the Middle East to secure vital supplies of this crucial drug for the Allies before they were captured by the enemy. For three weeks after his arrival in Jakarta on 2 February 1942 he co-ordinated negotiations with Netherlands East Indies authorities to get quinine reserves to Australia.[1] His efforts culminated in the cash payment by the Australian government for 130 000 kg of the drug.[2]

On 22 February Fairley embarked on the liner *Orcades*, which was carrying the 7th Australian Division from the Middle East in one of the last convoys to escape the Japanese invasion. Next day one of the officers on board told him that separate shipments of quinine, amounting to some 50 000 kg, had been loaded onto two ships at ports in Java for Australia. One ship was never seen again but the other, the SS *Klang*, sailed into Fremantle at the end of March.

By this time Fairley had arrived at Army Headquarters in Melbourne and had been appointed Director of Medicine for the Australian Army. He and his colleagues at the Medical Directorate had been anxiously awaiting the quinine consignment so they were very elated to hear of the arrival of the Dutch ship.

One of the local army medical staff went to the *Klang* to ascertain the amount of quinine on board and to arrange for its rapid transfer to army stores. The captain of the ship confirmed that 20 000 kg of quinine had been taken aboard at Tjilatjap. However, before sailing for Australia the ship called into Jakarta, where Dutch officials came on board and ordered the whole supply to be taken off. It was left behind on the wharf when the *Klang* sailed.[3] The reason for this was not explained, though some of the Australians thought that enemy 'fifth column' agents were responsible for its removal. In any event this was a serious blow, because quinine was in critically short supply in Australia and there was no immediate prospect of getting additional stocks from elsewhere.

Steps were promptly taken to conserve the limited supplies in the civilian community for military use. Under national security regulations an order was made on 24 March 1942 to restrict quinine solely for use against malaria on a medical prescription basis. The chairman of the Medical Equipment Control Committee recommended to the Commonwealth Director General of Medical Services that all stocks of quinine held by the wholesale drug trade, with the exception of small amounts needed for the treatment of malaria in the civil population, should be purchased by the Army.[4] This recommendation was carried out. The wholesale drug firms were requested to assist the government by buying back surplus supplies from retail pharmaceutical chemists. They agreed to do this without any profit, and all stocks were promptly handed over to the Army.[5] Explanatory articles were published in the *Australasian Journal of Pharmacy* so that chemists would be fully informed of their duties concerning control of quinine. An editorial in the *Medical Journal of Australia* urged 'that every medical practitioner must understand the criminal folly of using quinine for any other purpose than to secure its specific action in the prevention or treatment of malaria'.[6]

The measures taken to conserve existing stocks of quinine were important, but they were not enough to make up the shortfall in supplies and something else needed to be done as a matter of the utmost urgency. Fairley knew that the nation was in a perilous situation. It was already known that daily use of quinine did not prevent troops becoming infected with malaria but it tended to suppress fever and enabled the Army to keep on fighting. If the supply failed, a force operating in highly malarious areas would soon be rendered incapable of action. At that time the Australian Army held less than 5000 kg of the drug.[7] The New Guinea Force was using 1000 kg of quinine a month, so the existing supplies would soon run out. Atebrin was also in dangerously short supply. Orders had already been placed in America to augment Australian stocks but, after lengthy delays, only small quantities had arrived. The ship carrying the first batch of two million tablets of atebrin and one million tablets of plasmoquine was sunk through enemy action. Unless new shipments were obtained from overseas all antimalarial drugs in Australian hands would be exhausted by the end of 1942.

The supply of mosquito nets and repellents was also inadequate. Many of the nets in use in New Guinea were unserviceable. A suitable type of fine netting to stop mosquitoes could not be produced in sufficient quantity in Australia as supplies of cotton for this purpose were not available. Australian looms at full capacity were capable of producing 5000–7000 nets per week if they had right kind of yarn, but it had not been possible to arrange for adequate supplies of this cotton from either America or England.[8]

There was an urgent need to conserve the quinine that remained by replacing it with atebrin as soon as possible. This was of paramount importance for Australia and the South West Pacific campaign, but it was equally important for all Allied forces operating in other malarious areas. Fairley attended a meeting of the Drug Subcommittee of the Australian Association of Scientific Workers at the University of Sydney in August when this problem was considered.[9] The subcommittee met regularly throughout the war to promote local manufacture of essential medical drugs needed to support Australia's defence capability. One of the members, Dr Adrien Albert, a research chemist of the University of Sydney, had made an intensive study of atebrin manufacture. He confirmed that its chemical synthesis was very complicated, involving more than 20 intermediate steps. It was clear that large-scale production was beyond Australian industry at that time, due to wartime procurement difficulties, as it would be necessary to import nearly 20 kg of raw materials to make 1 kg of atebrin. During the course of discussion Major H. K. Ward, Professor of Bacteriology at the university, suggested that Fairley should go to the USA and Britain with an expert chemist, preferably Dr Albert, to acquaint overseas authorities with the urgency of the situation in the South West Pacific and to advocate that essential drug supplies should be earmarked for Australia. Fairley promptly took up this suggestion by writing next day to the Director General of Medical Services with the proposal that

> a tropical specialist and a chemist working in association with the Drugs Committee ... should proceed to the USA and Britain without delay to present the case for Australia, and ensure that (i) adequate supplies of quinine as well as of atebrin and plasmoquine, and (ii) adequate supplies of standard mosquito netting be made available if this is possible.[10]

He did not say who should go and, indeed, it would have been superfluous for him to do so, as it was evident that nobody in Australia was more fitted to this task than Fairley himself—no one in the medical community rivalled his international standing in the field of tropical medicine.

Approval was rapidly granted through official military channels with the highest priority. The medical mission, comprising Fairley and Albert, left

Essendon Airport in Melbourne on 10 September 1942 for the USA. Their primary objectives were to present the magnitude of the malaria problem facing Australian forces in the South West Pacific and to urge that adequate supplies of vitally needed antimalarial drugs should be sent to Australia as soon as possible. Albert's main role was to ascertain whether America had the capacity in raw materials, personnel and plant to expand its production to the enormous extent required, and whether American manufacturers were likely to respond to increased wartime demand.[11]

American authorities were convinced of the gravity of the malaria problem by Fairley's presentation of data collected from recent and past malaria surveys of New Guinea and the Solomons. This was aided by a memorandum, illustrated by maps, which had been specially prepared by Lieutenant Colonel E. (Ted) Ford, who was then the Assistant Director of Pathology for New Guinea Force. The memorandum was highly regarded by the Medical Intelligence Branch of the US Army Surgeon General's Office in Washington, where many copies were made for distribution.

During the time of the visit to Washington, an enquiry was made through official channels from President Franklin Roosevelt to Sir Owen Dixon, Australian Minister at Washington, concerning diseases likely to affect Allied and Japanese troops in the South West Pacific. At Dixon's request Fairley prepared a statement on this subject stressing the overwhelming importance of malaria. Also, a copy of Ford's memorandum was given to Admiral McIntyre, Director of Medical Services for the US Navy, who was President Roosevelt's personal physician.

On 19 September Fairley met two friends and colleagues from Britain, Major General A. G. Biggam of the Royal Army Medical Corps and Professor Warrington Yorke of the British Medical Research Council. They were in Washington with Mr Warburton, Director of Medical Supplies in Britain, to discuss production and distribution of antimalarial drugs with their American counterparts. Fairley represented Australia at these discussions. On 24 September the British and Australians took part in a conference on atebrin at the American National Research Council, and on 2 October they met senior American officials including Leo Crowley, the Alien Property Custodian, who in effect controlled production of atebrin in the USA.[12]

It was estimated that Java was producing one million kg of quinine per year. Stocks held by England and America were between 500 000 and 600 000 kg, and once this invaluable reserve was exhausted there was no possibility of it being replaced from sources outside of Java during the present war. The prewar global use of quinine was 700 000 kg per year and it was estimated that this might increase by half under wartime conditions to approximately one million kg annually. The equivalent amount of atebrin (based on a comparative dose and weight ratio of atebrin: quinine = 1:5) was 200 000 kg. The quinine reserves were sufficient to sustain the Allied countries for almost a year, if stringent economies were imposed, so if atebrin production in the USA and Britain could be increased to replace quinine, it might seem that this would be a satisfactory solution to the problem. However, atebrin is excreted from the body much more slowly than quinine and is stored in the liver and skin, which it stains yellow. There was the possibility that troops taking large doses of atebrin over a long period of time might develop toxic features from a cumulative action of the drug. Fairley pointed out that atebrin had not been employed previously by a European army in highly malarious areas throughout the whole year for prophylaxis and, in consequence, its use in this way would have to be regarded to some extent as experimental. The Germans had used atebrin for suppressive treatment in the Balkans and Macedonia throughout the five months of the malaria season but not for the remainder of the year. If continuous use proved toxic to the troops through cumulative action, there would be two alternatives: to withdraw troops to non-malarious areas and cease taking atebrin; or to substitute quinine for atebrin for such time as might be deemed advisable. 'If it proved impossible or impracticable to withdraw troops from such an area and quinine were not available, a grave situation would develop which might readily lose the campaign in such fronts as Burma, the Solomons, or New Guinea'.[13]

It was agreed at the meeting in Washington that 200 000 kg of atebrin per annum were necessary to replace the one million kg of quinine lost through the fall of Java. At the time of the meeting, the USA was producing 60 000 kg per year, but Crowley estimated that this would rise to 100 000 kg per year by the following January, and he said that Merck, Winthrop, Monsanto, and possibly other firms, would attain an output of 150 000 kg by June 1943. Present and future atebrin production in Britain was reviewed in a report presented by Mr Warburton: current output from pilot plants (10 000 kg per year) would expand to about 17 000 kg per year by the end of 1942. Two new plants, one of 15 000 kg capacity and the other of 25 000 kg, were expected to come into operation about May 1943 'so that we may take it from the middle of 1943, the capacity of Great Britain for the production of atebrin will be in the neighbourhood of 50 tons [50 000 kg] per annum'.[14] On this basis it appeared that the required production target would be met by the co-operative efforts of both countries. Fairley reported to Australia that, before he left Washington, 'arrangements were recently made to fly 1,000,000 tablets of atebrin and 500,000 tablets of plasmoquine to Australia, and 17,000,000 tablets of atebrin were to be sent by sea. Should these supplies reach Australia anxiety for the time being will be allayed'.[15]

Fairley and Albert arrived in London during the second week of October. The malaria reports of the Australian Army Medical Services were supplied to the Director General of Medical Services of the British Army, as well as to other government agencies, including the Ministry of Health and National Council of Medical Research. Certain aspects of the reports reached cabinet level via the Australian High Commissioner in London, Stanley M. Bruce. Sir Charles Wilson (later Lord Moran), President of the Royal College of Physicians and personal physician to Winston Churchill, also received a briefing. In addition, while attending many government and military committees and subcommittees and during individual interviews with Army and departmental chiefs, Fairley emphasised the seriousness of the malaria situation in the South West Pacific. He also had discussions with senior executives in the British companies ICI, May & Baker, and Boots, which were involved in atebrin production. He learned that, because of wartime restrictions, there were difficulties in getting adequate financial aid and priority for obtaining materials needed for essential plant construction. Production in England was also handicapped by the necessity of importing certain chemical intermediate products from North America.

The situation was further exacerbated by the fact that the British firms were not fully co-operating with one another in the manufacture of a drug essential to the war effort. Fairley said that 'though ICI and May & Baker have given detailed information to the U.S.A. regarding their process of manufacturing atebrin, a similar exchange of knowledge has not been made between themselves'.[16] As a result of these problems, the projections for atebrin production were considerably less that those foreshadowed at the meeting in Washington. The measures being taken in Britain to conserve the dwindling reserves of quinine were of equal concern. Shortly after he arrived in London, Fairley learned that the use of quinine was limited by medical prescription, under wartime regulations, but a doctor could still prescribe it 'for coughs and colds, as a tonic, or for any medical purposes he fancies'.[17] This was in contrast to the situation in Australia and America where its sale was restricted strictly and solely for medical treatment of malaria.

Over the weekend of 24–25 October Fairley wrote 'an appreciation of the present grave position regarding anti-malarial drugs', which provided a penetrating analysis of the whole situation concerning atebrin, quinine and other essential supplies, as well as the steps that should be taken to maximise their availability for Allied troops operating in malarious areas.

> These objectives can best be obtained by the establishment of a common pool of anti-malarial drugs, the distribution of which would be controlled by an inter-allied or Anglo-American committee in USA. Dr Mote, British Ministry of Supply, Washington, regards this as the only possible solution to this critical malaria problem, and this opinion is endorsed by all authorities with whom I have had an opportunity of discussion.[18]

Mote also told Fairley that America would not agree to pooling its quinine supplies with the Allies until British regulations restricted its use and sale exclusively for the treatment of malaria.[19]

Fairley resolved to approach the Ministry of Supply to discuss the problems of atebrin production, and also to suggest that the quinine regulations be amended to bring them into line with those of Australia and America. But, before doing so, he decided to solicit support from the Ministry of Health. Accordingly, he had a meeting with Sir John Maud, the Minister of Health, and Sir William Jamieson, medical adviser to the Ministry of Health, on 9 November.[20] Three days later he met the Minister of Supply, Sir Andrew Duncan. When considering the problems of atebrin production in Britain Fairley urged that, if the 50 000 kg promised at the meeting in Washington was to be produced in six or even twelve months, it would be necessary to give atebrin production a priority similar to munitions; to commence building and plant construction immediately; and to have a round-table conference at which the manufacturing firms were represented, to pool technical knowledge essential for manufacture. Duncan heeded these arguments, and arranged a meeting of the various manufacturers of antimalarial drugs. This was held at Portland House, Headquarters of the British Ministry of Supply, on 17 November.

The meeting was chaired by the Director General of Supplies, Sir Cecil Weir. In his opening remarks he said that it had been called so that Fairley and Albert could take back to Australia a complete picture of what was being done about production and supply of atebrin. He explained that contractors had been invited to be present in order to clear up certain conflicting statements on production programs that had been made, on the one hand to the Directorate of Medical Supplies, and on the other hand to Fairley and Albert. Company representatives were then asked individually to provide forecasts of atebrin production. Those from ICI and May & Baker both said that their new plants, forecast to produce 15 000 and 25 000 kg per year from May 1943 in the Washington meeting, would not come into operation until September and would not be able to get into full production until early 1944. It was estimated that the total British production during 1943 would amount to only 27 000 or 28 000 kg—just over half the 50 000 kg promised in Washington.

The Ministry of Supply was obviously discomforted by this discrepancy. Weir 'expressed the strong desire that such approaches [by the Australians] should in future be made only through the directorate of Medical Supplies and he suggested to contractors that they should not disclose information about quinine substitutes unless with the concurrence of and through the Ministry of Supply'. However, if not for Fairley's pertinent enquiries to the companies, the true situation of the considerable shortfall in supply of atebrin would not have been revealed to the authorities at this crucial time when remedial action was urgently needed. In response to a request from ICI, Weir promised a high level of priority for the additional plant so that increased production could be achieved at an earlier date. The control of existing stocks of quinine was then considered. An official of the Directorate of Medical Supplies revealed that an order was about to be issued that would restrict its use to the treatment of malaria and would prohibit doctors from prescribing quinine except for cases of malaria. Finally, contractors were urged to approach the Ministry of Supply if they required assistance of any description, 'and particularly if they found their estimates of [atebrin] production were not being attained'. After the meeting the contractors met to arrange for continuing collaboration between their respective companies.[21]

Ultimately, the authorities in Washington and London responded very favourably to the strong representations of the mission to give Australia the highest possible priority for antimalarial drugs and other essential supplies. The 18 million tablets of atebrin ordered from America arrived by the end of 1942. Following a request from Fairley to the British Ministry of Supply, 6000 kg of quinine from the British stockpile that was held in South Africa also arrived in Australia in December. Despite shortages of cotton yarn in Britain, adequate quantities of mosquito netting to support the New Guinea campaigns were allocated to Australia. Supplies of pyrethrum, as well as the seed needed to produce additional stocks of this plant-based insecticide, were also provided. These shipments greatly relieved the malaria situation in the South West Pacific theatre.

Fairley's overseas visit in 1942 was of immense benefit to Australia's war effort but it also had a lasting impact on Allied technical and industrial co-operation in the provision of medical supplies. The way for this was cleared by the British decision, strongly advocated by Fairley, to restrict the use of quinine solely for malaria. Steps were then taken to pool the resources of the two countries by co-ordination between the Combined Production and Resources Board in the USA and the Commonwealth Supply Council in Britain.[22] Malaria was one of the first diseases to be considered, specifically the allocation and distribution of atebrin in order to conserve the remaining quinine supply effectively.

Lieutenant General Edward K. Smart, the Australian Army Representative in Britain recorded an authoritative overview of the mission. Smart was in Washington during September and returned to London later in the month. He was personally involved with high-level deliberations concerning this enterprise in both places, and so was able to appreciate its impact at first hand:

Colonel Fairley and Dr Albert have done excellent and painstaking work both in the U.S.A. and here [UK]. In my opinion they have done a great deal in clarifying the position and in focussing attention on the measures necessary both to combat malaria and to provide for the necessary drugs and treatment for its prevention and treatment. After careful research and enquiry had convinced him that the measures being taken were inadequate, Colonel Fairley pressed his conclusions with firmness and tact on Service and civilian authorities. As a result it is anticipated that all possible measures will be taken, and that S.W.P.A. [South West Pacific Area] will get its proper proportion of drugs and supplies.[23]

3

Our Worst Enemy

Within a few months of their attack on Pearl Harbor, the Japanese had captured virtually all of South-East Asia and were expanding into New Guinea and the surrounding islands. Fairley's concerns about the magnitude of the malaria problem in this region were soon confirmed. Before he left on his overseas mission he made a visit to New Guinea Force Headquarters, accompanied by a senior entomologist, Major (later Lieutenant Colonel) I. M. (Ian) Mackerras, to inspect medical units and to make an appreciation of the health problems facing military operations.

Port Moresby is relatively dry, with only 750 mm annual rainfall, most of which falls in the first half of the year. It is not highly malarious compared with the typical tropical jungle areas that extend throughout most of the island. Yet Fairley found the malaria rate among the Moresby garrison to be disturbingly high—the cases requiring treatment between January and June 1942 represented 15 per cent of the force. He considered that as many as 50 per cent might contract the disease by the end of the malaria season in August, and observed that 'New Guinea Force [was] not malaria minded': antimalaria discipline was poor; protective measures were inadequate; and mosquito control was hampered by lack of equipment and staff. *Anopheles* mosquitoes feed during the night so it was essential that troops in malarious areas wear long-sleeved shirts and long trousers to minimise the chances of being bitten.[1]

Fairley saw many unserviceable mosquito nets, and noted that men guarding airfields and other installations at night wore shorts and short-sleeved shirts. In a report on his visit he wrote: 'Even when every possible precautionary measure is taken, it is difficult to avoid contracting malaria at night in the jungle. To take liberties with the mosquito vector under circumstances such as exist in New Guinea is to guarantee malaria'. He also reported that antimalaria drug administration was grossly deficient: 'Quinine tablets are not given on parade but are generally handed out with food, and it is left to the individual to decide whether he will take it or not'.[2] Before returning to Australia Fairley had an interview with the commander of the force, Major General B. M. Morris, during which he outlined the malaria menace, and made recommendations aimed at reducing the number of infections in Australian troops. Unfortunately, his advice was not acted upon.

During July the Japanese landed on the north coast of New Guinea and advanced across the Owen Stanley Range towards Port Moresby. The outnumbered militia troops of 39 Battalion fought a series of desperate rearguard actions, but they were forced back from Kokoda. The enemy was finally stopped in the mountain ridges north-east of Moresby, and the 7th Australian Division, recently returned from the Middle East, renewed the offensive along the Kokoda trail to Buna. A survey of the track across the Owen Stanley Range, which is above 1000 metres in altitude, failed to reveal the presence of *Anopheles* mosquitoes so it was decided that daily quinine would not be given to the troops in this area. It had been anticipated that the malaria problem would arise on the northern side of the range from Kokoda to the coast where the altitude was less than 500 metres.

Requests were made for antimalarial drugs to be flown in so that the division could start taking the drug on 10 November, one week after their arrival in the Kokoda area. Unfortunately, the supplies did not arrive in time, so the advance continued without the benefit of suppressive treatment, and in the middle of November malaria became prevalent. By January 1943 casualties in the division were: 2500 killed in action; 2500 wounded; and 6500 sick. More than 6000 of the sickness casualties were due to malaria, and it was a complicating factor in many of the battle casualties. Attacks of fever were not automatic grounds for hospitalisation. Only those who were obviously anaemic, and who could not work for more than two hours a day, were evacuated sick. In spite of these criteria, engineer troops, who had suffered practically no battle casualties, evacuated approximately 75 per cent of their strength because of malaria during a period of six weeks. A similar incidence of the disease occurred in 2/4 Australian Field Ambulance, and in mid-December this unit had to be returned to the base area by air. It was reported that

> operations had to commence in a highly malarious area before adequate protective measures had been made available to the division ... If jungle fighting continues in hyperendemic areas of malaria it is probable that history will repeat itself and that the whole force will become infected and incapable of offensive action within 4–6 months.[3]

During the last week of August 1942 the Japanese attacked Milne Bay on the eastern extremity of New Guinea (see Fig. 3). This was a most important locality from a strategic viewpoint, as the airfields there were a vital resource to the Allies, and an Australian force comprising the 7th and 18th Infantry Brigades defended it vigorously. The enemy was decisively repulsed, and withdrew during the first week of September. This battle was the first defeat suffered by Japanese land forces since the war had begun nine months previously, but the Australian victory was soon overshadowed by the spectre of disease. Milne Bay was regarded as one of the worst malarious places in Eastern Papua. The base perimeter contained about 100 square km of wet, low-lying ground that provided ideal conditions for the breeding of malaria mosquitoes.

The disease caused some casualties before and during the fighting, but was not a major problem during the engagement as many of the troops had only recently arrived. They were committed to battle either before they became infected or during the incubation period of the disease, but the situation deteriorated rapidly in the following weeks. By the end of November more than 5000 men out of a total force of 12 000 had been treated at medical establishments, and the epidemic peaked at over 1000 cases in the last week of December. But the damage was much worse than this. The actual number of treated cases did not adequately describe the situation as most men carried infections that were barely held in check by quinine.[4] In a secret memorandum to the Director General of Medical Services Lieutenant Colonel (later Colonel)

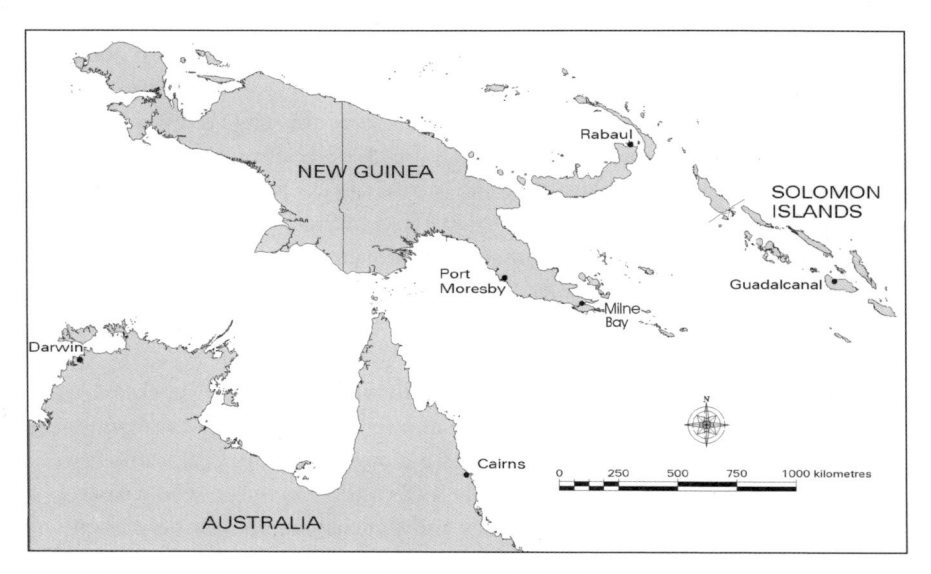

Fig. 3 South West Pacific theatre of operations, 1942–45

E. V. (Bill) Keogh, the Director of Pathology of the Australian Army Medical Services, wrote:

> In a few month malaria has, in New Guinea, reduced a first rate combatant force to an ineffective fraction of its original strength. It was known that malaria was hyperendemic in combat areas and that failure to appreciate its importance as a strategical factor in previous wars lead to military disaster. Knowledge was not translated into action.[5]

Keogh was especially critical of the failure to provide quinine in the advance across the Owen Stanleys on the advice of the senior medical officer of 7th Division and with the concurrence of the senior medical officer of New Guinea Force: 'In consequence practically 100% of wounded evacuated to Moresby have malaria. This was not due to shortage of the drug but to a deliberate decision of responsible administrative medical officers'.[6]

The Assistant Director of Pathology, Lieutenant Colonel E. (Ted) Ford, was the unofficial malariologist in New Guinea.[7] He had considerable experience of malaria in the country before the war and keenly appreciated what needed to be done. He realised that the malaria problem had developed to such catastrophic levels because

> practically the whole Force was utterly without a consciousness of malaria as a foremost menace to its success. From this arose a dangerous slackness in antimalarial discipline and an unconsciousness of the necessity for constant and vigorous antimalarial measures. This occurred from lack of training and of actual experience in hyperendemic malarial areas.[8]

Ford saw that the only way to avoid disaster was to provide an adequate knowledge of the details of antimalarial measures to all troops and especially to commanders. This had to be done while the force was engaged in protracted jungle warfare, and consequently it had to be carried out under conditions difficult for its adequate reception. Since no adequate organisation existed for this, and the situation did not allow of its rapid formation, the greater part had to be carried out by personal contact. There were relatively few officers who had experience of malaria under field conditions, but these gave great assistance by instructing their fellow officers and in educating the troops in practical measures to avoid malaria.

Ford himself took the lead in these activities. He was so shocked by the conditions in Milne Bay that he sought an interview with the Commander-in-Chief, General Thomas Blamey.[9] He told Blamey that, if this predicament were allowed to continue, it would inevitably lead to the loss of the whole force as a fighting body. Ford said that mistakes and deficiencies should be recognised promptly, for similar conditions would be encountered on almost any part of the South West Pacific islands:

Recognition must be full and rapid for it must lead quickly to a consciousness of importance of malaria and to a rigid malaria discipline. Without this a force is unfitted to campaign in such areas and success would be jeopardised from its inception. It was essential that every means be taken to instil into the minds of all ranks the awareness of malaria as a constant menace to the force.[10]

The enemy's attack at Milne Bay compelled the Australians to commence operations before the necessary equipment and stores for malaria control were available. There were adequate quantities of quinine for prophylaxis throughout the campaign but there were shortages of other antimalarial supplies including mosquito nets that were either lost by enemy action or left in the holds of the transport vessels when the men landed. These unavoidable deficiencies at the beginning of operations induced an attitude of hopelessness that was hard to dispel when the supplies did become available. The wearing of long-sleeved shirts and long trousers between dusk and dawn was often disregarded, and a bad example in this regard was set by some senior officers.

Blamey was suitably impressed by Ford's arguments, and he took action to ensure that the highest priority was given to antimalarial measures. He also wrote a short article for *Guinea Gold*, a service newspaper circulated to the troops of New Guinea Force, stressing that it was the responsibility of each man to protect himself against the malaria mosquito: 'Our worst enemy in New Guinea is not the Nip—its [*sic*] the bite'.[11]

The difficulties that malaria posed for Australian troops were also encountered by American forces in the South West Pacific. In March 1942 American troops landed on Efate Island, Vanuatu, to build an airfield. Within a short time more than 20 per cent of the force was going down with malaria each month. Later in the year US troops suffered five times as many malaria casualties as those resulting from combat during the battle for control of the Solomon Islands. The disease became a problem for the First US Marine Division. The men were then given quinine as well as atebrin for prophylaxis but, in spite of these measures, there were 5600 admissions to hospital (after two months on Guadalcanal) out of a force that at full strength was 16 000. By the end of the fourth month the Division could not march or attack and was only capable of defending a fixed position.[12]

Fairley was in the USA and England while these events were unfolding, but after his return he prepared a report for the Australian Prime Minister, John Curtin, that summarised the malaria situation in New Guinea. He emphasised that Australian troops faced the prospect of further years of jungle warfare in highly malarious regions, and that the ultimate result of the campaign might be determined by the ability of the army to keep malaria casualties at a low rate. This could only be achieved by high antimalarial discipline and training, as well as effective preventive measures: 'Success was essentially dependent on antimalarial supplies and equipment being given priority over guns, ammunition, tanks and aeroplanes'.[13]

The number of malaria cases in New Guinea Force during the first year of the war against Japan were alarmingly high but, unlike the debacle that followed the retreat from Rabaul, the death rate was very low. Early diagnosis, followed by prompt quinine treatment in military medical facilities, provided a crucial life-saving measure. However, men suffering an attack of malaria cannot fight and the continuing attrition due to the disease posed a serious manpower wastage on the forces committed to field operations. The Prime Minister was also Minister for Defence. In this latter capacity Curtin requested that, in view of the manpower problem in keeping the forces up to operational strength in tropical regions, the Australian Defence Committee should review the incidence of malaria and other tropical diseases in the forces in New Guinea.[14]

On 4 March 1943 the Committee considered a detailed report from the Director Generals of Medical Services for the Army and the Royal Australian Air Force (RAAF) on the manpower implications of battle and sickness casualties for maintaining the strength of the Australian Military Forces (AMF). Analysis showed that, if the wastage rates due to malaria continued at the levels experienced during the first year of the campaign, the existing rate of intake into the army would be insufficient to maintain the required force of 95 000 men in New Guinea. It would be necessary to eliminate two or three formations from the Order of Battle to make up the deficiency but, even so, that would only be sufficient to maintain the force at this level for about five months. The report concluded that, in view of all of the constraints indicated above, 'it is a matter of mathematical calculation as to the length of time in which the AMF will become exhausted under the prevailing conditions'.[15]

The Defence Committee made a submission to the War Cabinet that agreed with all of the major points raised in the reports by the services. Special reference was made to the following statement in the Army report: 'Before committing a force to any particular operation, it is regarded as essential that a detailed appreciation of the proposed operation, from the point of view of the effect of malaria, should be obtained early in the planning stage'.[16] These contemporary documents confirm that there was a very real concern in the highest levels of government that, if the malaria problem was not solved, the drain on the force due to the disease might outstrip the ability of Australia to find enough reinforcements to maintain the army in New Guinea.

The efforts of Fairley and Ford, with the support of Major General S. R. (Ginger) Burston, the Director General of Army Medical Services, were most successful in bringing the seriousness of the malaria threat to the attention of the authorities who were responsible for the conduct of the war. Antimalarial work received the utmost priority, and stores and labour for mosquito control measures were rapidly made available with the full authority of the Commander-in-Chief. Engineering works to reduce breeding of larvae, as well as oiling and treatment of breeding sites with Paris green, were co-ordinated by specialist malaria control units. The former treatment forms a film of oil on the water surface that cuts off access to the air and the larvae die of suffocation, whereas the latter involves applying a fine dust of copper aceto-arsenite (an effective stomach poison against *Anopheles* larvae). At the same time personal antimalarial measures were strengthened: the use of suppressive therapy and wearing of protective clothing at night (long trousers and long-sleeved shirts) were rigidly enforced by military discipline.

Administrative support for malaria control in New Guinea Force was co-ordinated in Australia by the Anti Malaria Advisory Committee (later called the Tropical Diseases Advisory Committee). This committee, which comprised Australian Army members (with Wing Commander A. H. Baldwin representing the RAAF), met in Melbourne at monthly intervals. Major Ian Mackerras reported to the committee on 10 March 1943 that, over the previous three months, the incidence of the disease in the garrison at Milne Bay had fallen from 80 to less than 10 cases per 1000 men each week. He attributed this improvement primarily to the work of the antimalarial control units, but Ford commented that General Blamey's name should be added to the credits for the astonishing change that had taken place.[17]

Fairley suggested to Major General Burston that there should also be a joint body with membership drawn from both Australian and US services to provide effective coordination of measures against tropical disease throughout all Allied forces in the South West Pacific Theatre.[18] This was a shrewd and timely move, as it set the stage for the strongest possible entreaties to be made for urgently required antimalarial supplies from America. Burston gave full support, and passed this proposal on to General Blamey, who recommended it to General Douglas MacArthur on 19 February 1943.[19] MacArthur replied favourably on 1 March, and the next day a directive was issued from General Headquarters (GHQ), South West Pacific Area, formally raising the 'Combined Advisory Committee on Tropical Medicine, Hygiene, and Sanitation'.[20] The committee included senior medical representatives from Australian and US Forces, with Colonel Fairley as chairman and another Australian, Colonel M. J. Holmes, as executive officer.

After the first meeting on 13 March, Fairley had a personal conference with MacArthur, who said that he did not wish the committee to consider minor problems or matters of academic interest. Concrete recommendations on essential medical measures were needed, and he stressed that the committee would always have his support.[21] The most pressing deficiency was atebrin, which continued to be in critically short supply despite the representations made by the Australian mission in Washington. By this time atebrin was the only prophylactic antimalarial drug used by Allied forces in order to conserve the limited supplies of quinine for treatment of acute cases.

In March 1943 the amount of the drug within the Australian Army was sufficient for only seven weeks, while the US Forces in the South West Pacific and the Marine Division from Guadalcanal were actually drawing on Australian stocks as they had not yet received adequate supplies from their own sources. There was a crucial requirement for sufficient atebrin to meet current needs and for a reserve to be built up for future emergencies. Shipping was scarce and vulnerable to enemy action. Following Fairley's interview with the Commander-in-Chief, a GHQ directive was issued granting the highest possible shipping priority for antimalarial drugs.[22] This overcame the acute shortage of atebrin and provided adequate maintenance of supplies to meet future requirements. Macarthur's favourable response to the formation of the committee and his unequivocal support for it may have stemmed from his personal experience with malaria. He was infected as a Lieutenant while on duty in the Philippines during 1904.[23]

Sir Earle Page, a prominent federal politician and medical practitioner before entering parliament, now entered the scene. He was critical of the medical administration of malaria in the New Guinea campaign and was concerned about the implications of the disease for the army and for the civilian population in Australia during and after the war. In April 1943 Page sought and was granted the approval of Prime Minister John Curtin to report on the situation.[24] Fairley was directed by Major General Burston to offer assistance and support. The terms of reference included consideration of measures to prevent malarial infection in the forces and also to prevent the disease spreading in Australia with the return of infected soldiers. During the last week of April Page attended a sitting of the Combined Advisory Committee in Brisbane. Major C. R. B. (Ruthven) Blackburn, an AIF medical officer with considerable first-hand experience of malaria in the present conflict at Milne Bay, was appointed to accompany Page throughout his inquiry. During the first week of May Fairley, Page and Blackburn visited Australian and US Army hospitals in Townsville, Cairns, and the Atherton Tablelands in this important Allied base area of the South West Pacific. Page and Blackburn then left for Port Moresby to inspect the malaria situation in forward operational areas, while Fairley remained in Cairns for several days to review the present position concerning malaria in the Cairns area and the danger it posed to troops stationed there.

During the first week of June, Fairley and Blackburn met with Page in his office at the Commonwealth Bank in Sydney, to assist with the compilation of a report.[25] A summary was prepared; recommendations were drawn up; and Page wrote a covering letter for the Prime Minister.[26] The report recommended that units or formations in malarious areas should be treated for malaria before leave to Australia was granted. Such men should not be posted to potentially malarious areas in Australia except in a military emergency. Over 3000 cases of malaria had already been treated on the Atherton Tablelands, where surveys had shown that malaria mosquitoes were not present so there was little danger of infected troops starting an epidemic among the civilian population. Moreover, the troops were also free from the risk of reinfecting one another. The report designated priority areas for treatment of malaria cases as: (1) New Guinea; (2) Atherton Tablelands; (3) southern Queensland. The report was accepted in its entirety by the Prime Minister, who sent it on to General MacArthur on 3 July. On 27 July Macarthur replied to Curtin that he agreed with all aspects of the report and that steps would be taken to implement all of the principal recommendations.[27]

Orders promulgated by General Blamey stated explicitly that the control of malaria was a military rather than a medical problem. 'The responsibility for malarial control rests on the CO of every unit and every individual soldier. Malaria can be controlled by the application of proven control measures under strict military discipline'.[28] Instruction on the nature of the disease, its effects on military operations and the methods of control were made an integral part of the training of all ranks. This included detailed and specific instructions in use of prophylactic drugs, personal protection measures with repellents, mosquito nets and protective clothing. Antimosquito squads were raised from the strength of every unit on the scale of one NCO and two other ranks per infantry company or equivalent. Their task was to control mosquito breeding in and around the base perimeters of unit lines.

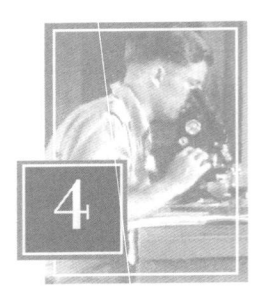

Anti Sweat

THE STEPS TAKEN to control mosquitoes by filling and draining of breeding sites caused a remarkable improvement around static base camps and fixed installations, such as at Milne Bay, but did not provide a complete solution to the malaria problem. There was still the dilemma of controlling the disease in current and future operations among front-line troops where it would be difficult (and often impractical) to implement antimosquito activities. Under these conditions the only feasible control method was the use of antimalarial drugs. Atebrin and quinine were both available but there was no clear evidence whether one was more effective than the other. It was known that they did not prevent infection, and informed opinion at the time was that their only action when taken before the bite of an infected mosquito was the temporary suppression of a clinical attack. This raised the question: Was there any other drug, including newly discovered or inadequately tested compounds, which might provide complete protection of fighting troops in highly malarious areas? Such a drug would make an enormous contribution towards winning the war for the Allied forces, and this was already an important goal of research teams in the USA and Britain. One objective of Fairley and Albert's overseas mission was to find out what research was in progress in this field. They were to 'ascertain if research work in England and America was being undertaken with the object of discovering a true prophylactic drug, i.e., one having a specific lethal action on the sporozoite'.[1]

Studies conducted in Britain and Europe during the 1930s provided new insights into the malaria cycle that had important implications for the development of antimalarial drugs. This information had already been published in the scientific literature. In 1917 Professor Wagner Von Jauregg, a Viennese psychiatrist, found that deliberate infection with malaria improved the condition of mental patients with advanced syphilis. The results were somewhat variable, but infection led to considerable improvement in about a third of cases.[2] The spirochete causing syphilis is killed by elevated temperatures, and it was originally thought that the high fever of malaria produced this effect. However, it is still not entirely clear why this drastic therapy was beneficial to syphilis patients—other methods cause high temperatures in patients but do not give the same results. Von Jauregg infected his patients by injecting blood from a person with malaria. This method of inoculation was later used by Warrington Yorke and J. W. S. Macfie, who commenced malaria therapy of mental patients in Liverpool, Britain, in 1922. Some of the English patients were also bitten by infected mosquitoes which had previously fed on malaria cases. It was found that quinine, given three to seven days before and after inoculation, completely prevented infections in all patients who were injected with blood containing vivax malaria. On the other hand, this drug treatment did not prevent natural infections by mosquito bites.[3]

The difference in quinine response produced by the two kinds of inoculation was difficult to explain. In the years following Ross's discovery of the mosquito cycle in 1897 it was observed that there was an interval of several days between the bite of an infected mosquito with sporozoites and the microscopic appearance of blood stages in humans. It was not known what happened to the parasites during this period, but most workers assumed that the sporozoites directly entered red blood cells. The German parasitologist Fritz Schaudinn reported in 1902 that he had observed this under the microscope, but it was not confirmed by other workers. Yorke and Macfie's results conflicted with this theory because, if the sporozoites penetrated blood cells, inoculation with infected blood and bites from infected mosquitoes should have produced the same result, and quinine should have had the same effect on infections derived from both methods of inoculation.

Another Englishman, Lieutenant Colonel S. P. James, made an important contribution towards resolving this puzzle. In 1931 he repeated Yorke and Macfie's observations and speculated that the sporozoites might enter some other cells, perhaps those lining the blood vessels or connective tissue, rather than the blood corpuscles.[4] In 1937 James and his co-worker P. Tate announced the discovery that malaria parasites of birds developed in body tissues (the reticulo-endothelial cells lining the organs) before entering the blood.[5] This raised the possibility that a similar cycle existed in human malaria.

Strong supporting evidence for this was obtained during the same year by M. Ciuca and his colleagues working with malaria-infected mental patients in Romania. They showed that the blood of patients was not infective to other humans for five days after the patients were inoculated with sporozoites of falciparum malaria.[6] This implied that the sporozoites developed somewhere else, rather than in the blood. If this were the case, it would explain the failure of quinine to prevent the development of mosquito-transmitted infections. The existence of such a cycle would also have important implications for future research into antimalarial drugs. It would obviously be of great benefit if a drug was found that could act as a 'causal prophylactic', that is, that could prevent the development of malaria by eliminating the parasites before they produced any clinical manifestations of disease. Such a drug would destroy the so-called 'tissue phase' or 'exoerythrocytic' stages before they entered the circulation. The search for a causal prophylactic became an important focus of research in Europe and the USA in the years leading up to World War II.

The German development of atebrin and plasmoquine at Elberfeld showed that screening synthetic compounds for activity against malaria parasites of birds could lead to the discovery of effective drugs for human malaria, and this stimulated the search for new improved malaria drugs in Europe and the USA. The results of this research were reported in the scientific literature throughout the 1930s. In the latter half of this decade the sulphonamides came under scrutiny, and many experiments were done using this group of drugs against malaria parasites of birds, monkeys and humans. After the start of World War II, publication of scientific advances in many fields was restricted, in order to deny this knowledge to the enemy. (In any case, there was usually a delay of a year or so between the discovery and publication of new research findings.) The visit of Fairley and Albert to leading malaria research centres in Britain and the USA during the latter part of 1942 provided an ideal opportunity for the Australians to learn of the latest advances in this field. Even before the visit Fairley was aware that this was an important research avenue, and his proposal to the Director General of Medical Services specifically mentioned that one objective would be 'to establish a closer liaison with research chemists working on the more recent sulphonamide drugs and other synthetic preparations antagonistic to malaria parasites'.[7]

Fairley and Albert visited the only two places for testing new antimalarials in Britain. At the University of Cambridge they visited Dr Ann Bishop, working under Professor Keilin, who was performing tests of various drugs on canaries using the bird malaria parasite *Plasmodium relictum*. The results were sent to the Chemotherapy Committee of the British Medical Research Council, which initiated pharmacological investigations of promising drugs in mammals. The other institution they visited was the newly established ICI pharmacological laboratories at Blackley, near Manchester. Very little had actually been accomplished in this facility by the time of the visit, but the laboratories were testing sulphonamides against malaria. One of this group of compounds, sulphamezathine, appeared to be very promising, but high concentrations in blood were required and it was considered dangerous to persist with such high doses for very long.

Fairley and Albert found that the set-up for synthesising and testing possible new antimalarial drugs in the USA was as well organised (and far more comprehensive in scope) as that existing in Britain. The work was co-ordinated under the auspices of the National Research Council (NRC) by a group initially called the Conference of Chemotherapy of Malaria—later the Board for the Co-ordination of Malarial Studies. Members of the group were senior medical scientists involved in malaria research from various universities and the US Public Health Service, as well as officials of the NRC, and representatives from the Army and Navy. The approach was to screen large numbers of compounds against bird parasites with the ultimate aim of undertaking preliminary evaluation of the more promising ones in humans. The program commenced somewhat slowly and tentatively, but the pace of the co-operative effort increased after the USA entered the war. The Board oversaw the antimalarial research being carried out in various parts of the country; received reports of work in progress; and funded projects of which they approved. By the time of the Australian visit the facilities for testing antimalarial drugs in experimental animals had been well developed and standardised in half a dozen separate US institutions.

The Australians visited several key laboratories where work was in progress and had discussions with the senior staff. They visited the National Institutes of Health facilities at Bethesda where Dr L. F. Small was in charge of the chemical work on malaria and Dr G. Robert Coatney directed the parasite studies. Coatney and W. C. Cooper carried out experiments with sulphaguanidine and sulphadiazine, which were administered to chicks exposed to bites of mosquitoes infected with the bird malaria parasite *Plasmodium gallinaceum*.[8] Although some chicks became infected on the former drug, none of the chicks treated with sulphadiazine developed malaria. This suggested that it had a causal prophylactic action against the parasite. This work was not published until 1944, but it was filed with the Committee on Medical Research in April 1942 and it is likely that these important findings were discussed with Fairley and Albert.

Fairley and Albert called at the Rockefeller Foundation, New York, where Dr L. T. Coggleshall had reported in 1938 that sulphanilamide prevented infection of primate malaria (*P. knowlesi*) in rhesus monkeys. Cases of human malaria were not cured by this drug but his findings raised the possibility that a similar compound would prevent malaria in humans. During 1941 Coggleshall and his colleagues John Maier and C. A. Best (working at the Gorgas Hospital in Panama) had published a report that the sulphonamides promin and sulphadiazine had a beneficial effect when used in clinical treatment of acute cases of human malaria.[9] Fairley and Albert had the opportunity to meet Dr Maier while they were in New York. Fairley's report of the visit stated that Maier's experience, 'which was borne out clinically by his colleague, Dr Coggleshall, was that the antimalarial activity of sulpha drugs was *exactly* parallel to their antibacterial activity'.[10]

Fairley was also aware of field experiments begun by Dr G. M. Findlay with British Army troops in West Africa during 1942.[11] Half of the personnel of certain units took atebrin (600 mg/week) and the other half took 500 mg daily of sulphapyrazine, sulphamezathine or sulphamerazine. Results in early 1943 were starting to look promising against infections of falciparum malaria. In comparison with atebrin controls, sulphapyrazine appeared to be more effective; sulphamezathine was equally effective; and sulphamerazine appeared to be somewhat less effective. There were many uncontrolled factors in this trial so it was not possible to determine whether the sulphonamides were exerting a suppressive or a causal prophylactic effect. Nevertheless, when the data from American, British and West African experiments were considered together, they provided a promising lead that one of this group of drugs might be able to prevent human malaria infections.

The possibility that there might be a drug that would act as a causal prophylactic was of vital interest to Australia. If this proved to be the case, it was imperative that it be made available to the troops as soon as possible. This would be absolutely crucial to the war effort because it would resolve the major medical impediment for the Australians in the South West Pacific. It would give the Allies an advantage against the enemy and this could significantly tilt the tide of war against the Japanese. The possibility that one of the sulphonamides might be able to act in this way was particularly attractive as Australia had the capacity to manufacture these compounds, unlike atebrin, and the country would not be dependent on overseas supplies, which had already caused serious problems in the war.

Sulphaguanidine, another sulphonamide, had been proved by Fairley and Colonel Boyd in the Middle East to be effective against all forms of dysentery. It was adopted for treatment of dysentery by Australian troops before it was used for this purpose by the British and Americans.[12] It would have been apparent to Fairley during his overseas visit that the civilian-based research institutions in both countries were devoting the bulk of their efforts to screening new compounds in animals and relatively few resources were available for clinical testing against human malaria. Under these circumstances the idea arose that an alternative approach to permit rapid evaluation of the causal prophylactic ability of sulphonamides would be for the Australians to undertake this work themselves using army volunteers in a unit of the Australian Army Medical Corps.

The chain of events leading up to the adoption of this plan is not entirely clear. The official history of the Australian Army Medical Services notes that the idea was due to H. K. Ward, Professor of Bacteriology at the University of Sydney, Lieutenant Colonel Bill Keogh and Major Ian Mackerras,[13] but the concept could not have been developed without input from Fairley at the very outset. After the first meeting of the Combined Advisory Committee on Tropical Medicine, Hygiene and Sanitation on 13 March 1943, General MacArthur told Fairley in a personal interview that he wanted the committee to investigate thoroughly all tropical disease problems. If it were considered necessary, this could include experiments with troops.[14] This latter suggestion was probably initiated by Fairley, as he knew that such experiments could determine whether the sulphonamide drugs acted as causal prophylactics of malaria and it is likely that he was already preparing the ground for the formation of an Australian Army effort to undertake this work. He fully understood the background and complexities in this field of research and was familiar with the latest scientific publications on malaria. His visit to the USA and Britain in late 1942 was most important in alerting him to the latest research developments overseas. He was the only Australian capable of assessing promising research avenues that might lead to the development of a causal prophylactic, and to identify this as a worthy goal for an Australian research team to pursue in search of an effective drug against New Guinea strains of malaria.

While in Sydney during May 1943, Fairley discussed the possibility of establishing a malaria research unit at the University of Sydney with members of the staff.[15] The subject of the unit clearly became a major topic at Army Headquarters around this time, as Keogh mentioned in a personal letter to Ford that Fairley had agreed to 'a tentative scheme for the great experiment'.[16] There is evidence that Keogh played a leading part in advocating that the plan be adopted as soon as possible. In another letter he wrote to Ford that 'I have been at him [Fairley] for the past months but he wouldn't tell me what it was all about and only a week ago gave me some of the dope. I tried to get some action but he just said that nothing could be done until he had finished with Earle Page'.[17]

After finalising Page's report in Sydney, Fairley returned to the university on 5 June, where he met Professor Harvey Sutton and Dr George Heyden to 'discuss in some detail the facilities for accommodating a malaria research unit'.[18] The question of constructing an insectary for rearing mosquitoes was raised with Heyden. The development of *Anopheles* larvae is dependent on temperature, and the survival of adult mosquitoes is strongly influenced by humidity. Also, the duration of the mosquito cycle of the parasite is extended at lower temperatures, and if it is too cold the cycle is arrested. The ideal rearing condition for most mosquito species is around 25°C, with relative humidity of 70–75 per cent. Winter temperatures in Sydney are well below this level, so the provision of a reliable air-conditioning system within a purpose-built insectary was an essential prerequisite. The estimated cost was less than £1500 ($3000), and Fairley observed in his visit notes that the enterprise 'should be entirely under Army control and this can best be achieved by financing it entirely'. The afternoon was spent in discussions with Professor Ward on possible siting of wards for the experimental work on the site of two old tennis courts 'adjacent to the pathological department where the biochemists and parasitologists [of the unit] would be located, and near to the School of Hygiene and Tropical Medicine where the proposed insectarium would be built'. Food could come from the kitchens of adjacent Prince Alfred Hospital and nursing staff could probably be accommodated at St Andrews—a residential college for students of the university.[19]

Despite these talks, it was decided to establish the unit in northern Queensland at Cairns rather than in Sydney.[20] In early official correspondence the scheme was described as the 'Malaria Experiment'; it was to be conducted at Cairns by specialist staff attached to 5 Australian Camp Hospital (ACH).[21] The reasons for choosing Cairns do not seem to have been documented but it is likely that a number of factors were considered. The idea of attaching the staff to an existing army unit was a convenient way of starting the work with a minimum of delay. Moreover, the tropical environment was favourable for rearing mosquitoes without the need to construct an air-conditioned insectary. An additional inducement for selecting Cairns rather than Sydney may have been the presence of Army Malaria Control units in north Queensland. They were immediately available to collect *Anopheles* larvae from the surrounding area for the experiment.

The identity of the drugs to be tested was kept secret for reasons of military security. Major I. J. (Ian) Wood suggested 'anti sweat' as a code name, and Fairley and Keogh abbreviated this to 'A-S' followed by a roman numeral for each drug within the series.[22] The drugs to be used and their codes were: A-S I = sulphamerazine; A-S II = sulphamezathine; and A-S III = sulphadiazine.

Reports from the USA indicated that sulphamerazine had a high rate of absorption from the intestinal tract and a relatively slow excretion by the kidneys. Following a single dose, blood levels of this drug rose more rapidly and were sustained longer than with sulphadiazine. Also, there appeared to be less risk of toxic symptoms with sulphamerazine, which was excreted more completely in urine than sulphadiazine. These characteristics suggested that it might be administered in smaller amounts and less often than other sulphonamides while, at the same time, maintaining effective blood levels for therapeutic purposes. For these reasons it was selected, as A-S I, for the first experiments at Cairns, and was subsequently subjected to more extensive tests than the other two sulphonamides. The possibility of manufacturing this drug in Australia was also explored.

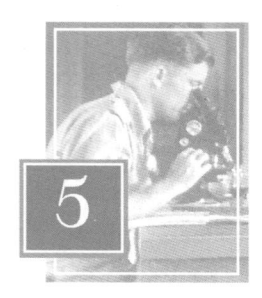

Priority Neill

THE AUSTRALIAN ARMY 'malarial experimental group' in Cairns included a physician (also Officer Commanding), a pathologist, an entomologist, a biochemist and supporting technicians, as well as nursing staff who were to be attached to 5 ACH.[1] Volunteers, who had never previously been subjected to the risk of malaria infection, were to be drawn from convalescent depots in southern Australia. Parasites were to be obtained from army 'donors' who had contracted the disease on active service in New Guinea. Local anopheline mosquitoes were to be reared by the entomology section and used to transmit infections from the donors to the volunteers who would take the various drug regimens to be tested. The Army moved quickly—the provision of additional nursing and clerical staff at 5 ACH to support the malaria experiment was authorised by Army Headquarters, Melbourne, on 22 June 1943.[2] At the same time movement orders for the first specialist staff were raised.

The Officer Commanding the Cairns research facility was Major (later Lieutenant Colonel) R. R. (Rod) Andrew, who was also responsible for the medical aspects of the work. Andrew, a physician, had already acquired considerable clinical experience of malaria in the war. During 1941 he was involved in investigations of malaria, first in Kantara in Egypt as a medical officer at 2/2 Australian General Hospital (AGH), and later with 2/7 Field Ambulance in Syria. After returning from the Middle East he was posted as physician (Major) to 105 Casualty Clearing Stations (CCS) in Port Moresby, and was later seconded to 2/1 CCS at Milne Bay. The major part of his work in New Guinea concerned malaria. He was mentioned in an official letter from the Assistant Director of Pathology of New Guinea Force, Lieutenant Colonel Ted

Ford, to the Director General of Medical Services as being among a small group of officers who gave great assistance in raising the malaria consciousness of the troops.[3] Andrew was a protégé of Lieutenant Colonel Bill Keogh who was behind the move for his appointment to the group at Cairns.[4] Keogh wrote to Ford at around this time that he was ' very bucked that Rod should be here very quickly and that he will run the show at Cairns'.[5]

The pathologist appointed at Cairns was Major T. C. (Clive) Backhouse who had excellent credentials in tropical medicine, including malaria. Before the war Backhouse had been the Government Pathologist in Rabaul, and had served as pathologist at 2/7 Australian General Hospital in the Middle East. Backhouse arrived in Cairns on 27 June with a trusted technician from his former unit, Sergeant (later Lieutenant) M. S. A. (Max) Swan.[6]

The site of 5 ACH in 1943 was North Cairns State School on Sheridan Street. The building was a single-storey structure on top of piles 2–3 metres high; the lower level was enclosed with makeshift canvas walls to turn it into several messes for officers, sergeants and support staff. Sleeping quarters and a mess for the other ranks were in tents erected in the playgrounds. Part of the building, which included a teachers' common room, was partitioned off for use by the malaria experimental group.[7] There were two large wards, able to take 35 and 25 patients, respectively, as well as two smaller wards and a laboratory. The area was mosquito-proofed to prevent the risk of malaria transmission from infected volunteers via local mosquitoes to the surrounding community. Four nursing sisters and another four nursing orderlies cared for the volunteer patients. The senior nursing officer was Captain B. E. (Beryl) Burbidge, with clerical support provided by Corporal R. E. (Rosemary) Gore.

Before undertaking the experimental work at Cairns, Fairley wished to be sure that long-term use of sulphonamide drugs would not produce toxic symptoms in men exposed to arduous conditions in the tropics. In order to exclude this possibility he arranged with Lieutenant Colonel R. V. Bretherton, OC of 9 Field Ambulance, stationed in Port Moresby, for 100 of his men to be put on 1000 mg daily of sulphadiazine, together with 100 mg atebrin, for six weeks.[8] The men worked hard and experienced considerable fluid loss by sweating. They were clinically monitored throughout this period, but none developed toxic manifestations.

A necessary criterion for selection of volunteers was that they had not previously visited or lived in a malarious area. This was important—'non-immunes' had no acquired immunity afforded by previous exposure to the disease and that might have obscured the effect of the test drugs. Men were accepted for preliminary investigation as volunteers if they were between 18–45 years; were physically fit (A1 in the army sense or unfit for front-line duties on account of certain disabilities, e.g. a missing limb or eye, but otherwise fit); and had no history of venereal disease, asthma, hay fever, auditory or optic nerve diseases, or jaundice within the previous five years.[9] All of the 'recipient volunteers' were infected with malaria by sporozoite-infected mosquitoes or by blood inoculation. They were classed as either 'test cases' who would receive drugs or 'controls' who were exposed to infection while not receiving drugs.

The 'donors' for the Cairns studies were men who had already been infected with malaria in the South West Pacific. Their essential attribute was the presence of gametocytes (the stages that infect mosquitoes) in the blood. Mosquitoes fed on these 'gametocyte carriers' would then transmit the disease to recipient volunteers. An important consideration was that the donors must be protected from being bitten by local mosquitoes that might transmit their malaria to the local population. In order to prevent this possibility they were housed at 2/2 AGH at Rocky Creek in the Atherton Tablelands, about 100 km from Cairns. There was no risk of local malaria transmission in this locality as surveys had shown it to be free of *Anopheles* mosquitoes.

Fairley's experimental plan for Cairns involved infecting volunteers using mosquitoes carrying sporozoites of vivax or falciparum malaria (see Fig. 4). These mosquito-induced infections were essential to determine whether the

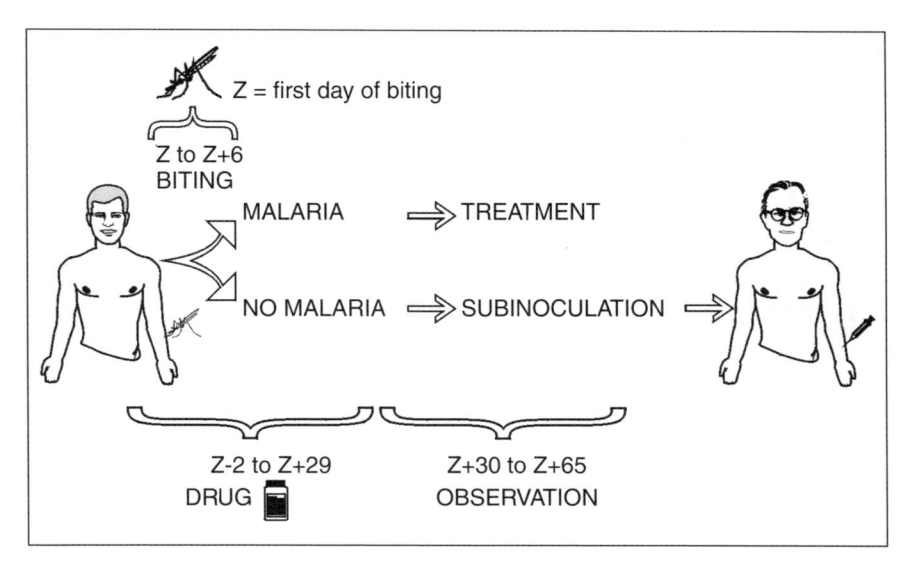

Fig. 4 Plan of experiments at Cairns for mosquito-transmitted malaria

This was the original plan devised by Fairley in June 1943. The numbers of tests and controls in each subgroup were subsequently varied according to specific experimental requirements. Subinoculation of test cases who remained free of overt attacks of malaria after the observation period was not always performed in subsequent experiments.

drugs acted as causal prophylactics by eliminating the parasites that developed from sporozoites before they invaded the blood.

Parallel experiments were carried out at 2/2 AGH, Rocky Creek, where volunteers received malaria by being injected with blood containing parasites from a malaria patient (see Fig. 5). In these tests the parasites bypassed the tissue stages (which are only initiated by sporozoites inoculated by the bite of an infected mosquito) and were restricted to the blood cycle. Lieutenant Colonel I. J. (Ian) Wood was in charge of this component of the work, which was designed to supplement the Cairns sporozoite-induced experiments by testing the suppressive action of the test drugs on the blood stages rather than their causal prophylactic action.

Clinical examinations of all volunteers receiving sporozoite inoculations at Cairns and blood inoculations at Rocky Creek were performed daily. Thick blood films were made each day and examined for the presence of malaria parasites. Blood and urine estimations of the quantity of the test drug were made on selected men in each group.

For each experiment the volunteers were divided into several subgroups of four men, in which three test subjects received the chemotherapeutic agent

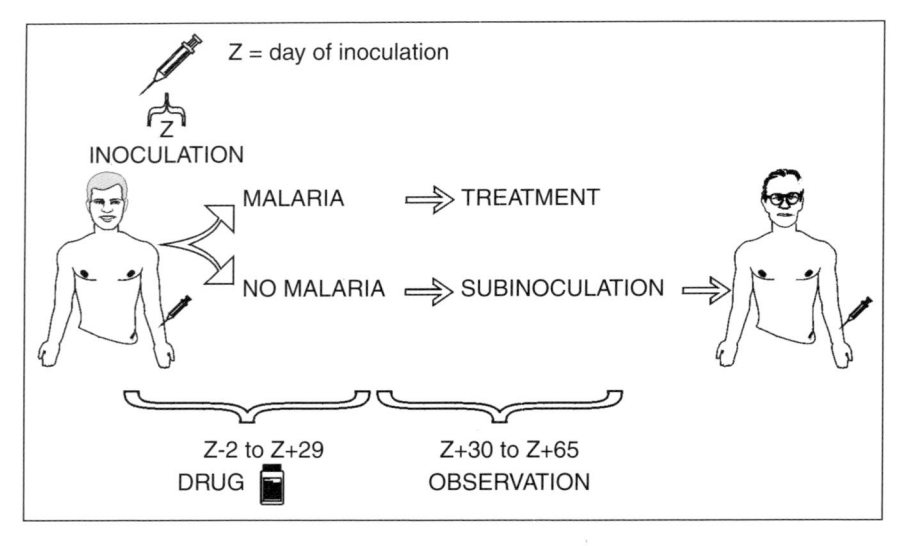

Fig. 5 Plan of experiments at Rocky Creek in the Atherton Tablelands for blood-induced malaria

In these experiments the volunteers were injected with 15 ml of blood containing malaria parasites on Z Day. The test subjects at Rocky Creek received the same drug regimens as the sporozoite-inoculated volunteers at Cairns (from day Z-2 until day Z+29). Subsequent observation, treatment and subinoculation procedures were the same as those adopted at Cairns.

being tested; one man of each subgroup received no drugs and acted as a control. The sulphonamide drug was administered to the test volunteers at a dose rate of 1000 mg daily for two or more days before they were exposed to infection. All four volunteers of each subgroup at Cairns were then bitten by *Anopheles* mosquitoes infected with sporozoites of either *Plasmodium falciparum* or *P. vivax*, over a period of seven days, during which time they received between 10 and 20 infective bites. The day on which the volunteers were first bitten was designated 'Z Day'. Drug administration commenced on Z–2 Day, biting occurred from Z Day to Z+6 Day inclusive, and drug administration continued until Z+29 Day (23 days after the last infective bite). This period of drug administration was chosen as it was considered adequate to cover the normal incubation period of South West Pacific strains of falciparum and vivax malaria.

Volunteers who developed overt malaria were treated with quinine, atebrin and plasmoquine therapy (QAP), the standard treatment regimen then in use by Australian forces. Those at Cairns who remained well throughout the 23-day period following exposure were transferred to 2/2 AGH, and observed there for a further five weeks. If the test volunteers remained well at the end of this period, 200 ml of their blood was 'subinoculated' (i.e. injected) into non-immune recipients who were not taking antimalarial drugs. Lack of development of overt malaria in the recipients over a 30-day observation period (during which daily blood films were examined) confirmed that the test subjects were free of infection at the time of subinoculation. If this occurred, their susceptibility to malaria was then tested by intra-muscular injection of blood from a patient with overt infection of the same species of parasite to which the test subjects were originally exposed by mosquito bite. After developing acute attacks of malaria the volunteers received the standard QAP antimalarial treatment at 2/2 AGH before being discharged from the experiment.

By mid-1943 many men who had been infected with malaria in New Guinea had returned to Australia, either by evacuation or normal rotation of their units. Those who reported for treatment of *P. vivax* relapses after their return from New Guinea to Australian base areas provided a convenient source of gametocytes for the experiment. On the other hand, *P. falciparum* does not relapse in humans after the initial blood infection is cured, and its prevalence in troops declined rapidly after their return to Australia. Some *P. falciparum* cases were obtained as donors from army hospitals in Queensland, and donors were also sought from troops serving in New Guinea.

Fairley visited Port Moresby during the last week of June 1943, and arranged for the evacuation of *P. falciparum* cases to Cairns.[10] It was decided that they would be evacuated by plane from Wau to 2/9 AGH in Port Moresby, where suitable gametocyte carriers would be selected and sent by plane either directly to Cairns or via Townsville. The selected cases were to be given just sufficient quinine to control their temperatures and clinical manifestations. As the flight time from Port Moresby to Cairns is only a few hours, this was considered to be a safe procedure. Nevertheless, falciparum malaria is a life-threatening disease if treatment is delayed unduly, and it was essential that these men should not be offloaded or delayed due to aircraft breakdowns or for other reasons.

On his return from New Guinea Fairley discussed this problem with air movement control officers in Townsville. It was suggested that a code word should be formally assigned so that the highest priority would be accorded to all transport matters concerning the Cairns experiment. Apparently Fairley's first name, Neil, was proposed but the code system required five letters so another 'l' was added.[11] This was the origin of the famous 'PRIORITY NEILL' adopted after Fairley met Major General Frank Berryman at Advanced LHQ in Brisbane.[12] It was initially used to assure immediate response from the military system for movement of personnel and urgently required supplies, but it also came to have a wider application as a code name for the entire malaria research project. It appeared on signals addressed to 'DIRECTOR OF MEDICINE. NEILL', and also on official correspondence headed 'NEILL EXPERIMENT'.

The first practical problem the group faced before the experiment could commence was to rear large numbers of mosquitoes continuously in the laboratory so that sufficient stocks of adult females were always available to transmit the parasite from donors to recipient volunteers. This required the services of an experienced entomologist. Captain (later Major) M. J. (Jo) Mackerras, who was assigned to this task, came from a famous family in Australian medical history. Mackerras, born Josephine Bancroft, was the granddaughter of Joseph Bancroft, the discoverer of the adult worm responsible for filariasis in humans. Her father, Thomas Bancroft, was also a distinguished medical researcher who, among other things, continued his father's research on filaria to include studies on the mosquito transmission of the disease. After graduating with BSc (Hons) from the University of Queensland, Jo Bancroft studied medicine at the University of Sydney. Soon after graduating in 1924 she married Ian Mackerras, another promising young medical graduate who also had a keen interest in entomology. From 1930 until the outbreak of World War II they both worked in Canberra as part of a research team (led by Ian) in the newly formed Division of Economic Entomology within the Council for Scientific and Industrial Research (the forerunner of CSIRO). Their work focused on veterinary entomology, with particular emphasis on sheep blowfly control . Both husband and wife subsequently joined the AIF. Jo Mackerras enlisted in February 1942, and was initially posted as pathologist at the Army Recruiting Centre in Sydney.

Jo Mackerras was well qualified for the position of entomologist at Cairns by virtue of her extensive experience in the laboratory rearing of insects. The ability of insects to mate in captivity tends to vary between strains and species. Blowflies (the subject of Jo Mackerras's previous endeavours) mate readily in captivity and are relatively easy to rear through successive laboratory generations. Some mosquitoes will also mate in the laboratory but, although there are some exceptions, it is notoriously difficult to get anopheline mosquitoes to mate in cages. In addition, there is no stage of the anopheline life cycle that can be kept alive for very long. The female mosquito needs blood to develop the eggs, which normally hatch two days after they are laid on the water surface. They can be stored on moist filter paper for several days and then induced to hatch by floating them onto water, but their viability is lost after about a week. The duration of the larval stages is usually 10–14 days and adults emerge from the pupae within one to two days. The females must remain alive for at least two weeks to transmit malaria, but it is difficult to keep them alive in captivity for more than three to four weeks.

Malaria is no longer endemic on the mainland of Australia, but it occurred in the tropical north of the country above 19°S latitude until the 1950s. Before this, epidemics occurred periodically in towns and Aboriginal settlements, particularly towards the end of the north Australian wet season when the density of mosquitoes was high. The disease was present in Cairns in the 1940s, and more than 500 cases were recorded in a local epidemic that started in March 1942. Dr G. A. M. Heyden incriminated the mosquito responsible for this epidemic, later identified by Captain A. R. Woodhill as *Anopheles farauti*, the major vector of malaria in coastal regions of the South West Pacific.[13]

This was a most important discovery as it permitted vector control activities to concentrate on breeding sites of this mosquito. This was done by members of the specialised Australian Army Malaria Control Units (AAMCU), which had been formed to carry out this role in the Pacific theatre. Small independent sections, called Australian Mobile Entomological Sections (AMES), which comprised an officer (entomologist) and two other ranks, were also formed to undertake vector surveys in malaria problem areas and to aid the AAMCUs in focusing their control activities as efficiently as possible. Both kinds of units were working in the Cairns area during 1943, and were available to assist the malaria experimental group.

Captain F. H. S. Roberts, an experienced Queensland entomologist, and Staff Sergeant P. O'Sullivan of 2 AMES were allocated to provide entomological support for the malaria experiment. With their help Jo Mackerras quickly set up a rearing system based on continuous field collections of larvae. The project was also assisted by 11 AAMCU staff who commenced systematic full-time collections of *Anopheles* larvae during June. It was found that an officer and 12 men were needed to collect six days a week in order to get sufficient mosquitoes for the experiment. Even with this large team it became necessary to go as far afield as the Daintree River, 80 km to the north, and a similar distance south to Innisfail to obtain adequate numbers of anopheline larvae, which are frequently scattered rather thinly over a wide area of water. Collectors waded into the water in gumboots, collected larvae from the surface using small scoop nets, and transferred them to pickle bottles and later to Winchester bottles. Collections were sent by truck back to the laboratory, where they were poured into enamel basins and reared to the adult stage by feeding on powdered baby food ('Farex' brand). Pupae were removed from dishes each morning and placed in cages where they emerged as adults.[14]

The entomological laboratory consisted of a mosquito-proofed room and verandah in a four-roomed cottage in Sheridan Street, Cairns, which was already housing the AMES and AAMCU staff who were working for the experiment. This accommodation soon proved inadequate, and the entire house was screened against mosquitoes. Two rooms and the verandah were taken over for the laboratory, the remainder of the house still being used as sleeping quarters. The laboratory was about 1 km along Sheridan Street from 5 ACH. Men who were gametocyte carriers were transported down to Cairns in small groups from the Atherton Tablelands, and were housed within mosquito-proofed wards in 5 ACH, where gametocyte counts of their blood were made daily. Cages of mosquitoes (at least two days old) were taken by truck between the laboratory and the wards where they were fed on the donors. Engorged mosquitoes were returned to the laboratory, and held for 10–14 days. During this period any dead or dying mosquito specimens were dissected, and the gut and salivary glands were examined for evidence of oocysts and sporozoites to confirm their suitability for transmission to the test and control volunteers of the experimental subgroups.

In Fairley's original outline for the experiment, donors were to leave Rocky Creek at 1500 hours and arrive in Cairns at about 1830, with the initial groups (each comprising three vivax gametocyte carriers) to arrive on 18, 21 and 23 June.[15] This tentative schedule was followed precisely as the first vivax donors arrived at 5 ACH on 18 June, and mosquitoes were fed on them on 20 June.

Initially, 'multiple feeds' were made, by pooling batches of mosquitoes fed on several donors. Batch no. 1, comprising mosquitoes fed on eight donors from 20–26 June, gave negative results as all of the 11 dissected mosquitoes subsequently proved to be uninfected. Pooled batch no. 2 (mosquitoes fed from 23–28 June on five donors) was not much better, with only one specimen out of 31 dissected being infected with oocysts.[16] Andrew recorded in his war diary that 'the results after the first fortnight are disappointing. Very few infected mosquitoes have been found after feeds on carriers'.[17]

Fairley went to Cairns on 3 July after returning from New Guinea. He arrived at 5 ACH in the late afternoon, and discussed difficulties in mosquito transmission with Captain Jo Mackerras, Captain Roberts and Major Andrew.[18] The next day he inspected the mosquito-proofed wards; saw the donors admitted as gametocyte carriers; and discussed, with Major Backhouse, the technique of counting gametocytes in blood slides.

The next two mosquito batches were fed on vivax donors during the last few days of June until 4 July, and were combined into one pooled batch. Salivary gland dissections showed that around 25 per cent developed sporozoites, and these mosquitoes were used to infect the first test and control patients for the first experiment with sulphamerazine.[19]

The initial groups of volunteers were recruited from Army Convalescent depots in southern Australia. The first group of eight men arrived in Cairns by train on 14 July, accompanied by Major A. Fryberg, the Deputy Assistant Director of Health in Brisbane, who was responsible for co-ordinating their movement. He told Andrew that the most suitable travel arrangements for future groups would be via the regular troop trains scheduled to leave Brisbane on Mondays, Wednesdays and Fridays. He needed five days' notice (preferably 36 or 48 hours before the actual time of departure) to get the men to Cairns.[20] One of the first group was rejected as he had a history of asthma, and a signal was sent to Brisbane advising that men with a predisposition to allergic manifestations should not be accepted for the experiment.[21] Major General Burston paid a short visit at this time and inspected the wards and experimental facilities.

Andrew's war diary for 17 July 1943 reports:

> The entomological section have some good BT [vivax infected mosquito] batches and today are ready ... The four men of subgroup i were taken to the entomological hut at 1900 hrs. They walked straight into the ambulance and were driven off immediately. The hut being screened, the chance of any stray natural infection is extremely remote. The first bite was recorded at 1915 hrs.[22]

The diary also records that considerable difficulty was experienced in getting some of the mosquitoes to bite. For these initial infection experiments, a suitable number of infected mosquitoes were placed in a small cage and the volunteer's hand was placed inside. This method proved uncertain, as it was difficult to see exactly how many fed on the subject, and there was the possibility that some infected mosquitoes might escape from the cage. For later infection experiments, mosquitoes were placed in a larger cage and a specified number were allowed to bite the back of the recipient's hand through the netting.[23]

Experimental transmission of malaria is not a simple exercise. Success is contingent on the harmonious association of the three biological components of the system: the parasite, the vertebrate (human) host, and the invertebrate (mosquito) host. Failure to complete the transmission cycle may be due to a number of independent or interrelated factors that are not always understood, even by experienced investigators. For example, gametocytes must be present within the human host for transmission to the mosquito to occur, but their presence does not always guarantee success. In some cases, these stages appear to be mature and viable but they may not be infective. *Anopheles* species differ in their ability to transmit the parasite. Moreover, it is common for only some mosquitoes in a batch of a susceptible species to become infected, even if all of those in the batch feed simultaneously on a human carrier with suitable infective gametocytes. The successful researcher working in this field requires dedication, patience, and a prodigious capacity for hard work. Clearly, Jo Mackerras and her assistants must have worked under immense pressure, knowing that the whole experimental program depended on their efforts.

Because the final decision on the location of the unit was not made until after 5 June, the first mosquito collections for the project could not have started in Cairns until after this date. The AAMCU and AMES staff were already on hand, but at least a week was needed before larvae collected in the field could be reared to the adult stage and be available for feeding on gametocyte carriers. It therefore seems incredible that sufficient progress in mosquito-rearing had been made to permit the first feed on gametocyte donors by 20 June. It is even more remarkable that, even though these first attempts to infect mosquitoes were not successful, better results were achieved with the next batches, which were promptly used to infect the first experimental recipients. This was an extraordinary achievement by Major Jo Mackerras and the entomology staff of the experimental group. Normal practice would have been to undertake a number of preliminary experiments, over several months, to optimise the transmission cycle from donors to mosquitoes before proceeding to infect the first recipients on the test drugs. The experimental work was driven by the urgency of the military situation, which precluded this sequential approach. In fact, the speed with which the experimental plan was implemented was probably without precedent for a scientific undertaking of this magnitude and complexity.

6

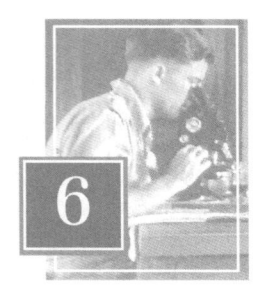

Neil Desperandum

ON 29 July 1943 indications of breakthroughs (i.e. malarial attacks during or shortly after drug administration) were seen in a number of the Cairns men on sulphamerazine, 12 days after they were bitten by mosquitoes infected with vivax malaria.[1] By 3 August all six test cases had overt infections. These results, which occurred while the test volunteers were still taking the drug, provided clear indications that sulphamerazine at a dose of 1000 mg/day did not prevent vivax malaria derived from fairly heavy natural sporozoite infections. Nevertheless, the drug did have some effect in moderating the initial course of the disease, as fever symptoms and parasites were much reduced in the test cases compared with the controls. Blood-induced infection experiments commenced at Rocky Creek on 14 July. The results were similar to those obtained at Cairns. All eight test cases inoculated with *Plasmodium vivax* blood stages developed malaria, five while they were still taking sulphamerazine, and three during the observation period after they had ceased taking the drug.[2]

The first attempt to infect mosquitoes by feeding on donors with *P. falciparum* gametocytes was made on 2 July.[3] The results were similar to the early feeding attempts on *P. vivax* infected donors—the infection rate was very low (only 4 of 59 dissected mosquitoes were infected) and the mosquitoes were not used for the experiment. Mosquitoes fed during the second week of July developed infection rates of 20–30 per cent and, on 24 July, they were used to infect the first *P. falciparum* subgroup receiving sulphamerazine. By the time the Tropical Diseases Advisory Committee met in Melbourne on 23 August, all of the volunteers in the first falciparum subgroup had completed their last dose of sulphamerazine. All were clinically well, though one 'had a persistent scanty infection for about ten days with mild intermittent symptoms', and a single parasite was seen in the blood films of the other two cases for one day only.[4] In summarising the initial progress of the malaria experiment, Fairley reported to the committee that a significant difference had already been seen in the effects of the sulphonamide drugs on vivax and falciparum malaria. He described the failure of sulphamerazine to suppress *P. vivax* infections, and gave a progress update on the more favourable initial results of this drug against sporozoite-inoculated falciparum malaria at Cairns. Fairley also mentioned the first results at Rocky Creek, which were similar to those at Cairns.[5]

Sporozoite-induced experiments with the other two sulphonamide drugs proceeded during August. The trend in the results for all drug regimens was apparent by the last week in September when all had completed their daily drug schedules for the 23-day period after receiving their last infected mosquito bites. All of the test volunteers subjected to sporozoite-induced or blood-inoculated *P. vivax* broke through with attacks of malaria, either while they were taking the drug or during the observation period after they stopped taking it. It was apparent that the administration of sulphonamides at a dose of 1000 mg/day offered little prospect for causal prophylaxis or adequate suppression of vivax malaria. Analysis of the *P. falciparum* experimental groups showed that 11 test subjects (four out of 21 from Cairns and another seven out of 24 from Rocky Creek) contracted clinical attacks of malaria either during or soon after the period of drug administration.

Fairley closely monitored the progress of the experiments by frequent visits to Cairns. He left for Melbourne after his first visit on 7 July, but returned again to north Queensland between 21 and 31 July, when he spent several days at 5 ACH; he called in again on his way to Brisbane on 13 August. The first cases of breakthrough of vivax malaria on sulphamerazine occurred during this period, and this was a source of considerable disappointment for the staff of the research team who were hoping for confirmation of the causal prophylactic properties of the sulphonamides. It would seem that this view was not entirely shared by Fairley. He appeared, at this stage, to be still optimistic about the sulphonamides and was already looking towards future experiments that might provide the desired results. Andrew said that this was expressed at the time as 'Neil Desperandum'.[6] Presumably, he was encouraged by the fact that there were 34 test volunteers inoculated with falciparum malaria (17 each from Cairns and Rocky Creek) who had not 'broken through' by the end of the observation period. Blood from these men was then subinoculated into recipients who, in all cases, remained malaria free. This demonstrated that the 34 test volunteers had been radically cured—their malaria parasites had been completely eliminated.

Fairley reported to the Tropical Diseases Advisory Committee meeting on 23 August that causal prophylaxis might still be obtained with higher sulphonamide doses and he urged that the project should retain its original priority.

At this point it still seemed that one of these drugs would be able to solve the malaria problem in the South West Pacific. If so, its local production would be expedited, and it would be adopted for use by Allied troops within a few months. Fairley said that the most promising lines to follow were a combination of sulphamerazine or sulphamezathine with atebrin, and said this should be the next series of experiments. Drug combinations were already being used for malaria therapy—the standard treatment for Australian troops at that time being QAP (quinine, atebrin and plasmoquine), but the idea of combining two drugs for causal prophylaxis or suppression was novel at that time. The study of atebrin plus sulphamerazine/sulphamezathine would require at least three months and 60–80 volunteers.[7] However, even if complete suppression was obtained, there could be cases of latent infections during which malaria persisted for a time without clinical symptoms, before relapsing at a later date. More volunteers would be needed for subinoculation experiments to prove freedom from such latent malaria.

Andrew received a communication from Fairley on 29 August outlining the experimental scheme for the 'combined series' in which 1000 mg daily of sulphamerazine or sulphamezathine would be combined with 100 mg atebrin taken six days a week.[8] As a comparison, some volunteers were to receive only atebrin without the other drug. Volunteers were to be infected with either *P. falciparum* or *P. vivax* by mosquito transmission at Cairns, or by blood inoculation at 2/2 AGH under the same conditions as those of the sulphonamide series. The period of sulphonamide drug administration (with Z–2 Day as day 1 of treatment) was also the same as the previous series, but atebrin (either alone or in combination) was to be given for three weeks before the first infective bite to permit adequate build-up of the drug in the test cases. The use of higher sulphonamide doses to further investigate the possibility of causal prophylactic activity, either by direct action on the sporozoites or on the undiscovered stages that developed from them, had already been mentioned by Fairley at the August meeting of the Tropical Diseases Advisory Committee. During September he decided to include additional test subjects for the 'combined series' who were to take sulphamerazine alone at a daily dose of either 3000 mg or 4000 mg, commencing on the day before the first bite and continuing until two days after the last bite. Andrew received a signal on 25 September advising that test volunteers on each of these dose regimens were to be added for both the vivax and falciparum groups of this series.[9]

Fairley returned to Cairns on 2 October, when the first vivax subgroup to include a subject on 3000 mg sulphamerazine was starting, and left for New Guinea via Townsville on 6 October.[10] He returned to 5 ACH on 14 October on his way back from Port Moresby and, on the following day, went with Andrew to visit 2/2 AGH. In the previous one to two weeks the first three subgroups (two vivax and one falciparum) had finished their biting period and the controls had already developed overt malaria infections. None of the test volunteers, who were still taking their daily atebrin and atebrin/sulphonamide regimens, had broken through with parasites in the blood, though two had mild fevers for a few days. However, the vivax subject on 3000 mg sulphamerazine over the biting period had just broken through, with the first parasites observed on 15 October.[11]

Andrew prepared an interim report on 31 October that outlined the initial results of the combined series.[12] The men in seven of the eight subgroups had been bitten by this time and the trends of the different regimens were already becoming apparent. None of the vivax cases on atebrin alone or atebrin combined with sulphonamides had broken through while on their drugs (see Table 1). This was in marked contrast to the previous series in which most vivax cases broke through with malaria attacks while they were still taking 1000 mg/day of a sulphonamide. This suggested that, even with the small numbers of cases observed, atebrin was superior to the sulphonamides in suppressing attacks of vivax malaria. It also seemed that atebrin alone was as effective as the sulphonamides against falciparum malaria, but the numbers were too small for definite conclusions to be drawn. Test and control volunteers, receiving the same sulphonamide and atebrin drug regimens as the combined series at Cairns, were infected by blood containing either falciparum or vivax parasites at Rocky Creek. None of the test cases taking atebrin combined with one of the sulphonamides broke through with clinical attacks of malaria.[13] The outcome of these blood-inoculated experiments reinforced the favourable results of the mosquito-transmitted experiments at Cairns.

Men in the last subgroup of the combined series finished being bitten on 3 November and, shortly afterwards, Fairley made a brief visit to Cairns accompanying members of a British Military Mission to inspect the work.[14] On 16 November Andrew sent some follow-up data to Fairley at Army Headquarters, Melbourne, when the observation period of the groups was about half-completed.[15] By then all tests on high-dose sulphamerazine had already broken through: one each *P. vivax* and *P. falciparum* on 3000 mg/day over the biting period; and two each on 4000 mg/day. This seemed to finally extinguish the causal prophylactic potential of the sulphonamides but, after the first breakthrough of the high-dose series in the previous month, Fairley decided to make one last experiment with sporozoite-inoculated vivax cases using sulphamerazine alone at 1000 mg/day.

This experiment, which was confined to one subgroup consisting of a control and four test subjects, commenced on 10 November. The experimental conditions were the same as the original sulphonamide series except that the volunteers received a single bite of a vivax-infective mosquito with confirmed

Table 1 Chronology of first series of Cairns experiments with sulphonamide drugs, and sulphonamides combined with atebrin

Experiment	Procedure	Results
A-S (Anti Sweat) series (*Plasmodium vivax*)	Original plan for sulphonamide experiments. Z day for first subgroup = 17 Jul 1943.	All test cases broke through while on drug or after drug ceased.
A-S series (*P. falciparum*)	Original plan for sulphonamide experiments. Z day for first subgroup = 24 Jul 1943.	Four test subjects broke through; 17 test subjects did not break through.
Combined series: A-S and atebrin (*P. vivax*)	Experimental conditions as for the original plan. 4 subgroups each of 5 men: 1 control; 2 on atebrin 0.6 g/week; 2 on atebrin 0.6 g/week, together with 1 g/day of an A-S drug. Z day between 24 Sept and 3 Nov 1943.	No breakthroughs in men on atebrin alone or in combination with A-S. All test subjects had vivax relapses about three weeks after drugs ceased.
Combined series: A-S and atebrin (*P. falciparum*)	Experimental conditions as for the original plan. 4 subgroups each of 5 men: 1 control; 2 on atebrin 0.6 g/week; 2 on atebrin 0.6 g/week, together with 1 g/day of an A-S drug. Z day between 28 Sept and 3 Nov 1943.	No breakthroughs in men on atebrin alone or in combination with A-S.
High A-S, 1 dose over biting period only (*P. vivax*)	Additional test cases added to the combined series. 1 test case on 3 g/day A-S 1; 2 test cases on 4 g/day A-S 1. Drugs given for 9 days only.	All test cases broke through between Z+15 and Z+23.
High A-S, 1 dose over biting period only (*P. falciparum*)	Additional test cases added to the combined series. 1 test case on 3 g/day A-S 1; 2 test cases on 4 g/day A-S 1. Drugs given for 9 days only.	All test cases broke through between Z+17 and Z+23.
A-S, series 2 (*P. vivax*)	One control; 4 test cases. Each man received 2 infective bites only. 1 g/day A-S 1 for 30 days after biting. Z day = 10 Nov 1943.	One test case broke through on drug; 2 test cases broke through after drugs ceased; 1 test case did not break through.

sporozoites on two successive nights. The rationale for this test was not explained, but the sporozoite exposure was considerably less than the normal procedure for vivax experiments (21 infective bites over seven days). It seems likely that Fairley wished to investigate the possibility that the sulphonamides had some limited effect against sporozoites that was masked when the volunteers received a large dose of inoculum. Perhaps a more favourable result would be seen if cases were exposed to only two infective bites rather than 21. However, this hope was soon eliminated when one test volunteer broke through with parasites 15 days after the first bite, even though he was still on the drug.[16]

With the failure of the sulphonamides as causal prophylactics, the original thrust of the experimental program had come to a dead end, but the progress of the combined series now suggested a promising new line of investigation. All of the falciparum and vivax test subjects remained free of parasites throughout the period that they were on either atebrin or atebrin/sulphonamide. Some men had minor clinical features of headache, malaise, or occasional mild fever associated with tenderness of the liver, but none of these symptoms were sufficiently severe to confine any of the test volunteers to bed. However, a difference between the two kinds of malaria was apparent when all of the subgroups had been transferred from Cairns to 2/2 AGH. None of the test subjects exposed to *P. falciparum* had malaria attacks after ceasing the drugs and volunteers subinoculated with their blood remained free of infection. On the other hand, all of the vivax test subjects broke through with attacks of malaria, 22 days on average after their last dose of atebrin.[17]

American scientists also continued their work on the sulphonamides during 1943 under their Board for the Coordination of Malarial Studies. At a Board meeting in Washington in April Dr G. R. Coatney, a senior malaria scientist at the National Institutes of Health, reviewed the work on sulphadiazine undertaken by the NIH laboratories in Maryland and South Carolina.[18] After finding that high initial doses of sulphadiazine for three or four days did not prevent infection, they discovered that in five cases 2000 mg twice daily for 11 days protected four out of the five men against *P. falciparum*, while a similar regime against *P. vivax* did not give protection. Experiments from there on were limited to the study of causal prophylaxis with the former parasite. Dr James A. Shannon of New York University, the director of the malaria research program at Goldwater Memorial Hospital, stressed that 'this [was] the most important lead so far available on causal prophylaxis and ... additional studies on causal prophylaxis in humans should be started in other places and the program pursued vigorously'.[19] The Service representatives Captain E. G. Hakansson (Navy) and Lieutenant Colonel P. F. Russell (Army) 'emphasised that nothing could be more important than causal prophylaxis and that every effort should be made to extend and expand it in every way possible'.[20]

Following a recommendation that the US Army should undertake field trials, tests of sulphonamide compounds were carried out in hyperendemic areas of the Pacific, the Caribbean and in India. Unfortunately, this work was started without proper planning and consultation with the scientists of the Board. Consequently, these trials were unable to provide an unambiguous indication of the comparative efficacy of the test compounds to prevent or suppress malaria under operational conditions. This was discussed at a Board meeting in October: 'It was emphasised that ... there is insufficient correlation between these studies and the fundamental clinical investigations from which they sprang and no careful integration to yield the specific answers which are urgently needed'.[21] Also, some of the tests were not properly controlled and produced misleading results. For example, the minutes of the same meeting state 'it was the consensus of those present that, on the basis of the data, [of US Army field tests] ... sulphamerazine in doses of [500 mg] daily would appear to be equal to atebrine in doses of [600 mg] weekly as a suppressive'.[22] The work with sulphonamides and atebrin then in progress at Cairns, soon demonstrated that this was not the case with South West Pacific strains of malaria. Even at a dose of 1000 mg daily sulphamerazine was unable to suppress vivax malaria and breakthroughs of falciparum malaria occurred.

One of the US Army trials was conducted on sulphamerazine in New Guinea under the direction of Colonel Maurice G. Pinchoffs, who was a US Army representative on the Combined Advisory Committee on Tropical Medicine, Hygiene and Sanitation.[23] The trial included two groups of 100 men, one group on sulphamerazine and the other on atebrin. Unlike some other US Army trials, the importance of including adequate numbers of untreated control subjects was acknowledged beforehand: 'The committee feels that it is highly desirable for conclusive proof that there be included a group who will live in the malarious area without any protection from anti-malarial drugs'. The malaria cases arising in this group (of 50 men) could then be compared with the test cases to determine the degree of protection afforded by the drugs being evaluated. A progress report on this trial was presented to the Combined Advisory Committee at a meeting on 17 August 1943.[24] By that time 68 per cent of the untreated control group had developed malaria. The malaria cases in the test groups were 36 per cent for sulphamerazine and 18 per cent for atebrin. It was clear that there were fewer cases of malaria among the men on sulphamerazine and atebrin than in the control group, but the relative efficacy of the two drugs was not obvious from the final results provided to the Committee by Colonel Pinchoffs on 3 November 1943.[25] At the same meeting Colonel Fairley gave a summary of the sulphonamide experiments and combined series at Cairns and Rocky Creek, which clearly pointed to the superiority of atebrin. At that time the American Board for Coordination of Malarial Studies was unaware of

Pinchoff's trial and the Australian work. This is evident from the Board meeting held in Washington on 22 December 1943. In reviewing the US Army trials of sulphonamides it was noted that no report had been received on sulphapyrazine sent for trial to the South Pacific. The minutes stated that 'It is believed that this drug was turned over to the Australians for investigation'.[26]

Later work by Coatney's group at NIH showed that sulphadiazine 'in dosages at the limit of tolerance . . . did not act as a causal prophylactic'.[27] The Board concluded that the radical cure of infections following long-term administrations could be explained by the action of the drug against the blood stages. In early 1944 Dr Shannon 'called attention to the experience with sulphadiazine in which over a year of time and a lot of human material were used to show that sulphadiazine is not a prophylactic in man'.[28] The equivalent data at Cairns was generated in less than five months, and this included the time taken from conception of the original plan to the successful implementation of a far more comprehensive experimental series.

During the second half of 1943 mosquito breeding areas tended to dry up along the Queensland coast around Cairns (due to lack of rain in the dry season) and the supply of local mosquito larvae for experiments became unreliable. The species obtained in the Cairns area (in order of abundance) were *Anopheles annulipes*, *A. farauti*, *A. amictus*, *A. hilli* and *A. bancrofti*. All of these mosquitoes were used for the early experiments.[29] In order to supplement the local supply, collections of *A. annulipes* were organised by the Commanding Officer of the School of Malaria Control, Brisbane, and also by the local AAMCUs at Townsville and Sellheim, both elsewhere in northern Queensland. Consignments of larvae from these collections were sent by air to Cairns. The larval supply situation became worse in all these localities during the last week of August.

In early September an army entomologist, Major Francis Ratcliffe, was sent with Sergeant D. A. Cameron to Milne Bay in New Guinea to investigate the possibility of supplying live larvae from there for the Cairns experiments. Ratcliffe reported that this was an ideal locality, and he arranged for Cameron to remain and organise the collection and dispatch of *A. punctulatus*.[30] Well-grown larvae were collected from natural breeding places in Milne Bay, transferred to pickle bottles, packed in crates, and sent by air to Cairns. Approximately 5000 larvae were sent in each crate of six bottles and, provided they were not more than two days in transit, a good yield of mosquitoes was obtained. This species lived very well in captivity. Regular collection in Australia ceased in October 1943, when adequate numbers from Milne Bay were assured.[31]

During the last week of September 1943 Major Backhouse was reposted to his previous position at 2/7 AGH, and Captain (later Major) T. S. (Tom)

Gregory took over as pathologist.[32] Later in the year the Malaria Experimental Group became an independent unit, the Land Headquarters (LHQ) Medical Research Unit. The War Establishment of the unit was issued on 17 November 1943 and notified in General Routine Orders on 26 November. This provided for a full strength of 33, all ranks. There were eight officers: a lieutenant colonel (physician) as commanding officer, two majors (entomologist and pathologist), two captains (pathologist and physician) and three lieutenants (one assistant entomologist and two assistant pathologists). There were four staff sergeants as laboratory assistants (two in entomology and two in pathology), eight other ranks (batmen, driver, general dutymen and ward orderlies), as well as nine Australian Army Medical Women's Service staff employed as clerks and nursing orderlies. In addition, a senior nursing sister and three sisters were attached for care of patients.[33] The establishment was later amended to convert the unit to the AIF.[34]

The work completed during the first six months of the project (late June to December 1943) set the stage for future experiments. Transmission of infections from gametocyte donors to recipient volunteers via mosquitoes had developed into a reliable routine procedure that was followed in subsequent experiments. For reasons of logistics in handling mosquitoes and volunteers, it was convenient to administer the range of test doses to subgroups of four to six men who were then bitten by a single pooled batch of infected mosquitoes. For each particular experimental series several subgroups were infected, as mosquitoes and volunteers became available over several days or weeks, to provide replicates of the various drug regimens to be tested. Preliminary indications of success or failure of individual tests usually became evident while the experiments were still in progress, either when the recipient volunteers were still on the drug in Cairns, or during the subsequent observation period after ceasing the drug at Rocky Creek. It was usual for later subgroups of individual experiments to be modified in the light of preliminary observations of earlier subgroups. The work proceeded in an atmosphere of urgency and, as the duration of each experiment was two to four months, the research team did not wait for the final results of one experiment before starting the next. New experiments commenced while others were still in progress, and it was common for subgroups of several experiments to be in various stages of completion at Cairns as well as at Rocky Creek.

7

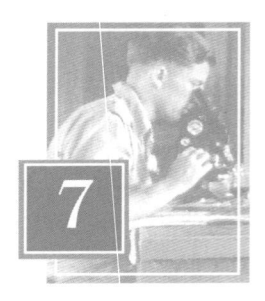

Atebrin

ATEBRIN IS A yellow acridine dye and its use for malaria prophylaxis led to a yellow discolouration of the skin and eyes. This was not injurious to health, but there were concerns that prolonged use of the drug might have some toxic manifestations. Nausea and vomiting sometimes followed the first doses of the drug. Such effects were usually observed to pass off, but doubts persisted as to its safety during long-term use. Dosage regimens of atebrin for prophylaxis (suppressive treatment) to be used by Australian forces were decided at a meeting of the Anti Malaria Advisory Committee in January 1943, when it was decided to adopt it as the prophylactic drug for the Australian Army in the South West Pacific.[1] Fairley stressed the need to hold stocks of quinine in case adverse side-effects of atebrin led to a switch back to quinine for prophylaxis. A cable was sent to London 'to keep the question of supplies of quinine to Australia alive in the minds of the British authorities'.

In highly malarious areas the dosage of atebrin was to be 100 mg/day for six days a week, excluding Sunday. In areas of low endemicity the dosage was 100 mg on three days a week: Monday, Wednesday and Friday. These recommendations were a reasonable compromise, considering what was known at that time. The extra protective effect of 600 mg/week in highly malarious areas outweighed the possible risks of toxicity of this higher dose. A weekly dose of 300 mg would have been a safer option, from the point of view of toxicity, and might have provided adequate protection in areas of low malaria risk. However, these recommended doses were not based on scientific evidence, as there were serious gaps in knowledge of the antimalarial activity of atebrin. It was not known what concentration was required to kill the parasites or to prevent them from multiplying in the blood. There was no clear indication of the efficacy of various dose regimens of atebrin for prophylaxis or for treatment of humans who had no immunity to malaria. People who live in malarious areas and suffer periodic attacks acquire partial immunity to the disease. This modifies the course of subsequent infections which are usually less severe than their initial attack. Doses of antimalarial drugs, which may be adequate to prevent clinical symptoms in these 'immunes', might be ineffective in 'non-immunes' who have had no previous exposure to malaria. Virtually all of the Australian and US troops committed to the South West Pacific theatre were non-immunes, so treatment and control were clearly of crucial importance to the Allied war effort.

The optimum dosage of atebrin for treatment of malaria cases was considered by the American Board for the Co-ordination of Malarial Studies. Dr Shannon studied a group of medical students who took atebrin in various doses for several weeks.[2] He was able to determine the relationship between the amount of drug ingested and the concentration reached in the blood using a photofluorimetric method developed in 1942 by the Americans B. B. Brodie and S. J. Udenfriend. This provided important baseline data but did not answer the essential question: what was the level of atebrin required for effective treatment following infection with malaria under field conditions? As the US Army representative on the Board, Brigadier General J. S. Simmons, said, 'This is the single most important problem confronting the [US Army] Surgeon General's Office'.[3] He agreed with Dr Shannon that it should not be decided by guesswork and urged that every effort should be devoted to accelerating a thoughtfully organised research program to give a prompt, definitive answer.

In response to this need for information on the effective blood levels of atebrin for treatment of malaria the Surgeon General sent a small number of US Army medical scientists to Australia to investigate this problem in the field.[4] They were First Lieutenant Frederick Bang (officer in charge), First Lieutenant William Trager, Second Lieutenant Nelson Hairston, and several enlisted men as technicians. The group was initially attached on temporary duty to 42nd US General Hospital in Brisbane, but reported directly to Colonel Maurice Pinchoffs.[5] This had the advantage of providing considerable autonomy and flexibility for their studies. They had a photofluorimeter from the USA, and used it to determine blood atebrin levels in malaria cases among American troops returned from the Buna campaign in New Guinea. Their work commenced in June 1943, about the same time that the Australian malarial research group was being formed in Cairns.

The results of the first month's work were summarised by Bang in a report dated 15 July. The photofluorimetric data suggested that the plasma atebrin concentrations needed for effective treatment of relapsing vivax malaria were around 30 µg per litre.[6] This was similar to the levels that Shannon had found effective against blood-inoculated cases of vivax malaria in New York. Bang concluded that the findings 'merely represent an orientation in the problem and no scientific conclusions can be made'. Nevertheless, the findings implied that inadequate dosage for prophylaxis could have been the cause of breakthroughs among troops in the field.

Fairley was in Brisbane in mid-July to chair a meeting of the Combined Advisory Committee. During this period he visited 42nd US General Hospital, in company with Colonel Pinchoffs, where Lieutenant Bang described the methods for atebrin estimation.[7] He received a typescript copy of Bang's report and passed it on to Andrew in Cairns.[8] These data would have been extremely useful for planning the initial atebrin experiments performed by the Australian research team.

After about three months with the 42nd General Hospital in Brisbane, the American malaria group moved to 6th Army Training Center in Rockhampton, where they continued their observations on atebrin levels in malaria cases among American troops returned from New Guinea. A fruitful liaison began between the Americans at Rockhampton and the Australians at Cairns. Lieutenant Bang visited 5 ACH on 25 August 1943.[9] Cordial relations were established, and Bang offered to perform atebrin estimations on some of the Australian volunteers. This visit occurred about one month before the start of the first 'combined series' on atebrin alone and with sulphamerazine. As the Cairns group did not have the ability to determine atebrin levels at this time, his offer was readily accepted, and arrangements were made for blood samples to be sent by air to Rockhampton.

The first experiments at Cairns showed that the rigorous experimental design devised by Fairley was admirably suited to evaluate the ability of antimalarial drugs to either prevent or to suppress infections in non-immune subjects. It was now obvious that the sulphonamides did not act as causal prophylactics of human malaria and, although they were reasonably efficient in suppressing *Plasmodium falciparum* infections, they were ineffective against vivax malaria. The combined series underscored the promise of atebrin for prophylaxis, both alone and in combination with sulphamerazine, against both kinds of malaria. Nevertheless, the numbers of test volunteers in this series were small, and there was the possibility that breakthroughs on the drug might occur in men fighting in hyperendemic areas, under conditions in which they were exposed to large numbers of infected mosquitoes over an extended period.

In order to investigate this possibility, it was decided to perform a second combined series with larger numbers of test cases subjected to mixed infections in which the volunteers were bitten by batches of mosquitoes infected with *P. falciparum* and by batches infected with *P. vivax*. Even though the previous results suggested that atebrin alone was just as good as atebrin combined with sulphamerazine, there was still a chance that the combination of the two drugs would have improved value for prophylaxis under more intensive infection conditions.

The drug combinations of this second combined series were essentially the same as the first series (see Chapter 6) except that atebrin doses were either 100 mg or 200 mg each day of the week. The high dose was included in case there were breakthroughs on the lower one. Each man was to receive 50 infective bites during 12 biting sessions spaced over a three-month period.[10] The men for the first three subgroups commenced their designated daily doses of atebrin on 14 November 1943 to provide a three–four-week 'build up' before being infected.[11] These men were subjected to heavy and sustained levels of infection. In highly malarious areas of the South West Pacific region sporozoite rates in the local malaria vectors are in the order of 1 per cent, so that 50 infective bites would correspond to bites from 5000 *Anopheles* mosquitoes. Over three months (100 days) this would be equivalent to 50 bites/night, which was considered commensurate with heavy mosquito attack rates in forward operational areas where mosquito control measures could not be implemented. This was the first group of clinical infection studies, which came to be known by the staff at Cairns as 'long-term experiments' or 'field-type experiments'.

In February 1944, while the atebrin experiments were in progress, Fairley was promoted to Brigadier. During the same month Andrew was promoted to Lieutenant Colonel and was appointed Officer Commanding the Medical Division of 2/2 AGH. This move ensured continuity of the complementary components of the work in Cairns and at Rocky Creek. Major C. R. B. (Ruthven) Blackburn was promoted to Lieutenant Colonel and was appointed Commanding Officer of the LHQ Malaria Research Unit. After graduating MBBS with first-class honours from the University of Sydney in 1937, Blackburn had worked at the Royal Prince Alfred Hospital, Sydney, initially as a resident medical officer and later as pathology/haematology registrar, where he completed a higher medical degree (MD) in 1939. In the following year he enlisted as a Captain in the Australian Army Medical Corps and embarked with 2/5 AGH for the Middle East, where he served in a number of medical positions. On returning to Australia in 1942 he was promoted to Major, and was posted as physician to 2/1 Casualty Clearing Station (CCS). He embarked with his new unit on the hospital ship *Manunda*, which arrived at Milne Bay on 6 September 1942, the day after the enemy conceded defeat and evacuated the last of their land forces from the area. As the senior physician in the area, Blackburn was soon immersed in the massive malaria problem that developed in the ensuing months. The unit held up to 500 patients and, under his direction, was one of the few to implement 13-day QAP (quinine, atebrin, and plasmoquine) therapy, with quinine administered intravenously to all malaria cases on the first two days of treatment. Towards the end of the year he contracted falciparum malaria, and was evacuated to Sydney by order of the senior medical officer, Colonel G. B. G. Maitland. After a period of recuperation and leave he returned to Milne Bay in early 1943. Soon afterwards he marched out of 2/1 CCS to take up a posting at 105 CCS in Port Moresby.

Sir Earle Page heard of Blackburn's experiences of malaria at Milne Bay while preparing to initiate his inquiry into malaria in the Australian Armed Forces and requested that he be appointed to assist the inquiry.[12] Major Blackburn was later summoned to Brisbane to accompany Page on his tour of Australian and New Guinea hospitals to observe the malaria problem in Australian troops at first hand. Blackburn had not met Fairley before this time, but had close contact with him during the preparation of Page's report. Page wrote in a letter to Prime Minister Curtin covering his report: 'We are also indebted to Major C. R. B. Blackburn, who has had a personal experience of malaria both from the point of view of the patient and doctor, and has had an extraordinary and successful clinical experience at Milne Bay as regards treatment'.[13]

After the completion of this secondment Blackburn was posted to 113 AGH at Concord in Sydney, where he worked under the senior physician, Lieutenant Colonel K. B. Noad. During this period he studied the effects of iron deficiency on anaemia in soldiers being treated for malaria. There is no documentary evidence for the reasons for his posting as CO of the Medical Research Unit, but it seems that this was attributed directly to Fairley. In the notes of his Sydney visit in June 1943 Fairley commented that 'Major Blackburn did excellent work throughout Sir Earle Page's tour'.[14]

Blackburn arrived in Cairns on 2 February 1944 for a few days' familiarisation at the unit, in company with Andrew, before assuming command on 9 February.[15] One of his first tasks was to see that the unit was brought up to the full strength of personnel authorised by the War Establishment. As the scale and scope of the research work had now increased considerably from that originally envisaged in mid-1943, Blackburn decided to institute a new numbering system based on roman numerals; this was applied to the experiments already completed or in progress, as well as to those still in the planning stages.[16] This formed the basis of a filing and record system for the case histories of the volunteers and for the collation of interim and progress reports of the unit that were sent to Fairley at the Medical Directorate in Melbourne.

The change in command of the unit occurred at an important time, as the men on the first three subgroups of the second combined series (designated Experiment V in the new numbering scheme) had then been subjected to multiple mosquito infections for two months. None exhibited any malaria parasites, though some had minor transient features similar to those of the first combined series.[17] The data accumulated to this time indicated that atebrin was capable of providing complete suppression of both falciparum and vivax malaria. In February Fairley pointed out the implications of this in some detail to Lieutenant Colonel Ford, who was then the malariologist of the New Guinea Force:

> [The results of] experiments at Cairns mean that volunteers who take [100 mg] of atebrin daily (preceded by a field build up of a similar dosage daily for 3 weeks) can be repeatedly infected with both M.T. and B.T. without a 'break through' occurring and without parasites appearing in demonstrable numbers in the peripheral blood. The volunteers are fitter than when they started the experiment ... An overwhelming amount of evidence is being obtained that if a man takes [100 mg] of atebrin *each day with invariable regularity* he should be very unfortunate if he develops fever even when infected repeatedly over a period of 3 months ... It seems more certain as time goes on and more data are accumulated that even allowing for fatigue factors etc. the reason for break through in jungle warfare is irregular taking of atebrin, and failure to get in 6 or 7 tablets per week.[18]

These predictions were borne out during the following month when the first subgroups completed their three months of repeated mosquito infections. None of the test volunteers developed clinical attacks of malaria while they were on atebrin. After the men ceased taking atebrin (one month after their last infected bites) it was found that falciparum malaria was cured in all cases, but all of the volunteers subsequently came down with relapses of vivax malaria.

The large number of volunteers involved in Experiment V and the need to continue their infection period for three months (rather than one week as in the original experimental plan for the Malaria Experimental Group) put a great strain on the improvised facilities. The bungalow used for the entomological section was now quite unsatisfactory, as it was far too small to rear the big numbers of mosquitoes required for the long-term experiments and to provide adequate laboratory space for dissections of infected specimens.[19] Also, it was about 1 km away from the rest of the unit and it did not have a telephone. The main part of the unit, including the wards for housing experimental patients, laboratory and office space, was in the original school building. In the four wards there were beds for 34 fit volunteers, seven gametocyte carriers, and six sick volunteers. This was grossly inadequate to accommodate the subjects for the long-term atebrin experiments, so extra beds were placed on the verandah, which had been earmarked as recreational space for the volunteers. The entire area was mosquito-proofed, and the volunteers had to remain inside between dusk and dawn to prevent experimental malaria infections being transmitted by the local mosquitoes to the people of Cairns. Because of these restrictions on the volunteers, it was considered essential that they have adequate recreational space, but this was not possible due to the overflow of beds on the verandah. It was clear that the unit had outgrown its accommodation at 5 ACH.

In March 1944 it was decided to construct a purpose-built facility at Jungara—7 km west of the original site in a canefield near Redlynch, at the base of the hills on the western side of Freshwater Creek. It was to be co-located with 116 AGH, a 600-bed hospital, which was also to be constructed on this site. Financial authority was granted in the first week of April, and the engineers promptly began building a collection of single-storey wooden frame buildings clad with 'fibro' (asbestos cement) walls and roof. There were three wards each 30 × 6 m and a recreation hut of the same size (see Fig. 6). These huts were built for the tropical climate, with wide eaves and walls. Glass windows were not fitted but large 'masonite' shutters were provided that could lowered in bad weather.[20] The unit moved in on 17 May 1944.[21] During the following week Blackburn wrote to Fairley that 'the move went well and we did not lose more than 3–4 hours work in all and the mosquito mortality was low'.[22]

The purpose of Experiment V was to test the efficacy of atebrin prophylaxis under conditions of active service. Volunteers in the first three subgroups had considerable recreational exercise, including walking, swimming, football

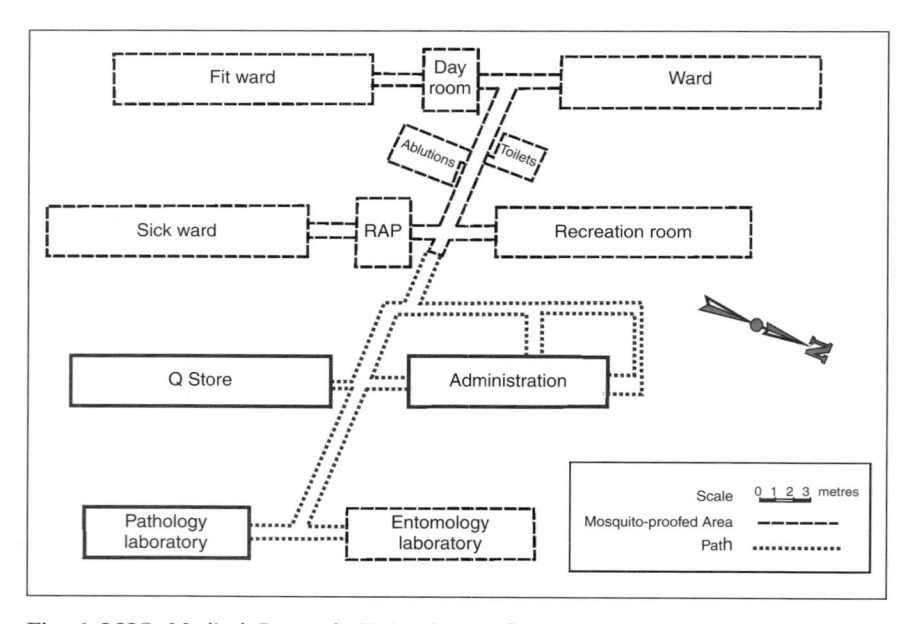

Fig. 6 LHQ Medical Research Unit, Cairns, floor plan of wards, laboratories and administration

and cricket. Nevertheless, it could be argued that, although atebrin was able to suppress malaria in men working under normal conditions, it might prove inadequate under the stresses and strains of combat. There was the possibility that breakthroughs might occur in men subject to the most arduous and hazardous conditions of jungle warfare, operating under conditions in which they were frequently exhausted, hungry, and subject to extremes of stress and nervous tension. Feedback from troops in the New Guinea Force had already suggested that this was, in fact, the case.[23] The likelihood of such breakthroughs had also been foreshadowed in a circular letter from the Office of the Surgeon General, US Army to American doctors.[24] It noted that 'in highly malarious regions, especially under the stress of combat, suppressive treatment [with atebrin] may fail to prevent clinical symptoms in a certain percentage of cases'. This was qualified by the statement that 'many instances of so-called break-through of clinical symptoms can be traced to failure of the individual to take the drug regularly', but the doubt remained. This issue was now addressed at Cairns.

Fairley 'decided to introduce factors in experiments which might lead to overt attacks of malaria while on suppressive drugs'.[25] He proposed that the men in the long-term experiments of Experiment V should have heavy exercise, and foreshadowed additional experiments 'to investigate some of the factors that may precipitate attacks of malaria'.[26] The first such trials to mimic physical stress commenced during April 1944.[27] This was done under the supervision of the unit CSM, Warrant Officer W. J. (Bill) Winterbottom, who had been attached to the unit for this purpose. Blackburn noted that Winterbottom seemed admirably suited for this job, and requested that he remain on permanent attachment.[28] Three of the fittest men in Experiment V undertook a program of heavy exercise. This included wood-chopping, and walking over the hills through the hottest time of the day. The men were closely monitored. None developed parasites in their blood or attacks of malaria.

Other factors outlined in Fairley's plan were also investigated during this period. First, there was the possibility that adrenaline secretion, associated with anger and fear, might induce breakthroughs of malaria. This was simulated by giving adrenaline injections to some of the volunteers on atebrin, but none showed subsequent appearance of parasites. Second, blood sugar levels fall in men suffering semi-starvation on a low-calorie diet. Some of the test subjects with malaria suppressed by atebrin were given insulin injections to reduce their blood-sugar levels, but the only symptoms observed were hunger, weakness or tiredness, and no parasites appeared in their blood. Third, the effects of cold temperatures were investigated with the aid of a freezing chamber in the local meatworks at Cairns. Volunteers were exposed for one hour to temperatures ranging from 0°C to –9°C, wearing only trousers, boots and socks, with only minimal movement allowed, but there were no symptoms or signs suggesting any activation of latent malaria, and blood films failed to reveal parasites. One volunteer who had parasites with minor symptoms was included in the group, but there was no detectable change in his condition.[29]

Blackburn felt that the various methods adopted for the first groups had been more in the nature of 'basal observations' rather than direct attempts to produce overt malaria.[30] In later subgroups it was decided to infect these volunteers more heavily than the earlier subgroups and institute very strenuous exercise throughout the day in the prevailing tropical humid climate of Cairns. The infections to which these men were exposed over the three-month test period ranged from 70 to 160 bites of mosquitoes infected with *P. falciparum*, as well as 30–130 bites of *P. vivax*-infected mosquitoes. These conditions represented considerably greater numbers of infective bites than would normally occur in nature, even in highly malarious areas.

At first, exercise consisted of wood-chopping and running, but subsequently long marches were given until the volunteers were exhausted. The marches were made in hilly country, and varied from one to three days, with only brief stops for meals and rest. One group marched 120 km in 36 hours. None of this produced attacks of malaria.

The unit was fortunate to receive the generous and timely assistance of the American malaria group at Rockhampton, who provided valuable data on blood atebrin levels to complement the clinical and parasitological observations of the test volunteers. However, as the experimental work expanded it became necessary to do these drug estimations at Cairns in order to accurately establish the relationship between the dose of atebrin taken by mouth and the actual blood levels required to suppress malaria. Specialised apparatus (a photofluorimeter) was required, and a technician would have to be trained in the method for estimating atebrin in biological fluids. In December 1943 Sergeant M. S. A. Swan was detached to 6th Army Training Center, Rockhampton, for six weeks' training in this procedure,[31] and a photofluorimeter was acquired for the Cairns unit. Lieutenant W. Trager came up from Rockhampton for a few days to help set it up.[32]

Additional useful information on blood atebrin levels was obtained from research undertaken in America by the Armored Medical Research Laboratory at Fort Knox, Kentucky, during the latter half of 1943.[33] This study extended the observations of Shannon in New York, and used a similar method in which men were not infected with malaria but were subjected to different prophylactic regimens of atebrin. The Fort Knox workers derived a simple formula from a large number of observations to assess the net change in plasma levels following drug administration. The actual blood level of atebrin was a function of daily dose, the pre-existing level, and the time interval since the last dose. The formula had considerable predictive value in determining the average plasma levels during suppressive therapy. The rate of decrease when drug administration ceased was about 10 per cent per day. Additional experiments to investigate the effects of simulated jungle climate were made in which one group of test subjects lived and worked in a hot room compared to another group taking the same doses of atebrin that remained outside in the prevailing temperate weather conditions. There were no differences in atebrin levels between the two groups.

The report on the Fort Knox work included a recommendation that field investigations be undertaken in hyperendemic areas to determine minimum plasma atebrin level required for prophylaxis. This was an objective of the American group at Rockhampton, who made important observations on this subject. However, there is a considerable element of uncertainty in studies relying on groups of men exposed to natural infections in the field, as the degree of infection to which individuals in such test groups were exposed cannot be determined. Such defects were not present in the Cairns experiments in which the timing and numbers of infected bites were precisely controlled. The atebrin data of these experiments afforded an ideal opportunity to accurately determine the plasma levels required to provide adequate protection from overt attacks of the disease.

A copy of the Fort Knox report was sent to Fairley in January 1944 by Colonel S. Bayne-Jones, Deputy Chief Preventive Medicine Service, Office of the US Army Surgeon General, before its review by the Commission on Tropical Diseases or acceptance by the Surgeon General: 'This copy is being sent to you at this time in order that the findings of the study may be made immediately available to those interested'.[34] Fairley replied that the report was much appreciated, as it 'is proving most illuminating and helpful, and explains many of the difficulties we have encountered in interpretation of the results of experimentally infected volunteers on atebrin suppressive therapy'.[35]

Plasma atebrin estimations were made by Lieutenant K. G. (Ken) Pope, the unit biochemist, and Sergeant Swan at regular intervals to determine the magnitude and variability of levels reached, the time required for equilibrium to develop, and the rate of reduction in levels after drug administration ceased. Blackburn wrote to Fairley on 6 July 1944 that they were doing large numbers of atebrin estimations and that 'Lieutenant Pope and I will have some sort of report on atebrin levels which we hope we will be able to compare with the Fort Knox figures'.[36] Part I of the two-part report concerned plasma atebrin levels associated with various dosage regimens, and Part II dealt with these levels in relation to prophylaxis and therapy of malaria.[37] In the first part, the levels determined from plasma samples taken from the Cairns volunteers were tabulated, and the frequency distribution of readings made from men on the same dose were plotted logarithmically. This confirmed the observation of the Fort

Knox group that a geometric rather than an arithmetic distribution was found in a given set of readings. Furthermore, the large variation in atebrin levels noted in the experiments at Cairns coincided closely with the range of individual readings made at Fort Knox. The second part of the report related plasma levels to malaria suppression in men infected in Experiments V and VI on atebrin regimens of 300, 400, 700 and 1400 mg of atebrin per week.

Analysis of the data showed that *P. falciparum* was suppressed and then cured when the mean atebrin level was 12.6 µg/litre throughout the period of biting and for 23–28 days after the last infective bite. None of the volunteers developed primary attacks of overt vivax malaria during prophylaxis on regimes of 300–1400 mg/week with plasma levels ranging from 4.1 to 62.1 µg/litre of atebrin. After drug administration ceased all of the men infected with *P. vivax* relapsed, and the final section of this report dealt with the timing of relapses and 'die away' of atebrin levels. By plotting the collated empirical data Blackburn showed that there was a linear relationship between the period of freedom from overt malaria and plasma atebrin level after stopping the drug. The data showed that for a mean plasma level of 20 µg/litre the period of freedom from malaria was 26 days; for a level of 40 µg/litre it was 61 days.

In addition to providing important information on the pharmacological evaluation of atebrin prophylaxis, the atebrin estimations made during the Cairns experiments provided an invaluable independent method of assessing whether the volunteers were actually taking their designated drugs. For example, one man on 1400 mg/week almost had an overt attack of falciparum malaria on Z+74 and Z+76 days. It had been noted for the previous fortnight that his colour was less yellow and his plasma atebrin was diminishing—the lowest level being 7 µg/litre. The nursing staff watched this man carefully at subsequent drug parades when the men lined up to take their drugs. This resulted in disappearance of his parasites, together with a concomitant rise in his plasma atebrin levels and increased yellowing of his skin. Questioning did not result in any admission that atebrin was being avoided, but a comment made by one volunteer to another (which was overheard) clearly indicated that he was not taking his atebrin.[38] The plasma atebrin level in another man fell from 37 µg/litre to nil over a five-week period while he was on prophylaxis of 700 mg/week. Parasites of *P. falciparum* appeared in his blood, and he developed a fever. Following close questioning about avoiding atebrin, fever and parasites disappeared and his plasma atebrin level increased. It was also observed that the men who were regarded as reliable tended to have higher plasma levels in relation to dose/kg/day than those regarded as unreliable. This reinforced the view that increased vigilance should be displayed by the nursing staff on atebrin parades, and more rigorous procedures were instituted to ensure that the drugs were ingested. The men were lined up, well spaced apart, and the atebrin was seen to be placed on the tongue. Half a mug of water was then drunk after which the men remained standing at attention for five minutes after the last volunteer had taken his drug. The whole procedure was personally supervised by either the CO, the CSM or a senior NCO.[39]

In experiments to determine the minimum effective dose of atebrin it was found that none of the volunteers taking doses of 300 mg/week developed attacks of vivax malaria. But breakthroughs of falciparum malaria occurred at this dose, so a higher dose was needed for complete suppression of this parasite.[40] If 100 mg (one tablet) were taken each day throughout the period of exposure and continued for a month after the last infective mosquito bite, it resulted in complete elimination of falciparum infections and a 100 per cent cure rate. On the other hand, all of the volunteers whose primary attacks of vivax malaria were suppressed by atebrin came down with relapses, usually within four to six weeks after they stopped taking the drug.

An RAAF report, considered by the Australian Defence Committee on 4 March 1943, mentions that

> despite the short supply of quinine it is considered necessary to use this drug for suppressive treatment of air crew personnel, as there is some evidence to show that the continued use of atebrin adversely affects air crew personnel who may be called upon to fly at high altitudes.[41]

Atebrin's side-effects on air crew were discussed by the Combined Advisory Committee on Tropical Medicine, Hygiene and Sanitation in Brisbane on 15 March.[42] Wing Commander A. H. Baldwin asked 'whether there was exact information available on the effects of atebrin on the aviator at high altitudes'. Colonel Fairley replied that British experiments had indicated that atebrin may induce adverse affects at high altitudes, but the evidence was not conclusive. It was agreed that, until further information was available, RAAF flight crews would continue to take quinine for prophylaxis in malarious areas.

During June 1944 the safety of atebrin at high altitudes was investigated as a co-operative effort between the LHQ Medical Research Unit and the RAAF. Eighteen test volunteers in Experiment V participated in decompression chamber tests to simulate the conditions of unpressurised transport aircraft operating in the South West Pacific Area. Baldwin, who was then RAAF Director of Hygiene and Tropical Medicine, arranged for these tests to be carried out at No. 1 Flying Personnel Research Unit, which was located within the Physiology School, University of Melbourne. The volunteers left Cairns by air on 25 May 1944 under the supervision of Max (now Lieutenant) Swan.[43] They had their last infective mosquito bites on the previous night, but their daily atebrin was taken under close supervision throughout their stay in Melbourne. A first series of altitude tests simulated 4600 metres for three hours and, in subsequent experiments, this was raised in 300 metre increments to 5800 metres. Oxygen was not provided, and temperatures averaged −2°C. On returning to conditions of ground altitude all of the men were capable of doing any duty that they could have done before the ascent. None developed any clinical manifestations of malaria while they continued to take their atebrin each day.[44] As a result of these tests, which showed no altitude-associated ill-effects from the use of atebrin, RAAF personnel operating in malarious areas changed from quinine to atebrin for prophylaxis.

The efficacy of atebrin had now been conclusively demonstrated, but what of quinine—the drug that it had replaced for prophylaxis? Despite the fact that this drug had been used against human malaria for two hundred years, its ability to suppress clinical attacks of the disease had not been adequately evaluated in non-immune humans. During a visit to Cairns in March 1944 Fairley summarised future experiments; these included an experiment to investigate the effects of quinine compared with atebrin.[45]

The aim of this experiment was to compare the efficacy of the two drugs when they were administered during the incubation period of malaria. The volunteers received mosquito infections of both vivax and falciparum malaria while they were taking daily prophylactic doses of quinine (at doses of either 325 mg or 650 mg) or atebrin (100 mg). The period over which drugs were administered was the same as the other 'short-term experiments' until 23 days after the last bite. Exercise was not strenuous, and no attempt was made to induce overt malaria. All of the men taking quinine developed overt attacks of vivax and falciparum malaria after the normal incubation period.[46] Their clinical symptoms were milder than those of untreated cases who took no prophylactic drugs, but all of them ultimately required therapy, the timing of which was determined by the clinical condition of the individual volunteer. None of the men had malaria while they were taking atebrin. In later experiments it was found that some, but not all, cases of vivax malaria were suppressed at a dose of 650 mg per day. This was the maximum dose that can be tolerated for long-term administration, but it was not sufficient to suppress falciparum malaria. Higher quinine doses of 1300 mg and 2000 mg per day were able to suppress both kinds of malaria, but such doses can only be administered for short periods for treatment of malaria attacks.[47]

The value of quinine lies in its ability to rapidly eliminate parasites and clinical symptoms in cases requiring treatment, and it still plays a vital role for treatment of severe and complicated malaria. The work at Cairns conclusively demonstrated that it was not a good prophylactic drug as it could not prevent clinical attacks in men who took the drug every day after being bitten by mosquitoes infected with New Guinea strains of malaria. Atebrin, on the other hand, could achieve this objective, provided that a tablet was taken each day

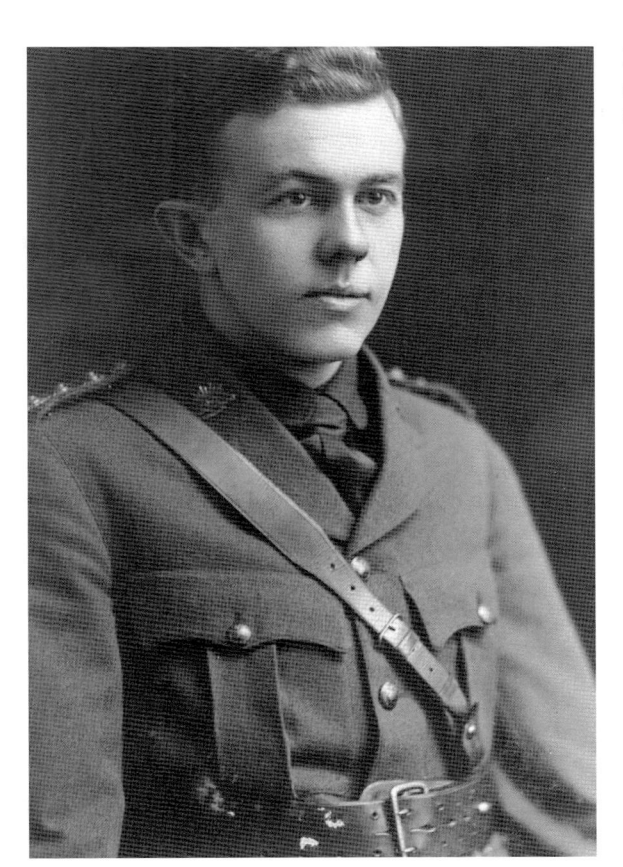

Neil Hamilton Fairley as a Captain medical officer in the First AIF during World War I

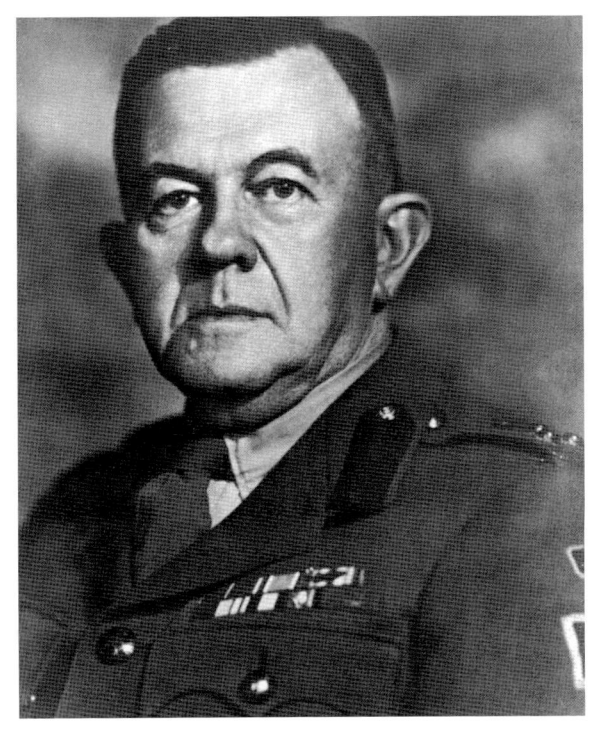

Brigadier Neil Hamilton Fairley, OBE, MID, FRS, as Director of Medicine Australian Army Medical Corps during World War II

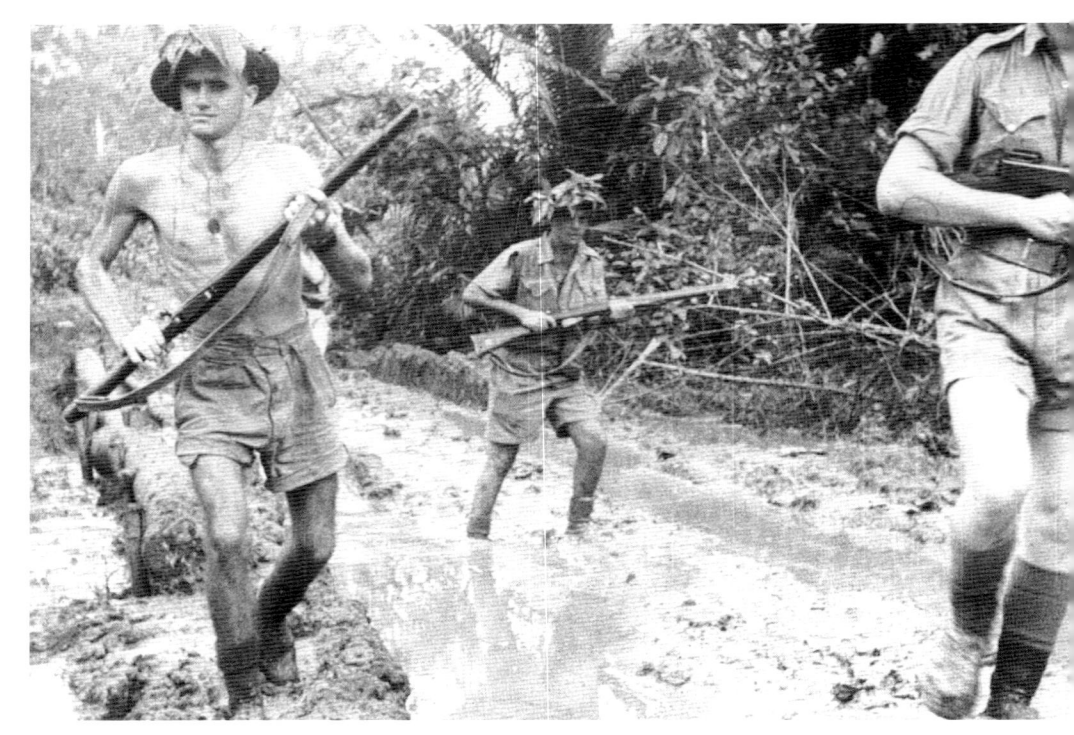

Australian infantry on patrol in the Milne Bay area. The muddy road pools provide ideal breeding sites for *Anopheles* larvae. To live and fight in such country without shirts and in shorts virtually guaranteed that troops would get malaria.

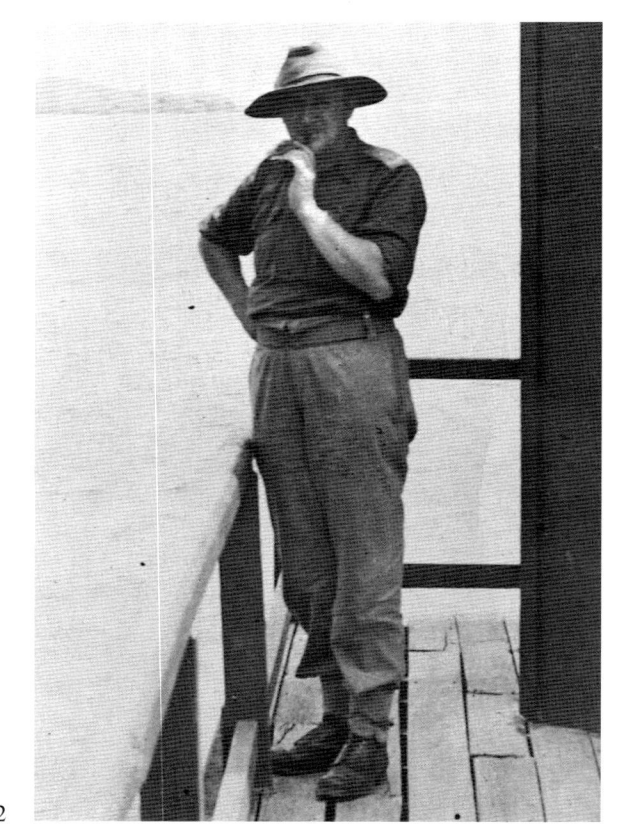

Lieutenant Colonel Ted Ford: as Assistant Director of Pathology for New Guinea Force he played a crucial role in alerting the Commander-in-Chief, General Tom Blamey, of the malaria threat in 1942

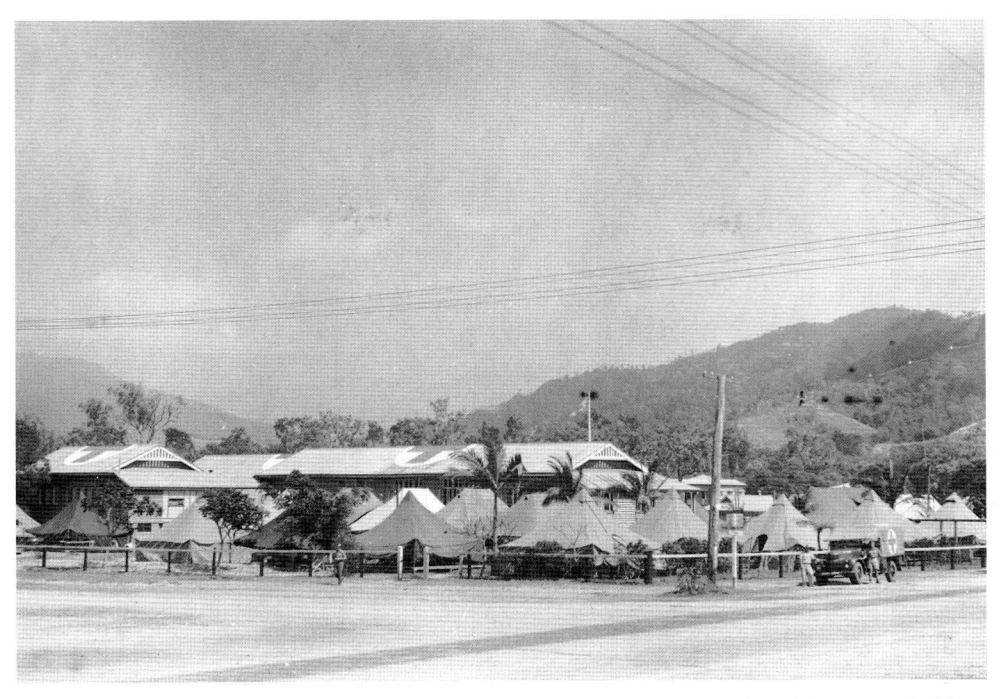

The buildings and tents of the Malaria Experimental Group at 5 Australian Camp Hospital in the grounds of North Cairns State School, Sheridan Street

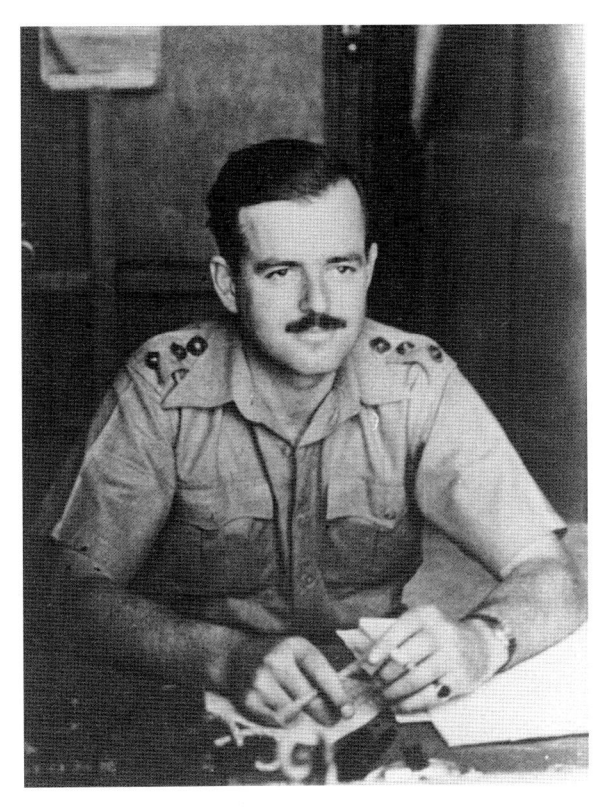

Major Richard Andrew, in the Middle East, when he was a captain

Major Jo Mackerras (oil painting by Nora Heysen)

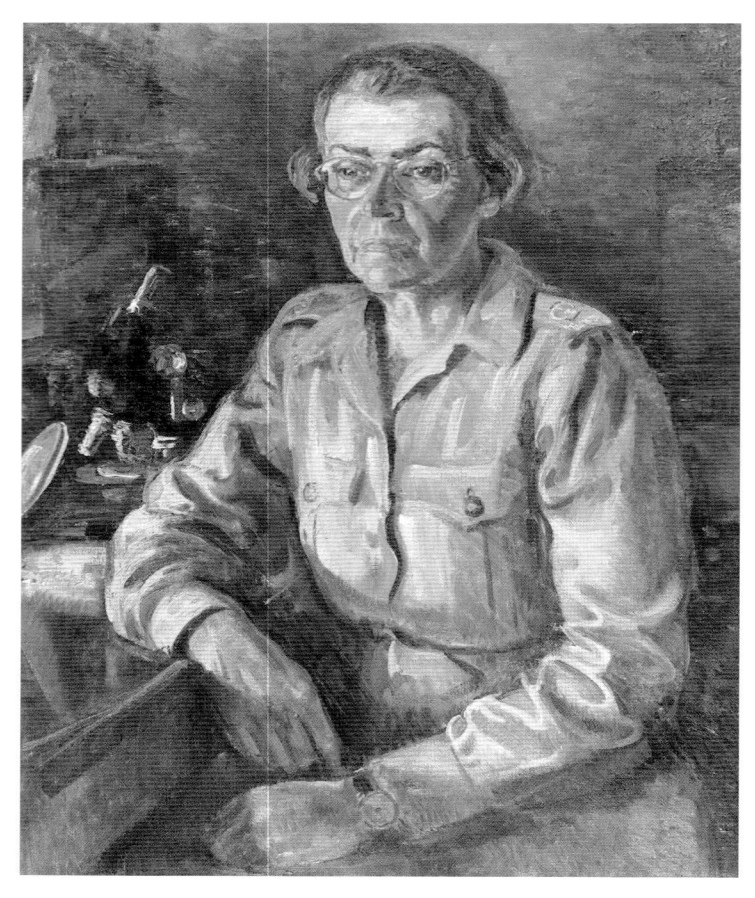

Lieutenant Colonel Ruthven Blackburn (oil painting by Nora Heysen)

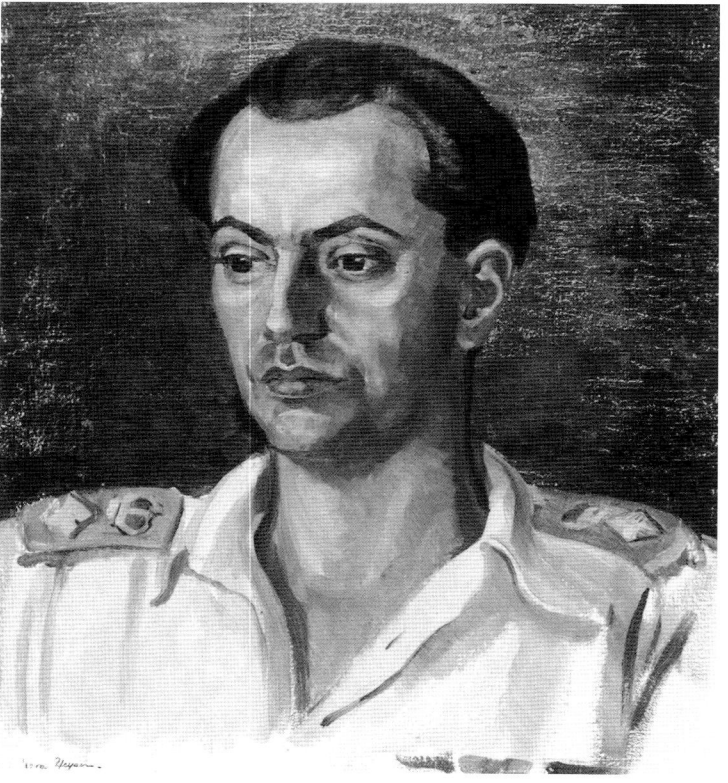

with absolute regularity. Such a result was unexpected at the time that atebrin was introduced to replace quinine in the South West Pacific theatre in early 1943.

Fairley continued to be concerned about possible toxicity from long-term use of atebrin as a prophylactic, particularly if there was a need to increase the dose to two tablets (200 mg) per day. During the New Guinea campaign in late 1943 the malaria rate soared to unacceptable levels among 2 Australian Corps, and it was decided to put the troops onto this higher dosage. It was felt that under the conditions of mobile warfare they were frequently neglecting their atebrin, and it was thought that this might compensate for the inadequate standard of atebrin discipline. In a personal letter to Ted Ford, Fairley asked whether there was any evidence that the increased dosage caused a decline in the 'break through' rate or induced toxic symptoms.[48] Fairley discussed the whole matter with General MacArthur, and pointed out the possibility that toxic effects could be produced. MacArthur replied that these troops could not be replaced and that such risks must be taken.[49]

During the Buna campaign a new variety of 'jungle rot' was observed, in which itchy red or purple patches developed on the skin. It was named 'atypical lichen planus' by US Army dermatologists who were convinced that it was a side-effect of atebrin, though the incidence was less than 0.3 per cent. Some patients developed a later stage in which raised scaly patches appeared on the arms and legs.[50]

In June 1944 Brigadier J. Steigrad, Deputy Director of Medical Services, New Guinea Force, wrote to Major General Burston on the subject of atebrin toxicity. He provided case histories on two patients admitted to 2/7 AGH with possible atebrin psychosis. Both men had been taking excessive doses of the drug.[51] In a lengthy reply on behalf of the Director General of Medical Services Fairley wrote that very large doses (2000 mg in 48 hours) could produce psychotic symptoms, but there was no statistical evidence that such symptoms had increased since the institution of atebrin prophylaxis.[52] It was later accepted that lichen planus and psychotic disturbances could be caused by the long-term use of atebrin, but such conditions were rare and of little consequence in comparison to the dangers of malaria.[53]

During the last year of the war it became evident that, as well as being more effective against malaria, atebrin was also a much safer drug than quinine. Blackwater fever is a complication of chronic falciparum malaria, characterised by breakdown of the blood cells and, as the name suggests, red or dark-coloured urine. It was a serious condition in highly malarious areas before the war, with an average case mortality of about 25 per cent. The close correlation between quinine and blackwater fever was long recognised, as it tended to have a sudden catastrophic onset following the administration of quinine treatment to malaria patients. The nature of the condition is not fully understood, but it is thought that intolerance or idiosyncrasy to quinine may be a precipitating factor.[54] Malaria was uncontrolled in the local population at the start of hostilities in New Guinea in 1942. Quinine was the only antimalarial drug in widespread use and blackwater fever was sufficiently prevalent among former tropical residents who joined the Army to cause considerable anxiety.[55] Despite the presence of devastating epidemics and severe malarial casualties among Allied forces in 1942 and 1943, blackwater fever was only occasionally encountered. There were no cases amongst the volunteers at Cairns. Following the substitution of atebrin as the prophylactic drug in early 1943, blackwater fever virtually disappeared with the elimination of chronic falciparum malaria cases inadequately suppressed by quinine.

The Atherton Conference

DESPITE THE LESSONS learned from the disastrous experiences at Milne Bay, malaria continued to be a most serious problem for Allied troops in the South West Pacific throughout 1943 and during the first half of 1944. Fairley visited 2 Australian Corps in the Atherton Tablelands before it was committed to battle in New Guinea. He had an interview with the commander, Lieutenant General Leslie Morshead, on 6 July 1943 during which antimalarial discipline and the proposed malaria experiments at Cairns were discussed.[1] Subsequently, this force suffered heavy malaria casualties during the Markham–Ramu and Huon Peninsula campaigns. The 9th and 7th Divisions had over 19 000 men evacuated sick with malaria at some time during the period September 1943–February 1944. This was 65 per cent of the average posted strength, and was more than six times the battle casualties inflicted over this time.[2] A further 25 per cent of these troops suffered from other tropical diseases, principally dengue, dysentery, and scrub typhus. The need to provide reinforcements to replace this wastage from sickness presented great manpower difficulties for the army.

The experiments at the LHQ Medical Research Unit provided overwhelming evidence that atebrin was able to provide complete protection against malaria in the field, but there was an urgent need to persuade the fighting forces that this was so. These considerations prompted the convening of a conference 'on certain aspects of prevention of disease in tropical warfare', which was held at Atherton, Queensland, on 12–13 June 1944.[3]

Fairley arrived in Cairns two days beforehand, and went over charts of the experimental work which were specially prepared at the unit for his presentation at the conference.[4] The conference was chaired by Lieutenant General V. A. H. Sturdee, GOC, First Australian Army, and was attended by senior officers, including formation and unit commanders of the 3rd, 6th, 7th and 9th Australian Divisions. The Adjutant General, Major General C. E. M. Lloyd, opened the proceedings with a succinct summary of casualties due to sickness in troops under the command of the New Guinea Forces. He foreshadowed certain medical evidence relevant to prevention of malaria and other tropical diseases that would be produced during the course of the meeting, and concluded by saying that 'it is necessary to consider it, and if it were accepted as valid, to work out an appropriate course of action to reduce the high incidence of tropical illnesses and minimise the loss of manpower by prevention of casualties'.[5]

This set the stage for a superb presentation by Fairley entitled 'Malaria, with special reference to atebrin suppression in the field'. He commenced by reviewing the Australian wartime experience of the disease in the Middle East and South West Pacific. The original forecasts of the gravity of the situation in the latter theatre had been borne out during 1942 and 1943. The US Marines at Guadalcanal, no less than the Australians at Milne Bay, were intensely infected, with incidence varying from 90 to 99 per cent of the forces involved. Fairley considered the factors responsible to be: (1) inadequate personal protection; (2) non-availability of essential antimalarial supplies; (3) late institution of adult and larval mosquito control; and (4) ineffectiveness of quinine suppression and irregularities in its usage. He described the establishment of LHQ Medical Research Unit, and provided an outline of the rationale and methods for the experimental investigations of prophylaxis and cure of malaria using various drug regimens in volunteers at Cairns and 2/2 AGH:

> As the experimental malaria infections are better controlled, and are conducted on a larger scale than has ever been previously attempted, the results obtained can be accepted without reservation as giving a clear answer to what these drugs can achieve in troops infected with New Guinea strains of malignant tertian and benign tertian malaria parasites.[6]

A summary of the initial trials with the sulphonamides was provided, with emphasis on sulphamerazine that gave reasonably good results against falciparum malaria (suppressed 95 per cent of cases, and cured 80 per cent). But the activity was much less satisfactory against *Plasmodium vivax* infections—parasites broke through and fever developed in all test cases, in many while they were still taking the drug. Fairley then described the more recent work with quinine by relating that a daily dose of 10 grains (650 mg) failed to suppress falciparum infections, but was successful in suppressing a proportion of vivax cases. A daily dose of 5 grains (325 mg) failed to suppress either falciparum or vivax, and treatment had to be instituted. He then went on to say that men on one daily tablet of atebrin (100 mg) did not develop malaria, despite the fact that they were bitten by infected mosquitoes from the same batches as those biting the men on quinine. Charts illustrating these experiments showed that the suppressive action of atebrin was much superior to quinine in heavy infections with New Guinea strains of malaria.

In presenting the detailed results of the atebrin series Fairley stressed that all cases of both falciparum and vivax malaria were suppressed while taking the drug. He described the conditions of the 'field type' experiments, in which volunteers were repeatedly bitten by many mosquitoes infected with falciparum malaria, as well as by other mosquito batches infected with vivax malaria over a period of three months. Falciparum malaria was cured when atebrin prophylaxis was continued for four weeks after the last bite. Extensive blood inoculation tests showed that these volunteers were not suffering from latent malaria and were not naturally immune: 'The only possible conclusion is that suppressive atebrin taken over a sufficient period of time cures malignant tertian malaria'.[7] On the other hand, all men infected with vivax malaria suffered relapses after prophylaxis ceased.

Factors that had been suggested as likely to precipitate overt attacks of malaria in individuals with latent infections included conditions such as physical exhaustion, exposure to cold and wet, anoxia and chill induced by high-altitude flying, blood loss, anaesthetic and surgical operations, alcoholic excesses, and malnutrition. It had also seemed possible that 'strong emotions of fear and anger, associated as they are with excessive adrenalin output in the blood, might act in the same way'.[8]

Fairley explained the measures used to simulate the above conditions in volunteers at Cairns and the RAAF experiments to simulate high-altitude flying, which were still in progress at the time of the conference. He conceded that it had not been possible to subject these volunteers to the same degree of physical and mental stress and strain as inevitably must accompany jungle fighting. Nevertheless, different groups had been subjected to conditions that would be expected to cause breakthrough of latent malaria in the vast majority of cases were they not taking a suppressive drug. Such breakthroughs were never observed. It was concluded that, if the blood and organs of the body have an adequate atebrin content, it is not possible for breakthroughs to occur even though the individual has malaria in latent form, and is exposed to factors that would otherwise induce an overt attack.

Fairley then touched on the results of research conducted in the USA that showed that it took six weeks for the level of atebrin in the blood to reach maximum equilibrium levels in men taking six tablets per week:

> These data were of military significance as they indicate it was possible, by increasing the dosage to 2 tablets per day, to attain atebrin equilibrium in 7 days. They also indicate the necessity for invariably maintaining the daily dose, for a day missed here and a couple of days missed there will so reduce the level that sooner or later parasites break through and an overt attack of malaria ensues.[9]

There was a widespread belief among Australian troops in New Guinea that atebrin caused impotence or sterility. Fairley addressed this issue by first stressing that it was a far less toxic drug than quinine. The yellow discolouration of the skin was due to staining with atebrin, and had no relationship whatever to jaundice or deleterious effects on the liver. He then demolished the unfounded rumours of its supposed deleterious affects on virility:

> Atebrin has no effect on spermatozoa and would be quite useless as a contraceptive. Similarly it could not conceivably produce impotence which arises from psychological causes in at least 90% of cases. Any disease, like malaria, which produces debility and anaemia, will decrease the physical vitality of the individual and to some extent his sex urge. By controlling malaria, atebrin will prevent this happening. Complaints of impotence in troops who have been subject to the mental stress and strain of war are not uncommon. They occurred in France in the Great War and after Tobruk, where neither quinine nor atebrin suppression were used. Troops need assurance on this subject for in the past it has been a contributory factor to their not taking atebrin, both in New Guinea and in Australia when on leave. Several deaths from cerebral malaria have recently resulted in troops on leave who have failed to take atebrin for one month after coming out of New Guinea.[10]

A final point was the crucial importance of ensuring complete compliance with suppressive therapy in the field:

> Atebrin should be given under strict supervision. It is not sufficient merely to hand out the atebrin at a meal or on parade. It must be observed to be swallowed. If, as in the case of small units, an officer cannot be present, responsibility should be delegated to the sergeant or corporal. It is specially important during jungle fighting that the officer or NCO should be responsible for ensuring that atebrin is taken daily, for unless the taking of atebrin has become a confirmed habit, the practice will break down at this critical juncture just when it is most needed ... Atebrin tablets are coated with a layer of shellac varnish and contain starch granules in order to make them disintegrate readily in the stomach and facilitate absorption. Medically this is advantageous but it makes it necessary to prevent atebrin tablets from coming into contact with water, sweat or fluid of any kind, otherwise disintegration ensues and the tablets are destroyed. In New Guinea where there is a high rainfall, it is essential that atebrin be carried in a watertight container, and not loosely in their cellophane covering in shirt pockets. Furthermore, a reserve of atebrin should be carried by every individual soldier for emergency purposes, in case supplies fail to arrive or lines of communication be cut.[11]

In his concluding remarks Fairley said:

> If these experimental data be correct, it follows that any force of non-immune troops who have built up and maintain an adequate concentration of atebrin in the blood throughout the period of exposure and for 4 weeks thereafter, can fight in

highly malarious country with an absolute minimum of malaria casualties ... When the force leaves the highly malarious area, returns to Australia and stops taking atebrin, relapses of benign tertian malaria will begin within a period of 3–4 weeks. The percentage of relapses in the force will depend on the efficacy of those measures of personal protection, such as use of the mosquito net, correct clothing and application of mosquito repellent lotion which prevent mosquitoes biting the individual. If anti-larval measures and adult mosquito destruction have been carried out and if anti-malaria discipline has been effective, the incidence of B.T. malaria will be low; if there has been laxity, the rate will be high. Atebrin suppression is vital but these other anti-malarial measures are equally important and must never be neglected if it is humanly possible to carry them out.[12]

The proceedings of the conference state: 'In the course of discussion the general opinion was that Brigadier Fairley had made an irrefutable case for the efficacy of atebrin'.[13] Brigadier W. J. V. Windeyer pointed out that fatigue and mental stress during action probably led to men forgetting their atebrin and caused increased malaria wastage. In support of this view Lieutenant General F. H. Berryman said:

In the Huon Peninsula campaign ... there was a relationship between the incidence of malaria and the physical condition of the men. With lowered physical condition it is probable that the men did not make the same effort to take precautions as they did at the start of the campaign. In the stress of battle malaria discipline relaxes and supervision of troops in close contact suffers. Our men are malaria conscious and have a high standard of personal hygiene. When the successful results of proper atebrin treatment are impressed upon them, there will be a big improvement. It is now the duty of commanders in all grades to intensify their efforts until the taking of atebrin becomes an ingrained habit. ... Disease must be considered an enemy, and the same energy and thought must be put into our training to overcome it as is put into our efforts to defeat the Jap.[14]

Major J. C. English, Malariologist, 1 Australian Corps, then made a presentation on the prevention of malaria in the field, with emphasis on personal protection against mosquitoes and on mosquito control. Major C. E. Cook, Deputy Assistant Director of Health, 1 Australian Corps, reviewed the control of intestinal diseases, particularly dysentery and cholera. This was followed by a general summing up and discussion by the Director General of Medical Services, Major General S. R. Burston, who commenced his talk by briefly summarising the contribution of the Australian Army Medical Corps to the saving of life and manpower during the present war. After outlining the use of sulphaguanidine against dysentery and measures taken to produce penicillin in Australia for military and civilian use, he highlighted the purpose of the conference—to discuss problems relating to the prevention of preventable diseases and particularly malaria:

> The role of the medical services in this respect is advisory. We also ensure that everything necessary to implement our advice is available to you but it is entirely your responsibility to ensure that our advice is carried out. We have in the Medical Directorate and on the staff of all major formations, officers of wide experience in active service, with the highest academic qualifications whose advice is sound and always practicable ... In my opinion they have not been used in the past as they should have been by many commanders. In fact they have had an extremely uphill fight. They have frequently been in the position of knowing what should be done and could be done, but their urgent representations have fallen on deaf ears. I am firmly of the opinion that a Commander who, by disregarding advice from the specialists who are there to advise him, allows his force to unnecessarily suffer large numbers of casualties from preventable diseases, is equally blameworthy as a Commander who, through his inefficiency, leads his troops into an ambush and suffers a similar number of battle casualties ... Finally we come to malaria. Brigadier Fairley and Major English have told you all there is to know about the control of this disease which up to now has been a far greater producer of casualties than the enemy. It has been amply demonstrated to you that the control of this disease is in your own hands; that if you follow our advice malaria should cease to be a problem of major importance as a casualty producer, and that not only will you have no deaths from malaria but your wastage should be negligible during active operations. It is purely a matter of training and discipline in all anti-malarial measures, particularly the taking of atebrin. The medical service has done its job. It has shown you the way and has provided you with all the material necessary to implement its advice. I have no hesitation in saying, most emphatically, Gentlemen —THE BALL IS NOW IN YOUR COURT.[15]

The chairman (Lieutenant General Sturdee) in closing the conference thanked the Director General of Medical Services (DGMS) Brigadier Fairley, and Majors English and Cook for the valuable information they had placed before the conference, the success of which had surpassed his expectations. The proceedings of the conference noted:

> There was no doubt that many officers came with little enthusiasm, if not hostility. However, in a very short time DGMS and his assistants had completely convinced all present of the seriousness of the position and of the need for the whole hearted co-operation of all ranks. So successful had the conference been, especially on anti-malarial measures, that commanders and staffs present now appeared to be desirous of pressing the medical services further even than the latter were prepared to go.[16]

One week after the Atherton Conference, the background to an official press release on malaria from General MacArthur's Headquarters was explained by Colonel Maurice Pinchoffs at a meeting of the Combined Advisory Committee in Brisbane.[17] Incredibly misinformed statements regarding malaria and other tropical diseases in American troops had been reported in US newspapers, along with strong criticism of the Army for the conditions alleged to exist. General MacArthur decided to counteract these misrepresentations by releasing facts to the press that would indicate the true situation, and to point out the success of control and treatment methods that were currently employed throughout the South West Pacific Area. However, as it had been decided previously not to permit press publication of malaria data on the grounds that it could be a source of useful information to the enemy, Australian authorities were advised of this decision. The reasons for this action were explained to Major General Burston by telephone before the statement was released.

In his role as chairman of the committee, Fairley responded by saying that this early advice was much appreciated by the Medical Directorate at LHQ as it coincided with the necessity to prepare information for the press regarding malaria in the Australian Army. This was required to explain the large numbers of cases of vivax malaria occurring in Australia after troops ceased taking atebrin on their return from New Guinea. He said that dissemination of information within the Army, on methods of malaria control, treatment of cases, and the results of research, was a valuable means of obtaining intelligent co-operation from the Services. Fairley then mentioned his recent address at the Atherton Conference during which 'the facts in relation to malaria control, particularly in respect to the effectiveness of suppressive atebrin, were placed fully before the officers. He was sure from the reaction obtained that a greatly enhanced co-operation of all arms and services could be relied upon'.[18]

The relaxation of press censorship concerning malaria prepared the way for an article published in *Salt*, the Army education journal.[19] This magazine, aimed at the general reader and illustrated by photographs and cartoons, was issued fortnightly and distributed free of charge to all ranks in Australia and overseas. In addition to items on the war, it included topics of historical interest, current affairs, and letters from servicemen. The article in question, entitled 'This was our longest and dearest campaign', was based on Fairley's presentation at the Atherton Conference. It provided factual information in a straightforward style on the threat posed by malaria and how it could be avoided: 'Experiments have decisively shown that, no matter where in the SWPA the Australian soldier may now be sent to fight, the only way he can be sure of avoiding malaria is to take atebrin: and that if he doesn't take it he may die'. The major points of Fairley's address at the Atherton Conference were summarised, including the disastrously high malaria casualties in New Guinea that stimulated the experiments at Cairns, and the results of research that showed the ability of atebrin to prevent breakthroughs of malaria in volunteers subject to extremes of physical stress and other arduous conditions. Particular emphasis was given to 'furphies' circulating among the troops in New Guinea: 'quinine taken by mouth never causes impotence or sterility and atebrin won't either. The Medical Corps boasts many "atebrin daddies"—M.O.s who went home

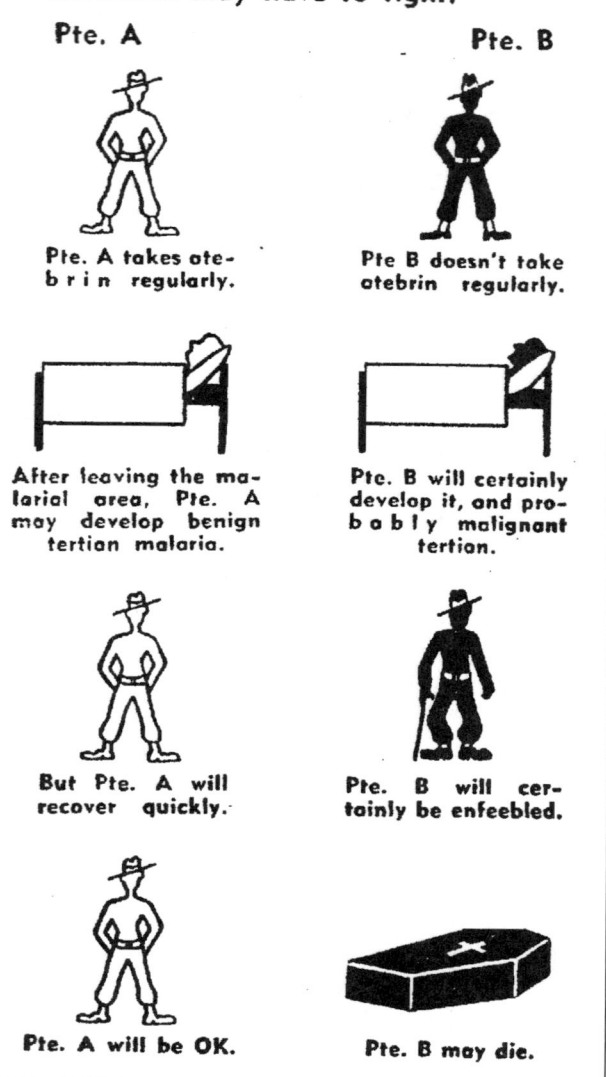

Fig. 7 Illustration from 'This was our longest and dearest campaign'

on leave, kept taking atebrin and are now fathers'. Rumours that it caused yellow jaundice were refuted, as was the proposition that 'certain types of Australians are "he-men" naturally immune to malaria, no matter how often they are bitten by infected mosquitoes'. The case for atebrin was effectively illustrated by drawings showing the story of two soldiers: Pte A takes atebrin regularly and, even though he may develop vivax malaria on returning to Australia, he will recover. On the other hand, Pte B, who does not take the drug regularly, will certainly develop vivax malaria, and he may die from falciparum malaria (see Fig. 7). It was pointed out that 'Several troops on leave recently have died—from cerebral malaria (affecting the brain) because they did not take atebrin for one month after leaving New Guinea'. The article concluded: 'Australia can be sure her sickness casualties will be far lower than before—but only if atebrin goes with, and into, the troops'.

The measures taken to educate the army about malaria and to spread the good news about atebrin had a very positive effect. The Atherton Conference motivated the commanders to mobilise their troops against the disease, and this was rigorously enforced by disciplinary measures. The article in *Salt* ensured that the message was carried down to the rank and file. This was reflected by a dramatic reduction in sickness casualties in 1945. For example, during the period November 1944 to October 1945 the incidence of malaria in Australian troops on operations on New Britain was less than 2 per cent.[20] This was the same area in which, just three years previously, the disease had decimated the survivors of the 2/22 Battalion in the retreat from Rabaul.

9

Subinoculation

THE CAIRNS EXPERIMENTS on sulphonamides, atebrin and quinine, as described by Fairley at the Atherton Conference, were of direct practical significance to the control of malaria. However, a full understanding of the action of the drugs was hampered by lack of knowledge of the complete cycle of malaria in humans. The sequence of development in the blood was well understood, but there was considerable uncertainty about the early course of the disease during the incubation period before clinical symptoms occurred. Few workers at this time thought that Fritz Schaudinn was correct in believing that he had seen sporozoites directly enter the red blood cells (see Chapter 4).

In 1937 M. Ciuca had demonstrated that the disease could not be transmitted by blood transfer from a donor to a recipient during the first five days after the donor was bitten by an infected mosquito.[1] This implied that the parasites were not present in the blood during this period. It was presumed that the sporozoites entered some part of the body other than the circulating blood, where they either remained dormant or underwent a process of development in a 'tissue phase' before invading the red blood cells.

Colonel S. P. James and A. Tate had shown that avian malaria parasites developed in the reticulo-endothelial cells,[2] and many contemporary workers thought it likely that a similar cycle of development also occurred with the human malaria parasites. But even if this view were accepted, there were still pertinent questions remaining to be answered: For how long did the sporozoites remain in the circulation after the bite of an infected mosquito? When did the first parasites emerge from the 'tissue phase' to enter the bloodstream? The answers to these questions were of direct relevance to appreciating how drugs acted on the various stages of the parasites in humans.

The second question needs to be viewed in numerical terms. The symptoms of malaria are similar to other diseases, including some viral or bacterial infections, and the only way to conclusively determine that someone is suffering from a malaria attack is to observe the parasites microscopically in blood taken from the patient. The procedure involves smearing a drop of blood on a microscope slide; staining the slide to differentiate the parasites within the blood cells; and examining the slide with a compound microscope. This is laborious work as it takes about an hour to scan all of a 'thick blood film' (containing the smear of a whole drop of blood) under the microscope. The volume of this drop is 1 cubic millimetre (1/1000 ml). There are 5 litres (5000 ml) of blood in the average adult so the examination of one thick blood film is equivalent to scanning 1/5 000 000 of the total blood volume. If it is assumed that the malaria parasites are randomly scattered amongst the blood cells, they will only be observed with a high degree of probability when their number exceeds 5 000 000. The practical implication of these numerical considerations is that there may be several million parasites within the blood before any are seen under the microscope.

The subinoculation experiments in which blood was transfused from an infected to an uninfected volunteer was a unique and inspired component of the Cairns work conceived by Fairley. It involved transfer of 200 ml or 500 ml of whole blood from the test volunteer to a suitable non-immune recipient with a compatible blood group. This procedure was initially carried out at 2/2 AGH by Captain E. M. B. (Bobbie) Fenner (née Roberts) using a manually operated, rotary pump, direct-transfusion apparatus developed by Dr Julian Smith.[3] The recipients were observed closely for a month afterwards. Daily procedures included a thorough clinical examination, and the whole of a thick blood film was scrutinised thoroughly for parasites. The development of malaria in the recipient confirmed the presence of parasites in the blood of the donor. Previous workers rarely used more than 10 ml of blood in experimental blood transfer of malaria parasites. The rationale for the large volume used at Cairns was to ensure the best chance of transferring parasites, even if they were present in very small numbers. A blood volume of 200 ml is equivalent to 200 000 drops of blood. Thus, this technique permitted the Cairns researchers to confirm the presence of malaria in men with extremely low levels of parasites—many times less than those that could be seen microscopically. During the sulphonamide and atebrin experiments this procedure was used for volunteers infected with mosquito-transmitted malaria who remained well after a five- or six-week observation period after drug administration had ceased.

This initial phase of the malaria cycle in humans was also investigated at Cairns using the subinoculation technique. The blood of volunteers exposed to mosquitoes infected with vivax malaria was subinoculated into uninfected recipients to determine the earliest possible time that malaria could be transferred by this method, and to find out the type of malaria that developed in the recipients. The first part of this study, Experiment XIII, commenced on 25 February 1944.[4] Half a litre of blood was transfused from a donor into an uninfected volunteer (recipient 1) several minutes after the donor was bitten by mosquitoes infected with vivax sporozoites (see Fig. 8). One day later a further transfusion was made from the donor to another volunteer (recipient 2). The first recipient came down with vivax malaria after the normal incubation period, whereas the second recipient remained uninfected. The positive result in the first recipient indicated that malarial parasites were able to pass rapidly through the pulmonary circulation to the periphery as different arms of the donor were used for biting and giving blood.

Lieutenant Colonel C. R. Blackburn considered that

> It seems probable that the malarial parasites [responsible for initiating malaria in the first recipient] were sporozoites as 7 minutes must be considered too short a period for any appreciable developmental changes to have taken place. With the passage of time evidence may be obtained from the behaviour of [the first recipient's] vivax infection as to whether it was sporozoite or trophozoite in origin'.[5]

The trophozoite-induced malaria experiments undertaken at 2/2 AGH had already provided information on the type of malaria that might develop from blood-inoculated vivax parasites. The donors for these experiments had infections naturally acquired in New Guinea. All of the blood-inoculated controls of the sulphonamide and atebrin experiments developed typical overt attacks of vivax malaria requiring therapy. None of them developed relapses after the primary attack was cured. Thus, if trophozoites were transferred in the Experiment XIII subinoculations, a primary attack of vivax malaria should develop in the recipients but subsequent relapses should not occur. On the other hand, if sporozoites were transferred, relapses should be seen after an appropriate time interval following the cure of the primary attack. The medical documents of all volunteers who received vivax malaria at Cairns were endorsed so that any relapses could be followed up and reported to the LHQ Medical Research Unit. Additional meticulous instructions were given to permit rigorous follow-up of any recipients developing primary vivax attacks following subinoculations. The first donor of Experiment XIII relapsed 85 days after the infective bites and the seven-minute recipient had a relapse after 291 days.[6] The recipient was not exposed again to malaria infection after his subinoculation, so this provided convincing evidence that his relapse was induced by transfer of sporozoites.

Fairley visited Cairns during 17–20 March 1944, and proposed further groups for Experiment XIII to be carried out in April and May.[7] This included a subinoculation at the time of biting. Blood from one arm of a donor was

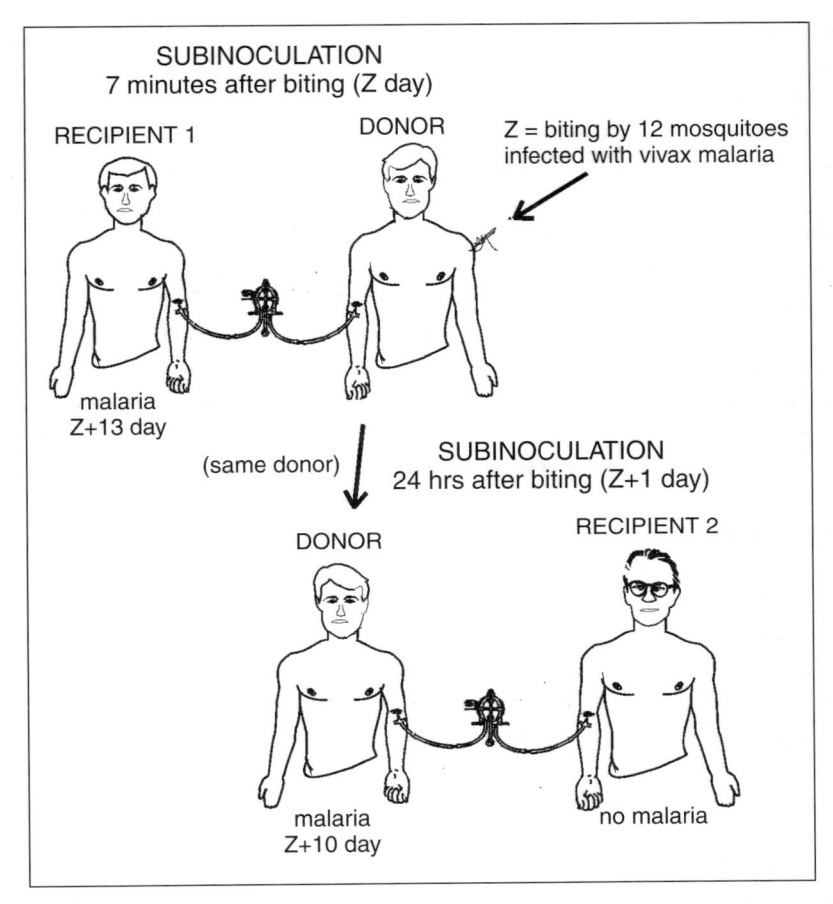

Fig. 8 Experiment to investigate the length of time that sporozoites remain in the bloodstream after the bite of a malaria-infected mosquito

The donor was bitten on the left arm by 12 vivax-infected mosquitoes over an eight-minute period, and 500 ml of blood was transfused from his right arm into Recipient 1 between seven to 12 minutes after biting ceased. A further 500 ml was transfused from the left arm of this donor into Recipient 2 24 hours after biting. The donor developed overt malaria on Z+10, whereas the seven-minute recipient had a slight headache with fever and parasites on Z+13, which subsequently developed into a typical attack of vivax malaria. However, the 24-hour recipient remained well, with no evidence of malaria for the entire 35-day observation period.

transfused to a recipient at the same time that vivax-infected mosquitoes were biting his other arm. Both donor and recipient subsequently developed overt vivax malaria. Several other subinoculations of vivax malaria were performed at various time intervals during the first hour after biting. Similar blood transfers were made to recipients from donors bitten by falciparum-infected mosquitoes.

The results indicated that viable sporozoites of vivax malaria circulated in the blood for at least 30 minutes after biting, and that falciparum sporozoites remained in the blood for at least 60 minutes. A consistent difference was noted in the course of infections between donors who received sporozoites directly by mosquito bites and the recipients who were inoculated with blood from the donors that contained circulating sporozoites. Microscopic levels of parasites were observed earlier in the blood of the donors than in that of the respective recipients. It was thought that this difference could have been due to the smaller dose of sporozoites received by the latter.[8]

Daily clinical examinations were made on all test and control volunteers at Cairns from the time that they received their first infected mosquito bites. The clinical data of controls of the sulphonamide experiments and the 'first combined series' of sulphonamides and atebrin were summarised in an interim report prepared by Major Andrew on 26 November 1943.[9] Parasites were first seen in blood smears of vivax controls between days Z+11 to Z+13 and between days Z+9 to Z+16 in the falciparum controls. There was considerable variation in the 'premonitory symptoms' (the first clinical signs that preceded the onset of malarial attacks) in these men. These initial symptoms sometimes coincided with the appearance of parasites, but in some volunteers signs and symptoms were noticed several days before the first parasites were seen. The earliest sign noted was a tender liver in one vivax case on Z+4, and in three cases of falciparum malaria between Z+4 and Z+6. Slight rises in temperature, headache or malaise were also noted in some of the volunteers before microscopic levels of parasites occurred.

Full-blown attacks of malaria did not occur in any men taking a daily tablet of atebrin, but occasional symptoms were recorded in some of these volunteers. These phenomena sometimes occurred over the same time period that premonitory symptoms were noted in untreated controls. This suggested that the symptoms in men on atebrin may be associated with early development and multiplication of the parasites, but the infections did not develop further as the trophozoites were dealt with by the drug. Fairley conceived the idea of using the subinoculation technique to investigate the action of atebrin during this early phase of infection before the parasites reached microscopic levels. It was hoped that such experiments would also throw light on the uncertain elements of the human malaria cycle during the incubation period.

An experiment designated 'Experiment VII—designed to demonstrate that atebrin suppresses then cures MT [malignant tertian] malaria'—commenced in Cairns on 9 March 1944.[10] This involved six men who received 10 infective bites of falciparum malaria. Three were on atebrin, 100 mg/day, and the other three were taking 1000 mg/day of sulphamerazine. It was planned to subinoculate 500 ml of blood into recipients, with a different man on each drug being used as a donor on days Z+9, Z+11 and Z+13. This work was to be done at 2/2 AGH under the direction of Lieutenant Colonel Andrew. Unfortunately, there was a lack of sufficient recipients of suitable blood groups in the volunteer pool at 2/2 AGH at the time, so it was not possible to complete all of the subinoculation regimens of this experimental group. The first two atebrin subinoculations were completed successfully on Z+9 and Z+11, but compatible recipients for the other donors were not available. Blackburn referred to this in a letter to Fairley on 4 April with the comment: 'This will not occur again'.[11] Steps were taken to ensure an adequate supply of suitable recipients before commencing any further subinoculation experiments.

The recipient from the atebrin donor subinoculated on Z+9 developed typical falciparum malaria nine days after the subinoculation.[12] The recipient from the man subinoculated on Z+11 subsequently showed no evidence of latent or overt malaria. Blackburn reported that this experiment 'has not been an unqualified success' owing to the lack of compatible recipients, but he realised that the positive result in the first recipient was most significant. On the day of this subinoculation the donor had malaise, as well as a tender liver and spleen. These were typical signs of malaria, but parasites were not detected in the examination of his daily blood films. His clinical symptoms lasted for only a few days, and he remained well for the duration of the experiment without developing an attack after drug administration ceased.

This successful subinoculation clearly demonstrated that, in this man at least, the phenomena of suppressed malaria was associated with a parasitaemia that was too low to be observed by microscopic examination of the patient's blood. This provided direct evidence that the minor clinical phenomena in men taking atebrin could be associated with low densities of parasites. It also suggested that the drug did not prevent the formation and liberation of stages from the 'tissue phase' nor the presence of trophozoites in the circulation, but that it acted by preventing their multiplication so that the parasites were not seen under the microscope and malarial attacks did not occur. The inference was that continued administration of atebrin suppressed, then eliminated, all of the blood parasites, and this resulted in complete cure of falciparum malaria.

Additional groups of Experiment VII were tested during the latter half of 1944 and during 1945 to pinpoint the time at which the blood stages first appeared in the circulation.[13] It was found that subinoculations made from donors between one and six days after biting by falciparum-infected mosquitoes invariably failed to infect recipients. However, blood transfused from donors between $6\frac{1}{2}$ and $8\frac{1}{2}$ days produced typical attacks of falciparum malaria in all recipients. These studies were also extended to vivax malaria and, in these infections, subinoculations produced negative results in recipients between one and eight days after biting. Transfusions made between $8\frac{1}{2}$ and $10\frac{1}{2}$ days after biting always yielded vivax infections in the recipients. The donors in these experiments were exposed to between two and 100 mosquitoes, but this did not affect the time during which the blood remained free of parasites. This implied that these intervals ($6\frac{1}{2}$ for falciparum malaria, and $8\frac{1}{2}$ days for vivax malaria) were biological characteristics of each parasite.

The subinoculation experiments also clarified the clinical and parasitological significance of recurring bouts of malaria following the initial attack. The return of fever within eight weeks of recovery from the primary attack was defined by the British malariologist, Colonel S. P. James, as a recrudescence, whereas fever returning between eight and 24 weeks after the primary attack was termed a relapse. He defined a return of fever later than 24 weeks as a recurrence.[14] However, the relationship between these clinical conditions and the concomitant behaviour of vivax and falciparum parasites in the human host was not fully understood. The data obtained during the first year of the Cairns experiments clearly showed that, in the case of falciparum malaria, relapses do not occur, and the infection is permanently cured when the parasites are eliminated from the blood. Infections of *Plasmodium falciparum* derived from sporozoites (by mosquito bites) or from trophozoites (by subinoculation) both behaved in the same way. This implies that the tissue phase does not persist after the blood stages are released in the primary attack.

Even though it had been known for many years that vivax malaria behaves quite differently to falciparum malaria, by relapsing at intervals long after the primary attack has ended, the essential features of this difference between the two human malaria species was not clearly appreciated. During the 1920s W. Yorke and J. W. S. Macfie showed that quinine could not prevent the primary attack of sporozoite-induced vivax malaria if it was only taken during the incubation period.[15] They also demonstrated that quinine was able to deal with trophozoite-induced malaria if the drug was administered for several days after blood inoculation of parasites.

The experiments at Cairns showed that daily suppressive use of atebrin could prevent the primary attack of both trophozoite-transmitted and sporozoite-transmitted vivax malaria. The former was radically cured by the drug, but relapses of sporozoite-transmitted vivax almost always took place several weeks after atebrin administration ceased. Parasites were not observed microscopically in the blood after the primary attack, and subinoculations during this period were usually negative, but subsequent episodes of fever associated with overt malaria ultimately returned. Thus, the tissue phase of falciparum malaria only gives rise to the blood stages causing the primary attack. If all of the blood stages are not destroyed after the patient is treated, they may persist for some time, at subclinical and submicroscopic levels, and subsequently increase again to cause another episode of fever and parasitaemia.

The term 'recrudescence' (or 'short-term relapse') is now restricted to this phenomenon in which secondary attacks are caused by multiplication of blood stages not eliminated after the primary attack. On the other hand, vivax malaria is characterised by recurrent attacks that may occur after prolonged absence of parasites from the circulation. In this case, parasites are released from the tissue phase to initiate the primary attack, and periodic subsequent releases from the tissue phase lead to later attacks. The terms 'recurrence' or 'long-term relapse' are used to designate attacks of vivax malaria that take place after the primary attack is cured.[16]

There was the possibility that some of the first generation of blood stages in the initial attack of vivax malaria might re-enter a tissue phase and subsequently re-emerge to cause relapses. If this were the case, subinoculations of the earliest blood stages (from donors bitten $8\frac{1}{2}$ days previously) should cause primary attacks and then relapses in the recipients. This did not occur, and there was no difference in the type of malaria that developed from early or later subinoculations, thereby indicating that all of the blood-stage parasites went through the same schizogonic cycle.[17] This provided indirect evidence that the tissue forms responsible for relapses are derived from the pre-erythrocytic stages and not from blood stages that re-enter the tissues.

The information obtained from the subinoculation experiments gradually emerged over a period of 12–18 months as the successive groups of Experiment VII bracketed key time intervals of the blood and tissue cycles. This component of the Cairns experiments proved to be of enduring and fundamental importance by shedding new light on the biology of the parasites in the human host. These insights also proved to be of considerable significance for the clinical evaluation of malarial drugs. Sufficient data had already been obtained by mid-1944 for this approach to influence the way in which all later work was done. As new knowledge accumulated it was progressively utilised to assist in planning and implementation of subsequent experiments. This set the stage for rapid and thorough evaluation of new compounds that emerged from the US and British programs for synthesis and development of new antimalarials. The subinoculation technique played a crucial role in revealing the mode of action of these new drugs and in assessing their efficacy as suppressive or curative agents of the disease.

10

Setbacks and Dilemmas in the US Program

AFTER THE VISIT of Fairley and Albert to the USA in 1942 the American malaria program went through a period of considerable expansion. Large numbers of compounds were screened against avian parasites, but there were difficulties in sustaining the momentum of the research effort to identify the most promising ones that could then be evaluated against human malaria. There was no clear consensus of opinion amongst the American scientists on what was the best way that this could be done. As the work continued, inconsistencies in drug action between bird and human parasites were found that threw into question the whole rationale of the screening program.

The background to these developments was summarised by Dr E. K. Marshall, a pharmacologist at Johns Hopkins University, Baltimore, at a meeting of the Board for the Co-ordination of Malarial Studies in October 1941.[1] He noted that there were few organic compounds with proven safety for administration to humans so it was essential that the bulk of initial studies be carried out on animals. The experimental screening systems used selected bird malaria parasites that produced consistent infections in a suitable experimental animal that could be maintained under laboratory conditions. *Plasmodium cathemerium* in canaries was one obvious choice for this purpose as it had been studied intensively in the laboratory since its discovery in 1927. However, as canaries are relatively small birds it was difficult to obtain sufficient blood to determine the concentration of drugs in their circulation. Another suitable parasite was *P. lophurae*; this had been originally found in pheasants, but it had been shown that ducks were very reliable hosts. Their larger size facilitated the estimation of drug levels in the blood. But the most promising experimental parasite appeared to be *P. gallinaceum*, which infected chickens. This species was not indigenous to the USA, and its importation was initially refused by the quarantine authorities who feared that local mosquitoes may spread it to domestic poultry farms. The desirability of obtaining permission for its introduction to designated laboratories was discussed at the first meeting of the Board in July 1941, and approval was granted three months later. Subsequent studies confirmed that *P. gallinaceum* was satisfactory for both blood-induced and sporozoite-induced infections, and it was chosen for screening tests of possible causal prophylactic agents.

There were two methods of pursuing this work. One involved examination of a representative sample of different groups of compounds to see whether any of them showed activity against malaria parasites. Marshall described this as the 'hit and miss' or 'miss and miss' method, with success being entirely dependent on chance. Another approach was to modify the structure of compounds already known to have some antimalarial activity, in the hope that this would result in an increase in activity and a decrease in toxicity. This latter method, which involved comparison of the therapeutic activity of different derivatives of a parent compound, had been used by the Germans in the development of plasmoquine and atebrin. However, adequate experimental techniques to make such comparisons in a quantitative way had not been devised. Both methods were used by the Americans as there was no clear indication as to which avenue might prove to be the most fruitful.

The most appropriate screening system would be one in which the response of the experimental parasite to drugs was similar to that of the human malaria parasites but it was not known, in the early stages of the program, how close any of the avian parasites came to meeting this ideal. In June 1942 Dr W. H. Taliaferro, who was then chairman of the Board, visited all of the supported research groups in the USA. He was gratified to see that efficient screening facilities based on avian parasites had been set up in a number of institutions. However, he pointed out that 'all of the "screening" tests in animals are open to the possible error that a drug may be effective in man but ineffective in lower animals'. He went on to note that 'it is, however, impossible to do other than assume that a drug effective against malaria in man will be at least partially active on the animal malarias—an assumption so far found to be true'.[2]

Another basic assumption of the avian malaria screening program was that compounds closely related chemically might have different orders of activity in avian and human infections, but the overall comparative activity of a related group of compounds was expected to be similar in both kinds of infections. However, as time went on there was a growing feeling among Board members that these basic premises may be in error. The experience of the first 12 to

18 months showed that it was difficult to estimate the promise of activity in humans because both the bird hosts and bird parasites differed widely in susceptibility to various groups of drugs.

By April 1943 over 3000 compounds (submitted by 62 institutions) had been screened against avian parasites. Antimalarial activity had been recorded in 10–12 per cent of the compounds, but some were active against one parasite but not another.[3] The observed differences in drug response in different avian parasites highlighted the deficiencies of the screening program, and demonstrated the importance of testing in humans. In order to do this it would be necessary to increase the number of tests in humans, but the clinical testing facilities available to the collaborating American institutions were limited and not capable of rapid expansion.

In December 1943 Dr R. F. Loeb took over as Chairman, and later in that month it was decided to reorganise the Board in an effort to promote better co-ordination of National Research Council-sponsored research. Board members were appointed to three specialist panels: the Panel of Chemistry, chaired by Dr W. Mansfield Clark; the Panel of Clinical Testing, chaired by Dr James A. Shannon; and the Panel of Pharmacology, chaired by Dr E. K. Marshall. In addition there was a Panel of Review, which included the chairman and secretary of the Board, Dr G. A. Carden, together with the chairmen of the three panels. The Panel of Review was initially set up as a fact-finding body with no independent authority to make decisions. It met to integrate the work of the three specialist panels so that promising leads could be correlated and submitted in a condensed report to the Board.

During the first two years after the USA entered the war there were only two institutions in the USA with the capacity to handle significant numbers of experimental patients for malaria studies. One was Dr Shannon's laboratory at Goldwater Memorial Hospital, New York, which had facilities for 20 patients per month receiving malaria therapy for syphilis. The work at New York, which was directed towards preliminary evaluation of drugs against the blood stages, involved injection of malaria-infected blood from donors to test subjects. The other institution was the National Institutes of Health laboratory of the US Public Health Service in Washington, where a research group led by Dr G. Robert Coatney and Dr W. H. Sebrell undertook trials with syphilis patients undergoing malaria therapy at Saint Elizabeth's Hospital. This was the only laboratory where mosquito-transmitted infections were used to investigate the causal prophylactic potential of drugs. The mosquitoes for this work were infected with either vivax or falciparum parasites derived from malaria therapy patients at the South Carolina State Hospital.

Both the New York and Washington units lacked the resources to rapidly increase clinical tests involving human patients. This problem was first raised at a Board meeting in August 1942. The minutes stated that 'Dr Shannon called attention to the fact that at the present time clinical studies on malaria were not sufficient to take care of the number of problems which needed to be studied'.[4] Unlike the work at Cairns, the US program was essentially a civilian enterprise. Even though there were representatives from the US Army and Navy on the Board, there appear to have been no plans or proposals to set up a clinical testing program in the USA using experimentally infected army volunteers.

Shannon suggested that new testing units should be established and, during 1943, strenuous efforts were made to find institutions where this could be done. A third facility based on the use of syphilis patients receiving malaria therapy was developed at the Gailor Memorial Hospital, Memphis, Tennessee.[5] These clinical studies, which were carried out under the direction of Dr Henry Packer and Dr Robert B. Watson of the Division of Preventive Medicine, University of Tennessee, were on a relatively small scale. Some suppressive tests with sporozoite-induced vivax malaria were made at Memphis on a few drugs. Other experiments involved administration of test drugs during the incubation period of sporozoite-transmitted falciparum or vivax infections. Members of the Board visited Connecticut to investigate whether a clinical unit could be formed at the State Hospital at Norwich, and it seemed for a time, in mid-1943, that the combined facilities in New York, Tennessee, Washington and Connecticut might be adequate to meet current needs. Unfortunately, a clinical testing program was not developed at Norwich, and plans to establish a clinical facility in Michigan did not eventuate.

A major impediment to an expansion of human experiments in the American research program was caused by a shortage of staff who could be employed for this work. The wartime requirements for medical personnel meant that it was almost impossible to obtain trained clinical staff from civilian sources.[6] The only means of resolving this difficulty was for such staff to be made available from the armed services. In June 1943 Brigadier General Simmons said that the Army would co-operate in helping him maintain personnel for this work.[7] However, by December the problem had become so acute that Dr R. F. Loeb and the Chairman of the Division of Medical Sciences of the National Research Council, Dr L. H. Weed, visited the Office of the Surgeon General of the US Army to discuss the personnel problem with senior staff officers.

Following this meeting, Dr Weed wrote to the Surgeon General in an effort to have military medical staff assigned to the clinical testing program. General N. T. Kirk replied that exceptions could not be made and no officers of the Medical Administrative Corps or Medical Corps could be assigned for civilian studies on malaria.[8] This decision was not reversed until submissions were made at the highest levels of the wartime government. This followed the personal intervention of Dr Vannevar Bush, the Director of the Office of Scientific Research and Development (OSRD). This was an umbrella agency with wide authority over all government science and service in the war, including the Committee of Medical Research and its subsidiary bodies such as the Board for the Co-ordination of Malarial Studies. OSRD provided the money to support the research activities recommended by the Board. Bush was a powerful figure in the wartime administration who reported directly to President Franklin Roosevelt. He negotiated the release of 12 medical army officers to participate in clinical testing of new antimalarials in February 1944, more than a year after difficulties with personnel to support the clinical testing program were first discussed by the Board.[9] This chain of developments was in contrast to the Cairns research effort where the highest priority was accorded to staffing and other essential requirements at the very outset, thereby vindicating Fairley's efforts to ensure that the enterprise remained under Australian Army control.

It became apparent that the numbers of patients undergoing malaria treatment for syphilis in the USA were not sufficient to support a substantial increase in clinical testing facilities and other avenues would need to be exploited to fulfil the wartime goals of the malaria research program. At a Board meeting in January 1943 Dr Shannon suggested that one way of overcoming the deficiency in clinical testing might be to seek development of civilian facilities in malarious areas of South America.[10] The most promising possibility appeared to be at Gulfito, Costa Rica, where the United Fruit Company offered the use of the company hospital for this purpose. A group of Board members subsequently visited South America to inspect potential field-testing locations. From information gained in Mexico City, Guatemala City, and San Jose, Costa Rica, they found that 'it was apparent ... that the high degree of natural immunity prevalent among the native populations of Central America eliminated these places as potential sites for clinical investigation'.[11] They considered that prospects were much better in Panama in the Gorgas and Clayton Hospitals that were both US Army installations. Drs D. P. Earle and J. V. Taggart, of Dr Shannon's group in New York, went to Panama at the end of 1943 to set up a clinical testing unit. However, it was found that very few cases of malaria were admitted to Gorgas Hospital during the following months, and it was decided to close this unit in April 1944.[12]

The withdrawal of staff from Panama was a serious setback for the expansion of clinical testing, but this was alleviated, to some extent, by more favourable developments in the USA. Dr G. A. Carden reported to the Board in December 1943 on a visit to the Massachusetts General Hospital in Boston to evaluate the facilities there for clinical and pharmacological tests in humans.[13] Tentative arrangements were made for pharmacological studies involving conscientious objectors, and this was approved in principle by the Board. New drugs identified in the screening program as being active against avian malaria parasites and not toxic to animals would be administered to conscientious objectors under carefully controlled conditions to confirm their safety to humans before being tested against the human malaria parasites. Plans were finalised in early 1944, and it was arranged for the pharmacological studies at the Massachusetts General Hospital to proceed in tandem with clinical studies on syphilis patients receiving blood-inoculated malaria therapy at the Boston Psychopathic Hospital Unit. A staff of four medical officers who were physically disqualified from Army service were obtained for this work, which functioned as an integrated unit under the direction of Dr Alan M. Butler.[14]

The clinical testing procedures adopted in Boston were very similar to those developed by Shannon's laboratory in New York and they provided a welcome addition to the human testing program. However, both these units were restricted to blood-inoculated infections, and were unable to evaluate the causal prophylactic activity of drugs, as this required sporozoite-induced infections initiated by the bite of infected mosquitoes.

During November 1943 the Board agreed that the US Public Health Service should be assigned the responsibility of maintaining adequate facilities for sporozoite-induced infections, and that they should promptly exploit any new facilities that might be available.[15] During the following month Coatney presented a contract proposal to the Board that was aimed at overcoming the bottleneck in clinical testing.[16] This arose from an approach to the Federal Bureau of Prisons with the suggestion that the inmates of one of the federal penitentiaries might contribute to the program of antimalarial drug testing. The prison authorities responded very favourably to Coatney's suggestion for the use of volunteer prisoners who would be subjected to mosquito-transmitted malaria for evaluation of new drugs.

In the following month Drs Sebrell and Coatney gave a report on facilities at the United States Penitentiary in Atlanta, Georgia. Detailed plans for the Atlanta project were drawn up and submitted to the Board for critical appraisal.[17] The unit was allocated a complete ward in the prison hospital, with laboratories, offices, and space for outpatients.[18] The malaria parasites used at Atlanta were to be derived from the bites of infected *Anopheles quadrimaculatus* mosquitoes reared and infected at the Malaria Research Laboratory of the National Institute of Health, at Columbia, South Carolina, by Drs Martin D. Young and Robert W. Burgess, with the co-operation of the South Carolina State Hospital. Preparations were rapidly completed and the experiments commenced in March 1944. The Board decided that the first trials were to be made with quinine as a standard of reference before experiments with other compounds commenced.[19]

The increase in human testing facilities in early 1944 did not produce an immediate solution to the shortcomings in the US program. By then clinical testing had lagged even further behind avian screening. Trials of representatives of promising drug series were needed to assess whether their human antimalarial activity was high enough and their toxicity low enough to justify further synthesis. The system almost bogged down for lack of direction and there was considerable debate among members of the Board about the most appropriate measures to overcome these deficiencies.[20] This situation was exacerbated by human drug trials conducted in the previous 18 months, which used up a large component of the available clinical testing resources and produced only negative or ambivalent results. The trials of sulphadiazine conducted by Coatney's group fell into this category (see Chapter 6), and a similar situation arose in the testing of two compounds developed by the National Institutes of Health (NIH) facilities.

The promise shown by the first of these (code named NIH 204) against avian parasites was considered sufficient to justify a limited trial in humans. This took two and a half months, involving the use of scarce human malaria subjects, only to discover that it was too toxic and too irregular in absorption from the gut to be of practical value. It was concluded that 'it is more toxic and less effective than atebrin and quinine, and, therefore deserves no further study'.[21] The second compound, NIH 700, was claimed to show similar promise on the basis of avian screening tests, but the clinical investigators were wary of committing it to human tests as 'a similar work up would require several months and [the use of] all our pharmacological and clinical facilities'.[22] These experiences underlined the need for the collaborating scientists to agree on what drugs should be subjected to human trial and at what stage in the development process such trials should commence.

At a meeting of the Pharmacology Panel in early 1944 there was 'a prolonged and lively discussion concerning the most efficient method of selecting a compound for trial in man'.[23] There was general agreement that a preliminary trial against human malaria should be done as soon as a compound was shown to be active in avian malaria and sufficiently non-toxic to justify such a trial. But from that point there was a sharp divergence of opinion between the US Public Health Service representatives from the NIH group in Washington, on the one hand, and other members of the panel. Most panel members felt that, if the preliminary trial of a new compound confirmed its activity against human malaria, then it was essential that it be subjected to detailed tests involving several avian malaria species to quantitatively document its toxicity in relation to its absorption and excretion. The rationale was that 'only in this way will it be possible to make a rational selection of one or two members of a large series as the most promising to warrant a careful evaluation in man'.[24] The group from NIH strongly disagreed with this approach on the grounds that such quantitative studies were more of academic interest than of immediate practical value. NIH representatives emphasised the need for haste, and argued that empirical evaluation of antimalarial activity in birds was sufficiently adequate to warrant clinical trial.[25]

The controversy and debate within the Board and its panels on pharmacological and clinical evaluation of new compounds was of fundamental importance, as it was obviously impossible to subject all active derivatives in a family of compounds to tests in humans. It was crucial that this matter be resolved as it would have direct influence on the direction that future work should take with the expansion of clinical testing facilities. As the members of the Board could not agree among themselves, it was decided to convene a conference to review the policies now being formulated 'in order that the Coordinating Board may effectuate an overall program which will lead to the most prompt and critical evaluation of active chemotherapeutic agents'.[26]

The Conference for a Review of the Malaria Research Program was held in the National Research Council Building in Washington on 29 March 1944.[27] In addition to members of the Board, it was attended by more than 20 'critical individuals prominent in the field of clinical investigation' from various research institutions in the USA, as well as by members of the Committee on Medical Research, the National Research Council, and representatives from the Army and the Navy. The Chairman, Dr R. F. Loeb, outlined the importance of the malaria problem in the war, the scope of the wartime program, and the aims of the conference. He pointed out that 'pressure of time necessitates the employment of research which might not perhaps be chosen in peacetime'. Dr Coatney made a presentation on the biology and life cycle of malaria, stressing the need for information on how drugs affect the various stages in humans. Lieutenant Colonel Francis R. Dieuaide described current malaria treatment measures in the Army and Major O. R. McCoy covered malaria suppression with atebrin in US forces. Dr E. K. Marshall then presented a review of the pharmacological program based on avian screening, chronic and acute toxicity in animals, and studies on absorption, excretion, and degradation of individual compounds in test animals. He believed that the quickest results would be obtained by the 'hit and miss method', and pointed out that there had not been a single sulphonamide discovered by a rational system of synthesis.

Dr Shannon, the final speaker, reviewed the clinical testing program. He remarked that many of the things that could be said about the pharmacological aspects of the program also applied to clinical evaluation. Shannon explained that a basic premise of the program was that a compound affecting the blood stages was also likely to have an effect on the tissue forms from which the blood stages were derived. Thus, it was thought that atebrin had an effect on the tissue phase, but that the intensity of its action was too low to destroy it completely. If this were true, a compound with a higher activity against the blood stages should also be more effective against the tissue forms, and thus possess the capacity to act as a true causal prophylactic. One of the arguments in favour of clinical testing based on blood-induced infections was based on this hypothesis. The work of Shannon's own group in New York had shown that such experiments produced highly reproducible results in a relatively short time. With this approach drug concentration in the plasma could be accurately related to antimalarial activity against the blood stages. Nevertheless, Shannon was well aware that this hypothesis might not be correct. He said:

> Such results may give one a feeling of false security since they reflect the activity of potentially useful agents against the asexual forms of the plasmodium rather than activity against the tissue phase or phases which is our ultimate goal. The situation may be somewhat analogous to one where an attempt is made to teach an individual how to swim by teaching him how to skate on ice, making sure that the ice is thick enough to preclude the possibility of his getting wet.[28]

The essential point of this apt analogy was that that these experiments (based on the injection of blood from a man with malaria) could not simulate natural infections initiated by sporozoites injected by mosquitoes. This experimental method bypasses the tissue phase, and the injected parasites cycle solely within the blood phase. The difference between the two methods of infection was crucial if compounds affected one phase but not the other. For example, in a testing program based on blood-inoculated infections, a new compound with causal prophylactic properties would be overlooked if it did not have activity against the blood phase. Conversely, considerable time and effort in the search for a causal prophylactic drug could be wasted by testing compounds against the blood stages if active compounds identified by this method had no activity against the tissue phase.

These deficiencies in experiments based on blood-induced infections were appreciated by the senior investigators involved in the American program, and it was hoped that this would be addressed by the experiments at Atlanta State Penitentiary that were then about to commence. Nevertheless, even with the expanded capacity for sporozoite-induced experiments in this facility, it would only be possible to evaluate a limited number of compounds for causal prophylactic activity in humans.

But how were such compounds to be selected for trial? Shannon alluded to this question in his address to the conference. 'Surely, one would have thought that drugs which completely cure falciparum malaria have a better chance to cure vivax malaria than drugs selected for trial on the basis of the avian infections'. However, American experience in the field had already indicated that atebrin could prevent and cure falciparum malaria but not vivax malaria. This implied that the two parasites differed in their biology so that they did not always respond in the same way to antimalarial drugs. He said: 'How much more irrational is the use of an avian infection, however used, as a screen for the selection of drugs for trial in the human infection'. As tests based on one avian or human infection had limited predictive value, it was essential that

> any series of chemical substances showing a moderate degree of antimalarial activity of one sort or another and having a relatively low toxicity should be tested for activity in the human infections by techniques which will demonstrate [causal] prophylactic, suppressive, and/or curative action.[29]

This was an undertaking requiring extensive clinical evaluation. Shannon mentioned that it was not known how long it would take for prophylactic tests. He thought it would probably take much longer than experiments based on blood-induced infections but, in any event, 'the final standardisation of the prophylactic test must await the development of a truly prophylactic agent'.

The presentations stimulated considerable discussion between Board members and the invited consultants. When adjourning the conference, Loeb asked each consultant to write to the Secretary, Dr Carden, 'outlining his opinion of the present program making any suggestions or changes which seemed desirable and including any approaches which occurred to the consultant after thinking this conference over'. These comments were subsequently added as an appendix to the minutes of the conference.[30] Regrettably, none of them were sufficiently innovative to stimulate a new approach or alternative line of investigation that might have led to a more efficient allocation of resources for the overall benefit of the program.

11

Captured from the Enemy

WHEN THE ANTIMALARIAL drug screening program was set up in the USA there were some initial difficulties in obtaining the full co-operation of research laboratories of US pharmaceutical and chemical companies because of concerns about commercial secrecy. These were overcome by the formation of an office of the Board known as the Survey of Antimalarial Drugs, under the direction of Dr Frederick Wiselogle of the Chemistry Department, Johns Hopkins University, Baltimore.[1] This office acted as an intermediary between the various chemical firms and testing laboratories. It received compounds synthesised by the chemists, and gave them to the pharmacologists for testing.

The Survey office also maintained a system for tabulating data on the various test compounds. This involved the use of survey numbers, 'SN', followed by digits, as identity codes for specific compounds. 'Survey Tables', summarising the results of screening tests in bird malaria, were circulated to suppliers and the co-operating laboratories to prevent duplication of effort and to provide information on whether a particular group of compounds was adequately covered. Nevertheless, the synthesis and evaluation of the compounds were essentially empirical in nature and, as the mass of data accumulated, it was easy to overlook those that merited further investigation. By an unfortunate series of incidents one group of compounds, originally discovered by the Germans before the war, was prematurely bypassed by the Americans, and this delayed the development of the most important drug that emerged from the US wartime malaria program.

After their groundbreaking discovery of atebrin, the German team working in the Bayer laboratories at Elberfeld continued synthesis and testing of potential antimalarials. Dr Kenneth Blanchard, a member of the Survey of Antimalarial Drugs, was sent on a mission to Elberfeld very soon after the end of hostilities in Germany. He interviewed Drs W. Kikuth and F. Schonhofer to find out what progress the Germans had made in this field during the war.[2] They screened approximately 1000 acridine derivatives related to atebrin, but none of them were superior to atebrin itself. They also investigated many other compounds, including some 4-amino-quinolines. One of these synthesised in 1934 was named resochin. Tests by Kikuth showed that it was as active against avian malaria as atebrin, but slightly more toxic. It was later administered to a limited number of blood-inoculated cases of vivax malaria by Professor F. Sioli in Dusseldorf but it was not subjected to an adequate clinical trial, as Sioli thought it was too toxic.[3] Following the decision to discard resochin, a related compound, sontochin (also known as sontoquine) was produced, which Kikuth found to be less toxic in animals. Human trials conducted in Germany by Sioli during the period November 1937 to May 1938 yielded very encouraging results against 16 cases of blood-induced vivax malaria. By 1939 more than 1000 cases had been treated with sontochin by German medical scientists. Resochin, sontochin and several other 4-amino-quinoline derivatives were patented in Germany in November 1939.[4]

Winthrop Chemical Company in New York had a cartel arrangement with Bayer in Germany, and received manufacturing directions for sontochin in May 1939. The German patent for the 4-amino-quinoline series was issued as a US patent in the name of Winthrop in March 1941. During October 1940 J. T. Sheehan of Winthrop synthesised a small amount of sontochin that was given to L. T. Coggleshall and J. Maier of Rockefeller Foundation for tests in lower animals. Maier reported to the company in January 1941 that the compound was active against bird malaria. Winthrop did not release this data at that time, and it was not passed to the Survey of Antimalarial Drugs until November 1942. It was then given the Survey Number SN-183, and further testing was recommended at a meeting of the Panel on Pharmacology on 20 January 1943. However, this was not done, as the Chairman, Dr E. K. Marshall, wrote to the Survey Office that this was not necessary. He mistook the structure of the drug for an 8-amino-quinoline, and said that there was no need to study additional derivatives of this group. Consequently, no other tests were carried out in the USA at this time, though the Germans had already proceeded with development of sontochin in Europe.[5]

Bayer promoted atebrin in the French colonial empire through the pharmaceutical branch of the firm Rhône-Poulenc. In July 1941 samples of sontochin and clinical data were provided to the French under this arrangement, and Dr P. Decourt, a clinical consultant of the company, took the drug to Tunisia for human trials. By July 1942 he had obtained good results against vivax malaria without adverse side-effects.

In the following month Dr J. Schneider joined Decourt in Tunis to expand the field-testing program. Trials were set up to compare sontochin with atebrin and quinine for treatment of acute cases of malaria. Field trials were also conducted in west Tunisia to compare sontochin with atebrin for malaria prophylaxis. Decourt returned to France, but Schneider remained until the Allied invasion of North Africa on 9 November 1942.

Allied forces arrived in Tunis in May 1943, and Schneider offered the remaining supplies of sontochin and a detailed report of his test results to the US Army on the understanding that the commercial rights of his company would be safeguarded.[6] The covering letter from Brigadier General F. Blesse, indicates that the material was sent from North Africa Headquarters to the Surgeon General in Washington on 8 July 1943, but a copy was not sent to the Board for the Co-ordination of Malarial Studies until 15 September 1943. So, after a delay of more than three months, Schneider's report and his samples of sontochin were finally received by the Board.

Dr W. Mansfield Clark made a brief statement to the Board on 2 September 1943 that it had been captured from the enemy in North Africa. He stated that its chemical identity had probably been established by Dr W. A. Jacobs at the Rockefeller Institute in New York, but he deferred making a final report 'pending its chemical comparison with a product under an old German patent which may be identical'.[7] At the next meeting Clark confirmed that the compound was identical with the Winthrop formula for sontochin, and advised the Board that preliminary data on its therapeutic activity and acute toxicity should soon be available.[8] On 4 November Dr E. K. Marshall reviewed the background of sontochin to the Board, and explained how it had been overlooked. The Rockefeller data, indicating that it was quite active against bird malaria, had been released by Winthrop 12 months previously, and the information had subsequently remained in the files of the Survey Office.[9] Dr G. Robert Coatney, who was present at this meeting, wrote later that 'this created havoc bordering on hysteria. We had dropped the ball and in so doing had lost valuable time in the search for a reliable synthetic antimalarial. Number SN-183 was declared dead and a new one—SN-6911—was assigned to it'.[10]

Marshall summarised preliminary tests that had already been conducted in his laboratory at Johns Hopkins University and by Dr E. M. K. Geiling's group at the University of Chicago. The results were very promising, as they showed that sontochin was considerably more active than quinine against *Plasmodium lophurae* infections in ducks.[11] The report that J. Schneider gave the Americans included a table of results and explanatory notes obtained from a prophylactic (suppressive) trial in which sontochin was administered in daily or weekly doses to more than 1200 people for three and a half months from mid-August until the end of November 1942.[12] There were deficiencies in the trial, as some

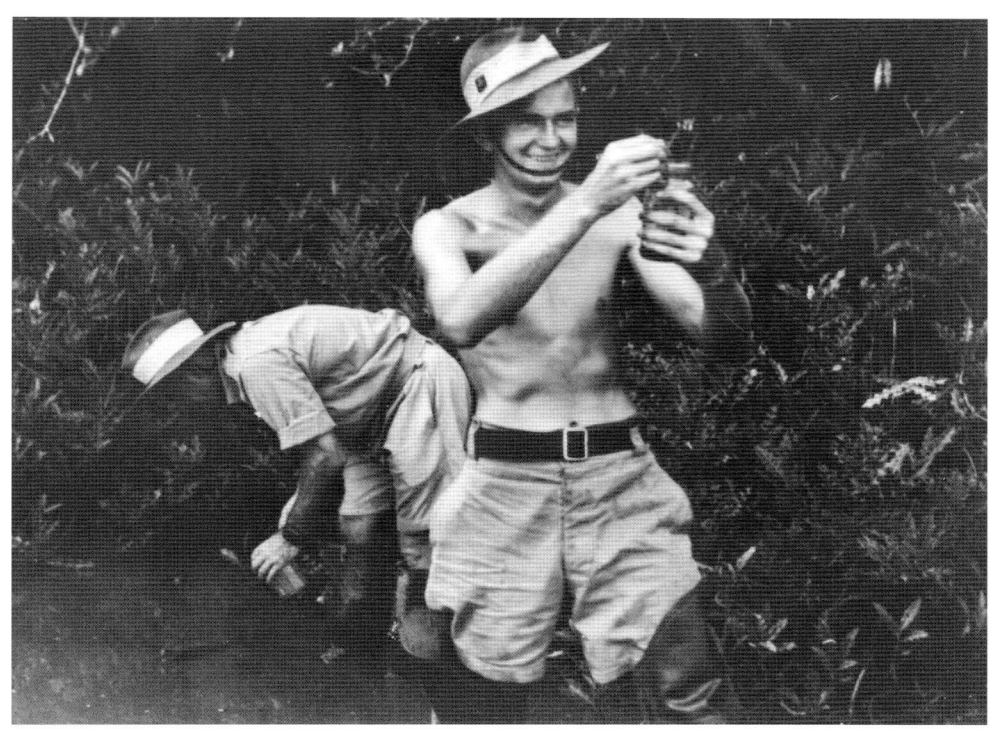

Collecting mosquito larvae in a swamp near Cairns for malaria experiments

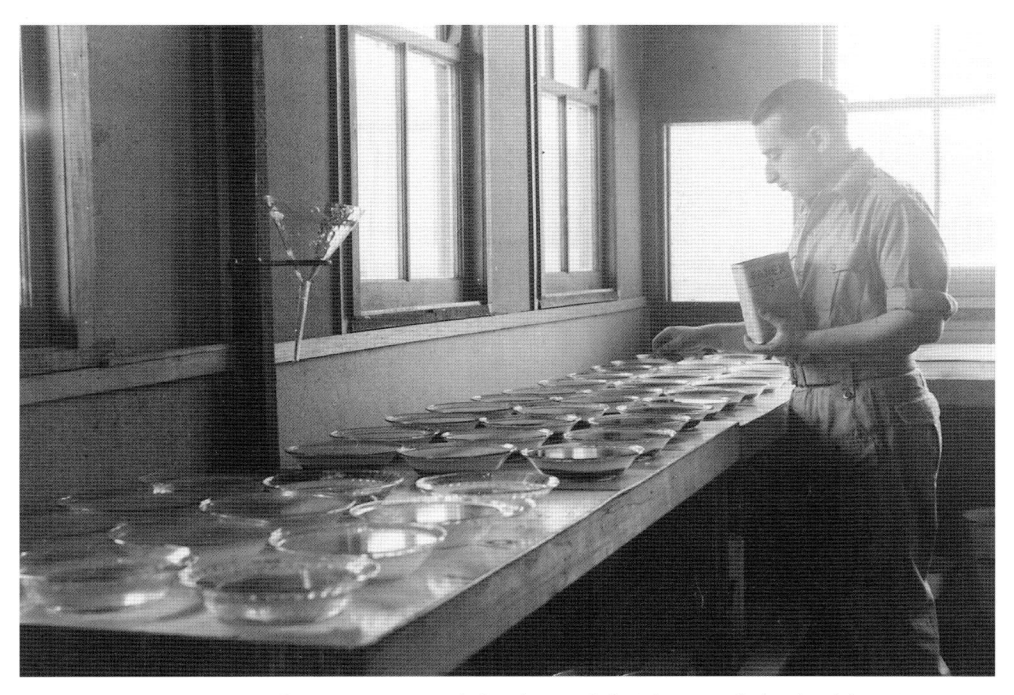

Field-collected mosquito larvae in rearing dishes being fed with Farex baby food by Private Hans Mannheim, a volunteer recruited from 8 Employment Company, who worked in the entomology section after completing his term as an experimental subject

Lieutenant Tom Lemerle (left), collecting mosquito pupae from larval rearing dishes; Private H. Mannheim (right) is adding apple pieces as food for caged adult mosquitoes (oil painting by Nora Heysen)

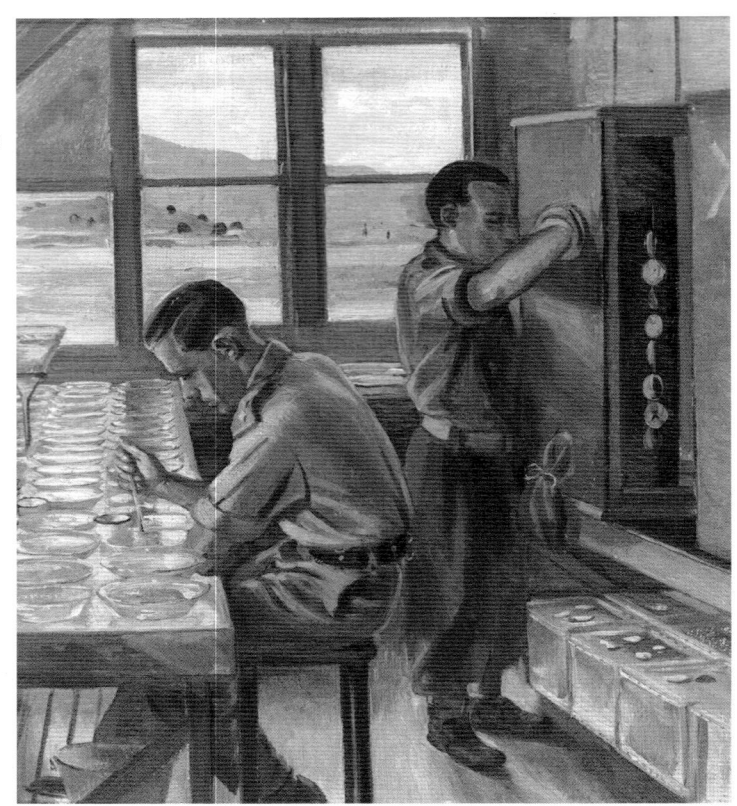

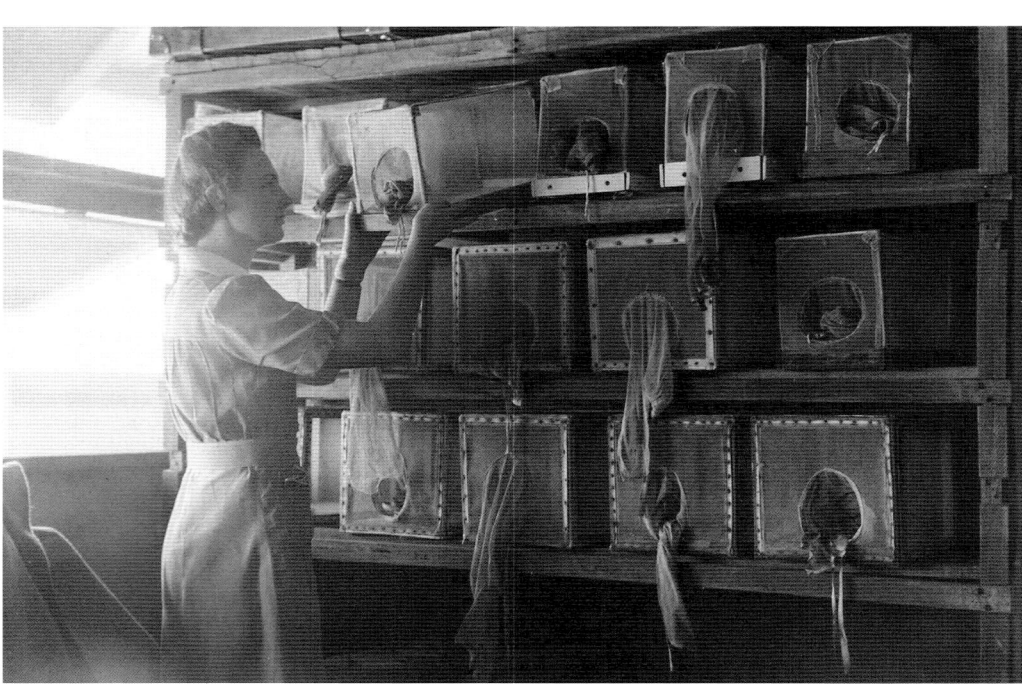

Private Patricia Johnson sorting mosquito cages used for feeding female mosquitoes on carriers and volunteers for experimental transmission of malaria

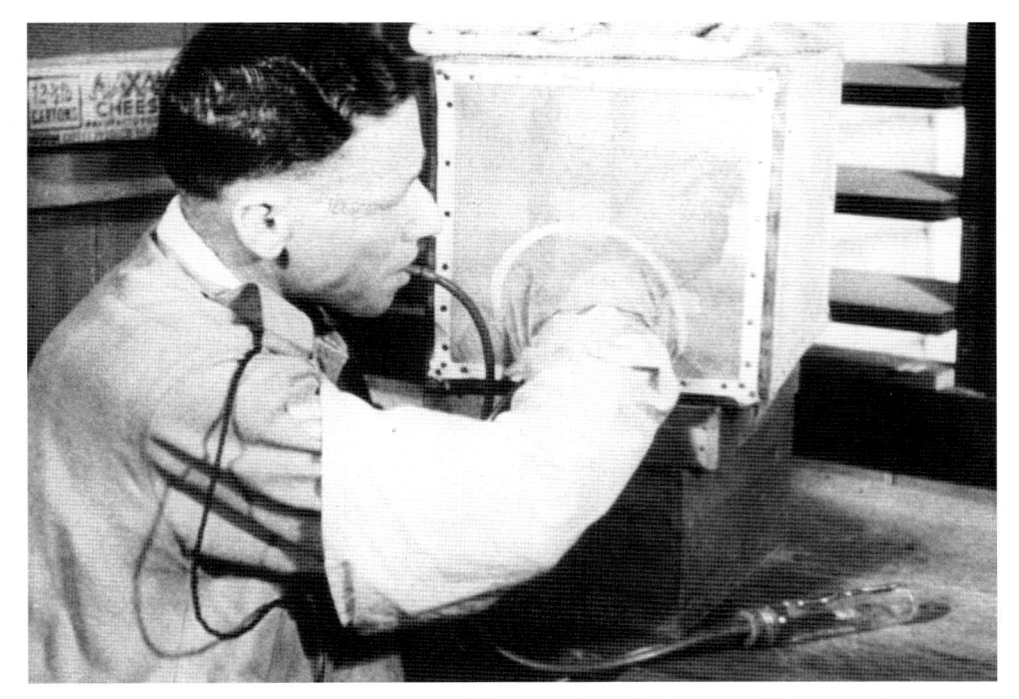

Staff Sergeant Jack McNamara removing adult mosquitoes from a cage. The mosquitoes are sucked from the cage with a rubber aspiration tube, and are drawn into the glass test tube on the lower right (still from movie film).

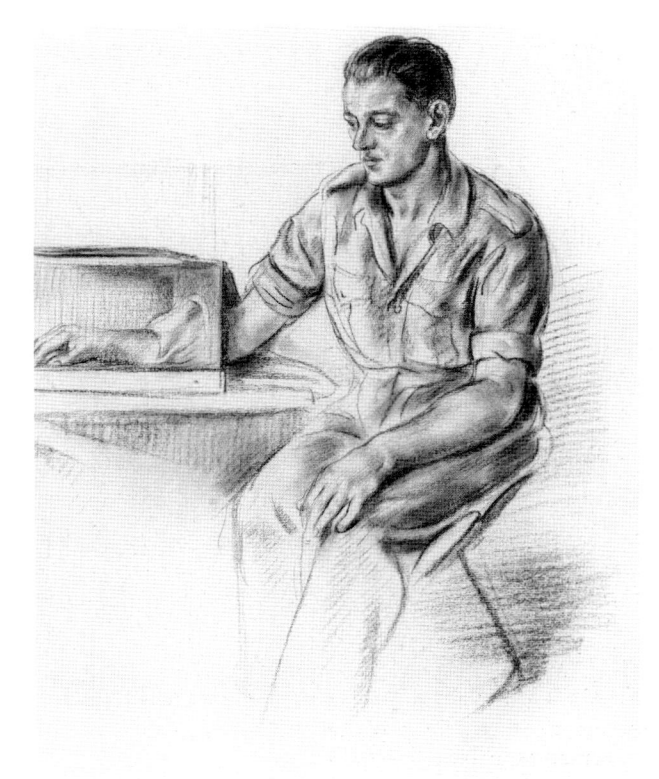

Gunner Gilbert Seaton, a volunteer who was also a donor (gametocyte carrier), infecting a cage of mosquitoes with his malaria (sketch by Nora Heysen)

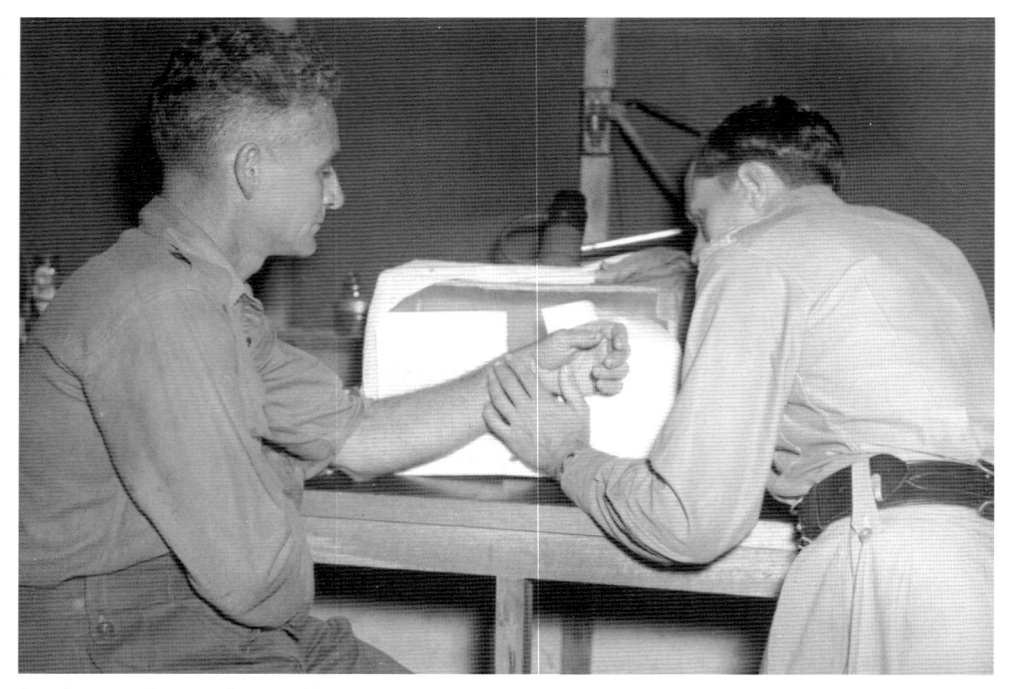

A volunteer, Corporal J. H. Clune, receiving a regulated number of bites from infected mosquitoes. The staff member, Lieutenant Tom Lemerle, is counting the number of mosquitoes feeding on the volunteer's forearm pressed against the outside of the cage.

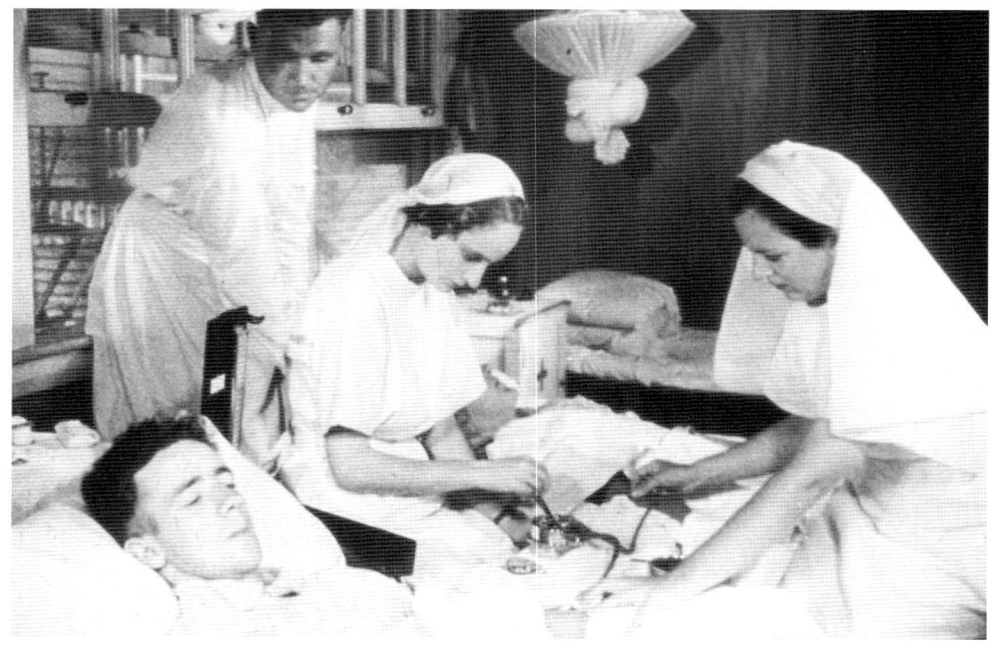

The subinoculation technique, involving transmission of malaria by direct blood transfusion from infected donor (right) to recipient volunteer (left). The nursing sister in charge, Captain Bobbie Fenner (far right), closely monitored both patients while the AAMWS orderly (centre) manually operated the blood transfusion pump (still from movie film).

subjects missed doses, but the overall results were most promising. In one group of 350 people, taking 100 mg of sontochin/day, the parasite rate fell from 21 per cent to zero.

Curative treatment with sontochin was also tested in malaria patients at the Contagious Diseases section of Ernest Coneil Hospital in Tunis. The results were very encouraging, as parasites and fever cleared within 48 hours. The report also noted a total absence of intolerance among subjects taking sontochin. Dr Marshall felt that, since Dr Schneider had given it a fairly extensive trial and found it less toxic than atebrin, it should be reasonably safe for testing in humans. However, for future reference it was decided that the drug should receive a prompt and thorough pharmacological work-up, such as was instituted on compound NIH 204.[13]

Schneider's report and the samples of sontochin arrived in Washington at an important stage of the US wartime malaria program. During the previous two years the co-ordinated efforts of the chemists, pharmacologists and clinical investigators had failed to identify any new compounds that might be developed for operational use against the malaria problem facing Allied forces. Considerable resources had been devoted to evaluation of the sulphonamides and several other compounds only to show that their initial promise could not be sustained.

New leads and directions were desperately needed. After their initial dismay at neglecting the Winthrop results, the collaborating scientists quickly focused on sontochin as a priority goal for accelerated evaluation. The Board recommended that 'When the work on the pharmacology of the various salts of sontoquine has progressed a little further, this drug should be promptly exploited in man'.[14] By early March 1944 it had been tested in 11 patients with *P. falciparum* and three with *P. vivax* by Shannon's unit in New York. The drug showed 'a high order of activity in relation to dosage and blood level and is without apparent toxicity'.[15]

Chronic toxicity studies in animals were instituted, and the Board asked Dr Clark to request more rapid production of the compound through Winthrop and, if necessary, from other sources. At a meeting of the Panel of Review on 18 April Dr Marshall reported that large doses were well absorbed in animals and that the maximum levels obtained in humans were considerably lower that the minimal toxic doses for dogs and monkeys.[16] During the same meeting it was mentioned that several kilograms of the drug were being tabletted for clinical trial.

On 29 April 1944 the Board recommended that SN-6911 should be subjected to controlled clinical trials in Army and Navy hospitals in the United States.[17] The purpose of these trials would be to investigate the relative effectiveness of sontochin compared to atebrin in preventing relapses in troops already infected with vivax malaria during previous service in malarious areas.

However, experience with similar trials conducted with the sulphonamides during the previous year in military establishments implied that this approach was unlikely to provide a prompt indication as to the true value of the new drug. Moreover, such tests could not evaluate causal prophylactic activity, which was a major objective of the American program. In spite of the efforts to expand human testing the scope of the clinical evaluation program was still inadequate to cope with all the demands placed upon it. The work at Atlanta had only just started and the first control experiments, using quinine as a standard against which other compounds could be compared, were still in progress. Dr Coatney advised that the quinine work was due to be completed in mid-May after which studies on SN-6911 (sontochin) could commence.[18] The Board endorsed the importance of undertaking causal prophylactic tests of the new drug by the Atlanta unit as soon as possible. Nevertheless, despite these plans there were still serious gaps in the capability of the various American groups to provide a rapid and yet exhaustive clinical evaluation of SN-6911 and related 4-aminoquinoline compounds.

The Americans first heard details of the Australian malaria research in January 1944, six months after the work at Cairns commenced. This consisted of a cable and letter extract sent from Fairley to London, which they then received from British sources. It comprised a two-page narrative summary of the sulphonamide and atebrin experiments and the results achieved to November 1943, and was circulated to American workers as Malaria Report no. 67.[19] The text stated explicitly that 'These sulpha drugs [sulphamerazine, sulphamezathine, and sulphadiazine are] not causal prophylactics in man'. After working for a considerably longer period the Americans had finally arrived at similar conclusions. For example, at a Board meeting on 4 November 1943 Dr Shannon was reported as being 'convinced that the sulphonamide compounds do not act as prophylactics in man, but that their action is purely one of suppression'.[20] However, even though the National Institutes of Health (NIH) work had shown that sulphadiazine was not a causal prophylactic, the Americans did not have the experimental evidence to show unambiguously that this was also the case with other sulpha drugs. The work at Cairns, which extended this finding to two other sulphonamide compounds, was therefore of considerable interest.

Fairley's letter mentioned the first atebrin experiments that were still in progress: 'After stopping atebrin, fever regularly developed in BT [benign tertian malaria] infections, whereas MT [malignant tertian malaria] infections generally remained suppressed. Proportion cured uncertain as results of blood inoculation tests not yet available.'[21]

Finally, the cable mentioned preparations for the long-term experiments in which test subjects would be exposed to large numbers of both falciparum- and vivax-infected mosquitoes for more than two months while the men were taking daily doses of atebrin alone or in combination with sulphamerazine. This latter regimen was also of particular interest to the Americans.

At the Washington Conference that reviewed the malaria research program on 29 March 1944 one of the consultants, Dr Hastings, asked whether atebrin and sulphadiazine had been tested in combination against sporozoite-induced malaria.[22] Dr Shannon replied that this had not been done extensively in humans. At a Board meeting four weeks later, the Chairman, Dr Loeb, expressed the hope that 'more information will be available on the sulphamerazine–atebrine studies being conducted by Brig. Hamilton Fairley in Australia'.[23]

Later in the meeting Loeb spoke about discussions that he and the Secretary of the Board, Dr G. A. Carden, had with Lieutenant Colonel Ian Mackerras, who was then in Washington on an official visit to the USA, and Colonel Ewen Downie, the senior Australian Army medical officer on the staff of the Australian Military Mission in Washington.

The purpose of Mackerras's visit was to 'exchange information on recent research in malaria and other insect-borne diseases with special reference to the practical field application in the South-West Pacific Area'.[24] Since his visit to New Guinea with Fairley in June 1942, Ian Mackerras had continued to be closely involved with the malaria threat facing Australian forces in the South West Pacific. As Director of Entomology he was responsible for the planning and organisation of the antimosquito component of malaria control activities in the Australian Army. His particular interest was operational research in the fields of epidemiology and entomology, which contributed directly to practical prevention in the field.[25] This involved co-ordination of the work of 5 Australian Mobile Entomological Sections in Australia and New Guinea, as well as experiments on DDT and mosquito repellents by Captain D. F. Waterhouse in Canberra and a taxonomic review of the *Anopheles* mosquitoes in the Australasian region (to assist field identification) by D. J. Lee of the Department of Zoology, University of Sydney, and Captain A. R. Woodhill.[26] Mackerras visited a wide range of institutions in the USA, Britain, Panama, Canada and west Africa between March and October 1944. During this period he spent more than three months in the USA visiting entomology and malaria research centres, including many collaborating laboratories associated with the Board for the Co-ordination of Malarial Studies.

Mackerras was an experienced medical scientist who understood the complexities of malaria and its control from both academic and military viewpoints. His overseas visit was very timely as he was able to provide a balanced picture of the situation facing the troops in the field at a time when the civilian members of the Board lacked a full appreciation of the malaria problem in the South West Pacific. Their lack of knowledge was exacerbated by misleading reports sent back to Washington from the Pacific. For example, an Office of Scientific Research and Development report in early 1944 stated that 'atebrin increases the resistance [to malaria] and fatigue and malnourishment decreases it ... Some of the strenuous forced marches which we have read about, particularly by Australian troops, has resulted in 100% succumbing ... to malaria'.[27] A further illustration of this misinformation was provided at a Board meeting in December 1943 when Captain Rivers, a US Navy representative, reported on his experiences on a recent extensive tour of the South West Pacific.[28] He stated that there was no unanimity of opinion about malaria suppression and therapy: 'Many believe that men should be allowed to have initial chills and only use atebrin after symptoms appear'. He was convinced 'that quinine and atebrine will never be the solution to the control and cure of malaria'. Rivers's ill-informed comments were not rated highly by the Board:

> Several members emphasised the misleading nature of the impressions gained from field visits, stating that such impressions have been the basis for much of the erroneous information on malarial therapy which has dominated medical thought for many years ... It was the feeling that without scientific data and documentation it is more harmful than helpful to generalise from field observations.[29]

Mackerras was invited to give lectures and informal presentations at numerous venues during his tour of the USA. His views, based on first-hand experience and backed up by firm scientific data, must have been of considerable benefit to the civilian investigators associated with the US program. But the major achievement of his visit was that it acted as a catalyst to stimulate a most fruitful collaboration between the Americans and the Australian research group at Cairns, which was of lasting benefit to the control of malaria by drugs. He was most impressed by the scientists he had met, by the work he saw at the participating laboratories, and by the way it was integrated and focused by the activities sponsored by the Board:

> The whole organisation is guided by a small group of keen, far-sighted men, the degree of co-ordination and the stimulus to enthusiastic work are of the highest order ... No one, who has had the opportunity to see the new drug research which is going on in America, could fail to be impressed both with its magnitude and its thoroughness. Nor could he fail to be equally impressed with the way in which workers in different fields and different institutions have been welded into a single team working for a single purpose on a single plan.[30]

On 26 May Mackerras attended a meeting of the Panel of Pharmacology and presented an overview of the facilities, staff resources and scope of the work at Cairns.[31] Although he was not a direct participant in the research, he was involved in setting up and staffing the entomology component. He had visited the unit on several occasions during the previous year and was thoroughly familiar with the experimental work and the remarkably rapid progress that had been achieved in the previous nine months. He indicated that the studies were based on freshly isolated strains of vivax and falciparum malaria from troops infected in New Guinea and that there were adequate supplies of non-immune soldier volunteers. During the previous six months 75 000 infected mosquitoes were used for sporozoite-induced experiments at Cairns, and there were additional facilities for blood-induced infections in the Atherton Tablelands. He then summarised the experimental plan for the short-term experiments and reviewed the results obtained with the sulphonamides and atebrin. The ability of a daily tablet of atebrin to provide complete suppression of both falciparum and vivax infections was confirmed, 'even when infection rates simulate that encountered in hyperendemic areas'. If the drug was administered during exposure and for three weeks afterwards, *P. falciparum* infections were eliminated. By the time of this meeting Mackerras had already visited the NIH unit at Atlanta Penitentiary, as well as the malaria laboratory in Columbia, South Carolina, where mosquitoes infected from malaria therapy patients were supplied for the Atlanta experiments.[32] He was aware that the American work on mosquito-transmitted malaria was much smaller than that being undertaken by the Australians, and that the scale of the research in Cairns exceeded the combined clinical testing facilities of all the collaborating institutions in the USA. Mackerras reported that the American difficulties were 'only partly relieved by the availability of paretics [malaria therapy patients] and convict volunteers, and are certainly not helped by the unwillingness of the authorities to permit experiments in the armed forces'.[33]

Both Mackerras and Downie were invited to attend the next meeting of the Board on 31 May.[34] Mackerras gave a detailed description of the Cairns results. His presentation had a very positive impact by informing the members of the extraordinarily thorough nature of the Australian research that encompassed both sporozoite-induced and blood-induced experimental infections as well as subinoculation procedures to determine whether the infections were cured or not. A report on this work had already been sent to London, and Brigadier C. Kellaway gave a copy to the National Research Council when he visited Washington.[35] This was circulated at the same Board meeting, and aroused considerable interest. It appears that the scientists of the Board did not grasp the complete significance of the account of the Cairns research described by Mackerras at this meeting. Downie's notes stated:

> During the subsequent discussion [of the experimental results at Cairns] Dr Shannon pointed out that in his opinion, although blood film and subinoculation experiments of M.T. patients may be negative after 23 days or more, he considered that specific sporulation of tissue forms may cause a breakthrough of the disease at a later stage. He further observed that he had noticed this to occur during experiments he had himself conducted. Dr Coatney supported this view.[36]

Fairley made a cryptic marginal comment on his copy of Downie's notes: '? How much more'.[37] In fact, the results of the atebrin experiments at Cairns were unambiguous on this point. Suppression and radical cure of falciparum infections were invariably obtained when men continued to take one tablet of atebrin for 23 days after the last infective bite. Subinoculations showed that parasites were cleared from the blood and recrudescences did not develop, thereby indicating that late release of parasites from the tissue phase do not occur in falciparum malaria. Presumably, the later breakthroughs noted by Shannon and Coatney were due to incomplete clearance of parasites produced in the primary attack.

The work that had already been conducted by the Americans on SN-6911 was reviewed at the Board meeting on 31 May. Tests against avian parasites had shown it to be a superior drug. Animal studies had revealed that it was not more toxic than atebrin, and in some animals it was less toxic. There was no evidence of gastrointestinal upset or liver damage in high doses and, unlike atebrin, it did not cause discolouration of the skin. Shannon had already administered it to humans in New York, and had confirmed the French Tunisian findings that it did not produce toxic manifestations. There were indications that it may be better than atebrin in controlling relapsing vivax infections, but it was not known if it would act as a causal prophylactic. The meeting agreed to allocate quantities to the US Army, Navy, and Public Health Service for clinical trials to assess its value for treatment of overt cases of malaria. However, the most important military need was for an antimalarial drug that would guarantee protection of troops operating in the field without producing any toxic symptoms. Ideally such a drug would act as a causal prophylactic and prevent infection but, failing this, it would completely suppress clinical attacks without any side-effects. The clinical testing facilities at the disposal of the US co-operative malaria program were not adequate to provide a prompt and definitive evaluation of these attributes. During the previous twelve months the Australian experiments had set new standards for clinical evaluation of antimalarial drugs. The approach pioneered for the atebrin series could immediately be adapted for the systematic and comprehensive testing of any other compound. This was immediately appreciated by the American scientists.

Drs Shannon and Marshall asked whether additional studies could be conducted by Brigadier Fairley at Cairns. The chairman of the Board, Dr Loeb, said that neither information nor supplies of SN-6911 had been distributed to anyone who was not working under the guidance of the Board. He emphasised that only limited supplies of the compound were available, but certain questions concerning its activity against human malaria needed to be answered, and he suggested that the Australians might be willing to try to find the answers. Colonels Downie and Mackerras were both sure that studies at Cairns could be carried out, and they felt that 'Brigadier Fairley would be willing to undertake those aspects of the investigation which the Board deemed of importance and which were not adequately covered by studies in the United States'.[38]

The chairman consulted the service representatives of the Board to seek their views on the advisability of asking the Australian representatives to communicate with Brigadier Fairley regarding this matter. They agreed that it would be highly desirable for the Australian group to investigate the drug against mosquito-induced infections in non-immune volunteers. Dr Marshall proposed, and the Board agreed, that sufficient drug for 20 patients be offered to Australia for suppressive trials at Cairns under the direction of Brigadier Fairley. After consultation with Mackerras, Downie tentatively accepted the offer, subject to approval of the Director General of Medical Services. At the same meeting a suggestion that some SN-6911 be sent to Britain for trial was vetoed by the Board, as the amount for experimental purposes was limited, and it was not considered that an adequate experimental set-up for a suppressive trial existed in England.[39] Later, when additional supplies became available, the Panel of Review agreed to send a sample of SN-6911 for testing in England.[40]

A signal was dispatched to Melbourne immediately after the meeting outlining the American offer and, on the next day, Downie followed this up with a letter to Fairley covering the agenda and minutes of the Board meeting together with brief comments on the new drug. He said that 'Marshall at Baltimore and Shannon of New York are both of the opinion it is at least as good as atebrin in treatment of B.T. and M.T. malaria'.[41] Fairley promptly agreed to test it at Cairns, and a signal to this effect was sent to Washington on 3 June.

Downie visited Marshall's laboratory three days later and received a thorough briefing on the history and development of SN-6911. The Americans clearly decided to take the Australians into their confidence, as Marshall admitted that SN-6911 was the same compound as sontochin but frankly added that, for political reasons, this was officially denied.[42] It appears from Downie's detailed notes of this meeting that Marshall neglected to mention the circumstances relating to the designation of this compound as SN-183 and how it was initially overlooked by the Americans. This is not surprising as it must have been a source of embarrassment to Marshall, who was himself involved in this oversight. Marshall outlined the details of its synthesis in Germany, its supply to Winthrop, and the French tests in Tunisia. He gave a copy of Schneider's report to Downie with the comment that it was of little value as a scientific trial but showed the drug to have been given to human beings without ill effect. Marshall said that enough drug would be available for Australia to try out on 30 to 40 patients, and that it would be delivered to the Australian Military Mission on 10 June. He thought that it might be tried as a causal prophylactic and as a suppressive in experimentally induced infections. Tests to be conducted in the USA would include trials on the relative efficacy of SN-6911 compared with atebrin in treatment of relapsing vivax infections in US Army and Navy personnel. Observations in service personnel would also be made to investigate its effects on the gastrointestinal system compared with atebrin.

An attempt to estimate its value as a causal prophylactic and as a suppressive was to be undertaken by the US Public Health Service under the direction of Dr Coatney. He went on to say that a meeting was planned within the next few days, between himself, Loeb and Shannon, to discuss the proposed trials and their views would be promptly communicated to the Australian Mission. Downie informed Fairley of these details in a letter on 7 June 1944, and made arrangements for priority air freight of the drug to minimise delay in getting it to Australia.[43]

Following the meeting of the American scientists, Dr Shannon prepared a draft proposal for Colonel Downie.[44] This was approved by the Panel of Review on 9 June.[45] The introductory remarks mentioned that 'the program of investigations covering the exploitation of SN-6911 in the United States will be aided considerably if the following facts can be ascertained with respect to the anti-malarial aspect of this drug as compared to that of quinacrine'. It was suggested that the two drugs should be administered at daily dosages of 100 mg 'with both of the two general experimental routines now in use by Brigadier Fairley at Cairns, i.e. short-term and long-term exposures to infected mosquitoes.' Downie communicated this information to Fairley by diplomatic air bag on Monday, 12 June.

12

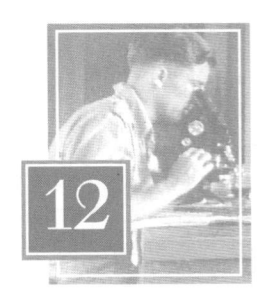

'SB'

THE AUSTRALIANS ACCORDED the highest possible priority to the American request for studies on SN-6911, and the research effort at Cairns was quickly focused on evaluation of the new drug. Fairley wrote to Blackburn on 1 July, advising:

> It should arrive at any time now, and we will need to get busy about it ... Sufficient is being supplied to test 30–40 cases ... In Marshall's opinion it is the first drug to be tested which in animal and toxicity tests can be regarded as equal to atebrin and possibly superior thereto. It may prove more effective in B.T. malaria. Therein would lie its value. Extensive trials in relapsing *P. vivax* infections are being made in USA. We will primarily compare [*sic*] our efforts to extenuating its value as a causal prophylactic and as a suppressive of M.T. and B.T. infection ... I will probably come up to Cairns about the 15th July to plan the experiment. In the meantime we should perhaps conserve our volunteers somewhat so as to avoid undue delay in initiating the experiment once the drug becomes available.[1]

Downie's letter containing the initial details of the new drug was sent to Cairns on the next day, and Blackburn confirmed their arrival on 6 July.[2] Fairley flew to Cairns a week later for discussions on the new drug, which was code named 'SB' for the Australian experiments.

At about the same time, a malaria mission from the USA, comprising two scientists associated with the American malaria program, Dr Robert B. Watson and Dr Fred C. Bishopp, arrived in Australia from Washington. Dr Watson was a member of the Panel on Clinical Testing of Antimalarial compounds of the Board for the Co-ordination of Malarial Studies and was a senior investigator involved in clinical trials of antimalarial compounds in syphilis patients undergoing malarial therapy at Gailor Memorial Hospital in Memphis, Tennessee.

Dr Bishopp, a senior entomologist, was chief of the Bureau of Entomology and Plant Quarantine, of the US Department of Agriculture. Their visit was initiated by a request from General MacArthur 'that a team of about five medical research men in civilian capacity be sent in the South West Pacific Area to conduct an intensive research program on malaria'.[3]

This request was considered at a meeting in Washington during April 1944, convened by Dr A. N. Richards, Chairman of the Committee on Medical Research, National Research Council (NRC), and attended by the Chairman of the Board for the Co-ordination of Malarial Studies, Dr R. F. Loeb, as well as Dr Francis Blake, of Yale University Medical School, and several senior Army officers.[4] The meeting agreed that 'it would not be profitable to set up a civilian laboratory in the field but that it would be exceedingly worthwhile to have a small group survey the problems and establish contact with units which are making, or are equipped to make, controlled field observations'. A primary objective would be to investigate possibilities for coordination of malaria research in the South West Pacific with that in the USA, with particular reference to the testing of new compounds of probable chemotherapeutic value in malaria. Dr Loeb proposed that the mission be led by Dr Blake (a specialist in the clinical aspects of malaria), with Dr Watson and a representative of Dr Bishopp's department to act as consultants on mosquito control, and with Dr Shannon as the consultant on chemotherapy of malaria. This proposal was approved by the Board, and it was recommended that the group should be sent as promptly as possible.

Plans were finalised by mid-June, but unforeseen developments prevented the participation of both Dr Blake and Dr Shannon. It was decided that Dr Watson would represent the clinical and chemotherapeutic aspects, and he and Bishopp left Washington on 4 July, arriving at General Headquarters, South West Pacific Area, a week later, where they had discussions with senior US Army medical officers, including Colonel Maurice Pinchoffs and Colonel Henry M. Thomas. They were also briefed on the Australian Army experience of malaria by Colonel M. J. Holmes, Secretary of the Combined Advisory Committee on Tropical Medicine, Hygiene, and Sanitation. It was decided that the mission should become familiar with malaria studies in Australia before going to New Guinea and they proceeded to Cairns, accompanied by Colonel Thomas, where they were met by Fairley on 17 July.[5]

During the next three days they inspected the facilities at the unit and had detailed talks with Fairley, Blackburn and Jo Mackerras on various aspects of the experimental work. The delegation visited the Atherton Tablelands to see the component of the experimental program involving the volunteers at 2/2 AGH and 2/1 Convalescent Depot. The mission then visited scientists and institutions in Sydney, Melbourne and Canberra before flying to New Guinea during the first week of August. The Americans received a very favourable impression of all that they had seen at Cairns. On 21 July Watson wrote from Brisbane to Shannon in New York:

> I have just returned after three days with Brigadier N. H. Fairley at Cairns where I have seen in detail his work on the suppressive action of atebrine in *falciparum* and *vivax* disease. This work I believe to be unique and the results unquestionably are most important from every standpoint. My only regret is that you could not have been present at the same time, and I still hope that it may be possible for you to see this work, particularly in connection with the use by Brigadier Fairley of the SN analogues. In the latter regard Brigadier Fairley received some time ago notification that SN-6911 had been sent and he has been expecting to receive it and has made all preparations for its testing. Today we dispatched a radiogram in an effort to trace the shipment. He is prepared to test this and other safe compounds immediately, and has, I believe, an almost unlimited supply of clinical material available for use.[6]

After their return to Washington Colonel Downie subsequently noted:

> The visit of Dr. Watson and Mr. Bishop [*sic*] has forged another link in a chain of good liaison which is developing between the Board for Control [*sic*] of Malarial Studies and Australia ... It is well recognised here by Marshall Shannon and others that there is nothing in this country to compare with the Cairns Research unit and that it presents a unique opportunity for the trial of new antimalarial drugs.[7]

The Americans originally thought that it was unnecessary to provide data concerning the plasma concentrations that might be expected with SN-6911, but they suggested to Colonel Downie that, if Brigadier Fairley wished to have this information, it could be made available at a later date.[8] However, the atebrin experiments at Cairns had already shown the crucial importance of relating drug levels in the blood to clinical and parasitological phenomena. Soon after receiving the initial request to test the new drug, Fairley sent a cable to Washington, asking for the technical details on sontochin, including blood concentrations and methods for estimating plasma levels.[9]

An even more important issue was the safety of SN-6911 for administration to humans in the doses proposed for clinical evaluation. The Cairns unit was not equipped for toxicological studies, and Fairley made a particular point of raising this matter with the American mission. Watson assured him that the compounds sent to him 'could be considered as reasonably safe at the recommended dosage; or, alternatively, toxicological data would be supplied from which he [Fairley] could arrive at a decision as to whether a drug could be used safely'.[10] In his letter to Shannon, Watson pointed out that 'this is an extremely important consideration from his [Fairley's] standpoint for the whole integrity of his program depends upon the well being of his clinical material'.[11]

This was a delicate matter for the Americans as it concerned the release to a foreign agency of commercially sensitive information about drugs supplied by American companies. The Australian government was not a party to the Co-operative Wartime Program, and had not been notified of the terms of reference for protection of commercial firms prepared by the Office for Survey of Antimalarial Drugs in July 1942. Nevertheless, it was recognised that all relevant knowledge should be made available to the leader of a laboratory working with a compound. Dr W. Mansfield Clark, in his position as Chairman of the Division of Chemistry, NRC, took the responsibility 'of defining Brigadier Fairley's researches in Australia as within the bounds of principle that pertinent information must be available to an investigator'.[12]

On 10 August Shannon wrote to Downie with detailed information on toxicity of SN-6911 obtained during experiments at Atlanta by Drs Coatney and Ruhe.[13] This work involved five prisoner volunteers who took 400 mg of the drug for 10 days and another five men who received the same dose for 24 days. None of the first group showed any side effects, but all of the second group exhibited gastrointestinal symptoms, such as nausea and vomiting, which were attributed to the drug. The adverse symptoms coincided with an increased plasma levels of SN-6911 in these men during the last 10 days of drug administration. None of these manifestations were sufficiently severe to warrant withdrawal from the experiment, but Shannon thought that Fairley may wish 'to lower the dose to 0.3 gm if he plans a long term trial at a high dosage level'. Nevertheless, he believed that, on the basis of these results, the daily dose of 100 mg proposed for the experiments at Cairns, would not produce any untoward effects. The letter concluded 'I trust that [the information provided] contains the essentials of the facts available and will be helpful to Dr Fairley'.

In the original proposal, which Shannon gave to Downie, it was suggested that the effectiveness of the new drug as a suppressive and curative agent of both vivax and falciparum malaria could be investigated in the Australian experiments. Shannon thought that 'it will be particularly valuable if it is possible to run the experiments on suppressive therapy ... with both of the two general experimental routines now in use by Brigadier Fairley at Cairns, i.e. short-term and long-term exposures to infected mosquitoes'.[14] Downie also asked Marshall what trials he would suggest might be carried out at Cairns. Marshall said that, in his opinion, it might be tried as a causal prophylactic and as a suppressant in experimentally induced infections. He mentioned that causal prophylactic tests were to be undertaken by Dr Coatney's group at Atlanta and would involve administration of the drug for five days after biting.[15] This scheme was based on the rationale that the compound would only be administered during the incubation period of the disease to see whether it could destroy the parasites before they invaded the blood.

Before leaving Cairns on 22 July Fairley discussed the proposed program of experiments with SN-6911 with Blackburn and the senior scientific staff. The suppressive evaluation of the drug was comparable to the series already done with the sulphonamides and atebrin. This would involve short-term experiments in which a group of 12 men (eight taking SN-6911, two taking atebrin and two controls) were to be exposed to mosquitoes infected with vivax sporozoites and another similar group was to be bitten by falciparum-infected mosquitoes. Both drugs were to be administered at the same dose rates. The test volunteers would receive a 'build-up' (200 mg twice a day for four days); and would then take 100 mg per day during the period of biting; and for 23 days after the last infective mosquito bite. The clinical and haematological observations were to follow the same procedures as those used in previous experiments. The efficacy of SN-6911 as a prophylactic and curative drug when administered to volunteers repeatedly bitten by both *Plasmodium vivax* and *P. falciparum* infected mosquitoes was to be evaluated by long-term experiments. The men were to receive multiple biting sessions over a three-month period, during which they would be subjected to strenuous exercise and other stress factors (chilling, insulin and adrenalin injections, etc.) using the methods developed for Experiment V—the atebrin 'field-type' studies.[16]

If the new drug acted as a causal prophylactic it would eliminate the infection during the incubation period before it invaded the blood. The suppressive experiments were not designed to investigate this possibility as they could not discriminate between the effects of the drug on the tissue stages and on its action against the blood stages of the parasite. Subinoculation experiments (Experiment VII) were still in progress at the time that the SN-6911 series were planned, and the initial results were already revealing important leads into the early development of malaria parasites in the human host (see Chapter 9). The full implications were not yet apparent, but it was clear to Fairley and Blackburn that they had a direct relevance for understanding the mode of action of antimalarial drugs. It was initially proposed to include a 'causal prophylactic test' for the 'SB' experiments at Cairns, similar to that devised for Atlanta. The plan was for volunteers to take the drug for four days before biting and for five days afterwards.[17]

In a letter to Fairley on 28 July 1944 Blackburn said 'I have added a note to the remarks on causal prophylaxis setting out certain difficulties which may arise in interpretation'.[18] Blackburn estimated the expected decline of atebrin levels in the circulation of men after they stopped taking the drug. His calculations were based on data in the report from the Armored Medical Research Laboratory at Fort Knox, Kentucky, which indicated that the rate of 'die away' was 10 per cent per day.[19] He calculated that 20 days after they ceased taking the drug they would have the equivalent plasma level of men on 300 mg of atebrin per week. Experience at Cairns had already shown that one out of two volunteers infected with *P. falciparum* had been cured by taking 300 mg per week for four weeks after the last infected mosquito bite. Blackburn thought that 'any success in this experiment might well be attributed to trophozoiticidal activity [i.e. activity against the blood stages]'.[20] His comments stressed that, in the case of atebrin, the Cairns work had already shown that this experimental method would produce a misleading result, as the slow fall of plasma concentrations after drug administration ceased would result in activity against the parasites after they emerged from the tissue phase and entered the bloodstream. If SN-6911 (or any other drug) had similar characteristics of a 'slow die away' its effect on blood stages could be confused with causal prophylactic activity. He concluded 'with respect to SB the above argument may not hold—no pharmacological data are available here [but] by analogy with atebrin (the dosage appears to be the same as also the "build up") any results could similarly be open to criticism'.[21]

These arguments may have influenced the order in which the SN-6911 experiments were conducted, as it was decided to proceed first with the short-term and long-term groups, with priority accorded to commencing the long-term studies first in order to save time. Blackburn estimated that it would take six to eight months for the series to be completed. An important addition to the experimental protocol was the incorporation of the subinoculation method of Experiment VII into the short-term experiments by transfusing some test subjects on SB and atebrin on days Z+7, Z+8 and Z+9 'to establish that trophozoites develop but are later adequately dealt with by the suppressive drug'.[22] In contrast to the original American plan for investigating causal prophylactic activity, the subinoculation technique (when used in this way) provided a unique tool to determine the mode of action of antimalarial drugs.

The new drug arrived in Cairns on 27 July 1944, and Blackburn notified Fairley that it was decided to defer the long-term experiments for some time, even though they originally had first priority, due to shortage of mosquitoes received from field collections. Instead, a short-term group receiving 20 infective bites of *P. vivax* infected mosquitoes commenced on 1 August (Experiment XXA). The build-up followed the original scheme, but the prophylactic dosages of the drugs during biting and for the next 23 days were changed from 100 mg in the original plan to 200 mg per day in this group. During the following week it was reported that, although it was too early to say anything about their suppression, the men themselves remained well and no clinical phenomena were observed that could be associated with the drugs. Both controls had developed overt vivax malaria by 21 August, but parasites were not seen in any of the men while they were taking atebrin or SN-6911, and they remained fit and well.[23] However, all of the test subjects on the two drugs showed minor clinical and laboratory features of suppressed malaria between the 9th and 14th days after their first infective mosquito bites.

On 7 August Blackburn said that 'Owing to lack of larvae for several days recently, we are unable to start a [short term] falciparum group till about the middle of the month'.[24] The collections flown each week to Cairns from Milne Bay were adequate to meet all experimental requirements for a period of 10 months from September 1943. Between January and July 1944 a weekly average of 10 000 pupae were recovered and from these 2000 to 3000 mosquitoes were fed each week on gametocyte carriers. These supplies were sufficient to provide thousands of infected mosquitoes for all of the atebrin short-term and long-term experiments, as well as the other tests involving mosquito-transmitted malaria that were conducted over this time. However, breeding in the Milne Bay area declined during July 1944 following a prolonged dry spell, and in August the position became acutely unsatisfactory.[25] This shortage delayed the start of the long-term SN-6911 experiments in late July, and it had the potential to seriously disrupt the evaluation of the American-supplied drugs.

Fairley returned to Cairns on 22 August for discussions on current and future work, accompanied by another visiting American from Washington, Lieutenant Colonel Francis R. Dieuaide, a malariologist on the staff of the US Surgeon General and an Army representative on the Board for the Coordination of Malarial Studies.[26] The seriousness of the mosquito position was appreciated, and arrangements were made to send Lieutenant T. H. (Tom) Lemerle of the Entomology Laboratory to Milne Bay to investigate the situation to ensure adequate future supplies.[27] If necessary, he was to reorganise collection and transport of the larvae or, if this site now proved unsuitable, to arrange for collections from some other locality in New Guinea. Lemerle left by air from Townsville the following week, and within a few days signalled back to LHQ MRU from Milne Bay: 'Breeding negligible. Starting artificial pools. Larvae may be available 15 Sep. Collect moluccensis [now known as *Anopheles farauti*] in Cairns area'.[28] Jo Mackerras discussed the latter proposal with the staff of the malaria control units in the area and was informed that the local collection of *A. farauti* was not very practical at that time as there was no appreciable breeding between Innisfail, 80 km south of Cairns, and the Daintree River, which was the same distance to the north of Cairns.

After a careful appreciation of the local situation at Milne Bay, Lemerle attributed the current irregularity of larval supplies to limited breeding because of cold weather conditions, and to extremes of wet and dry periods.[29] Nevertheless, he felt that adequate numbers of larvae could still be collected in the local area and that current collections in muddy sunlit pools on a village track provided ideal breeding conditions for *A. punctulatus*. Some crates containing small but healthy batches of larvae arrived from Milne Bay soon afterwards, which gave encouragement to the staff at Cairns and permitted the momentum of experimental infections to be maintained.

Lemerle received good co-operation from the US Army at Milne Bay, 'even to the extent of a suggestion by their malariologist to build concrete pools which would be irrigated by a pump supplied by them'.[30] These pools were later constructed, and they provided a source of some additional larvae during periods of dry weather. Until this time the local collecting team consisted of an NCO, carried as a supernumerary to 6 Australian Mobile Entomology Section in Cairns and stationed at Milne Bay Base Sub Area, together with two Papuan assistants. This team was sufficient when larvae were plentiful, but it was considered prudent to increase the Milne Bay staff to cope with the extra collecting effort required when larvae were scarce.

The mosquito collections were delivered to Australian Army Movement Control at Milne Bay. They were dispatched by direct flight to Townsville, and then transhipped by Movement Control on the first available service plane for Cairns. It appeared that delays in transport had recently occurred due to changes in air movements. The local Movement Control Office at Milne Bay had been closed down, and the regular plane service direct to Townsville discontinued. Also, flights from Townsville to Cairns were reduced to one civil flight by Australian National Airways each day. Alternative arrangements were made for flights via Port Moresby, with larvae being transhipped from Moresby to Townsville by daily courier and then by the civil flight to Cairns. Delays of two to three days in scheduled flights from Milne Bay to Moresby often occurred due to bad weather, and Lemerle stressed that 'standing instructions for high priority dispatch of the larvae be given through the proper channels to the various organisations concerned'.[31] Fairley himself later wrote to Blackburn 'Would you tell Major Mackerras I saw the Corporal personally at Townsville and he said they now had all the priority they needed to get the larvae on the first available plane. He understood the importance of doing this and I do not think you will have much unavoidable delay there'.[32]

During October the transport problem was alleviated somewhat as a number of shipments arrived by flying boat from Moresby direct to Cairns. The use of alternative collection areas were also considered. Localities with high densities of *A. punctulatus* larvae, which were well removed from areas controlled by malaria control units, were known in the vicinity of Salamaua and Dumpu on the north coast of New Guinea, but these sites were not close to airports. Fairley asked Lieutenant Colonel Ted Ford and Major Frank Fenner (another malariologist with considerable New Guinea experience) whether they knew of other possible collecting localities that met the requirements of consistently high larval densities and access to air transport.[33] They were unable to suggest suitable alternatives, and the Milne Bay collections continued. The measures instituted by Lemerle's visit proved sufficient to ensure continuity of mosquito supplies for experiments conducted during the next few months.

Jo Mackerras later attempted to establish a self-mating colony of *A. punctulatus*. She observed that the adult mosquitoes that emerged from the Milne Bay larval collections would not mate in small cages, so a large cage was constructed (base 0.3 metre square, and a height of 0.9 metre) to see if the larger space would induce natural mating. In February 1945 viable eggs were laid in the cage after the females were given a blood meal, and this permitted the establishment of a thriving colony after which it was no longer necessary to collect further specimens from Milne Bay.[34]

Despite the shortage of mosquitoes in August 1944 sufficient numbers were available to permit the commencement of the short term *P. falciparum* experiment with SN-6911. After the same 'build-up' conditions of the *P. vivax* experiment, this group (Experiment XXB) received 20 bites of infected mosquitoes on 22 August. A daily prophylactic dose of 100 mg of sontochin or atebrin was administered to the test volunteers during biting and for the next 23 days, as in the original proposal. It was also decided to undertake a comprehensive schedule of subinoculations from the control and test volunteers of this experiment. This involved transfer of 200 ml of blood to uninfected recipients using the method developed for Experiment VII. Subinoculations were to be made according to the following scheme: controls on Days Z+6 to Z+9 inclusive; test cases taking atebrin on Z+8 and Z+12; test cases taking SN-6911 on Z+8 to Z+11, inclusive. The nursing sister at 2/2 AGH in charge of using the direct transfusion apparatus for the subinoculation work, Captain E. M. B. Fenner, was attached to the Cairns unit for this purpose.[35] Care was taken to ensure that adequate numbers of recipients were available to match the blood groups of the donors for this important experiment, and all went according to plan except that neither of the controls were done on Z+9 as both had parasites at microscopic levels in the peripheral blood on this day. Also, one of the men taking SN-6911 was not subinoculated as he had a large fresh boil that might have produced adverse affects had his blood been inoculated into the recipient. A progress report on these subinoculations of 7 September records that the recipients of the controls inoculated on Z+7 and Z+8 had already broken through with overt malaria, but none of the recipients from the test groups had yet developed parasitaemia.[36]

On 12 September Fairley replied 'it is strange that none of the volunteers on either atebrin or SB gave positive subinoculations'.[37] However, a signal sent on the same day from LHQ MRU to the Director of Medicine, Melbourne, advised that 'all recipients from all donors subinoculated on days zero plus seven eight and nine have overt attacks'.[38] All of the above-mentioned donors were still receiving SN-6911 at this time and they were fit and well. None showed evidence of active malaria other than one man who had a solitary parasite in a blood film taken on Z+14. The positive subinoculations proved that all of these men had parasites in their circulation on the eighth and ninth days after receiving their infective bites. Subsequently none of them developed overt falciparum malaria while they were on prophylaxis, and there was no evidence of active infection during the observation period after drug administration ceased. This was a crucially important result as it provided the first direct evidence of how the new drug worked: it did not eliminate the tissue phase but acted on the parasites after they had invaded the blood.

Another signal was sent from Cairns to Fairley on 24 September advising that two test volunteers from the first *P. vivax* group (Experiment XXA) demonstrated parasites in their blood on 23 and 24 days after they ceased taking the drug.[39] This provided the first confirmation that SN-6911 was not a causal prophylactic against vivax malaria. Subsequently, all of the men in this cohort broke through within 31 days (average = 27 days).[40] These results implied that 200 mg per day of SN-6911 was adequate to suppress the primary attack of mosquito-transmitted vivax malaria, but the period of suppression after ceasing the drug appeared to be shorter than that obtained with atebrin at this dose level. The two men on atebrin had not yet broken through, and it was known from previous experiments that the average freedom from relapses was 60 days after ceasing atebrin at a daily dose of 200 mg per day.

It was decided to delay the start of the long-term experiment until there was a preliminary indication that SN-6911 could suppress falciparum malaria. None of the men taking the drug in the short-term falciparum group had developed indications of overt malaria in the first two weeks after they were bitten, so this experiment (XXIB) commenced on 7 September. After the same build-up as the short-term experiments, eight men taking SN-6911 and two men on atebrin (dosages for both drugs being 100 mg daily) were repeatedly exposed to mosquitoes infected with *P. vivax* and *P. falciparum* for three months. The men were subjected to heavy exercise on alternate weeks under the supervision of CSM Winterbottom. This included a 14-hour route march uphill from Jungara to Kuranda along the railway track and return by road, a distance of 50 km. The group also spent periods of an hour in the meatworks at −18°C and had injections of adrenalin and insulin.[41] These procedures followed the scheme devised for the long-term atebrin experiments and were designed to reproduce conditions encountered in jungle warfare in a mountainous tropical country like New Guinea.

In his letter to Blackburn on 12 September Fairley mentioned that 'It is likely that I will be going to USA and the UK sometime in October'.[42] This visit would afford an ideal opportunity for the Australian research results to be presented to key scientists and administrators in Washington and London who were influential in guiding the directions of medical research, as well as ensuring that the results of this research were translated into the health policy among

Allied forces in malarious areas. Fairley stressed in his letter that the work at Cairns should concentrate on the SN-6911 experiments so that he could present as much information as possible about the Australian findings on the new drug.

Another short-term vivax group, in which SN-6911 was administered at a daily dosage of 100 mg, commenced the following week, and Blackburn started the compilation of progress reports of the SB series.[43] Drafts summarising Experiments XX and XXI were prepared in time for Fairley's arrival from Melbourne on 27 September.[44] He remained at Cairns for a full week as there was much to be done before his departure overseas.[45] Plans for future work were discussed with Blackburn and senior staff. This included a conference on the Milne Bay mosquito situation attended by Lieutenant Lemerle who had just returned from New Guinea. Considerable effort during Fairley's visit was devoted to the preparation of a report on the sontochin experiments that was to be presented to the Americans in Washington. During July a draughtsman, Corporal Patrick Fitzherbert, was attached to the unit to assist with the preparation of graphs and charts to illustrate the experimental results. These were nicknamed 'see at a glance' by the unit HQ staff. This arose from Fairley's habit of saying 'Well, you can see at a glance' when referring to the charts to illustrate his briefings of visitors to Cairns.[46] Fairley devoted some attention to selection of charts for the report from those prepared by Fitzherbert with the assistance of Corporal Rosemary Gore.

The evaluation of drugs based on heavy metals was discussed by the Americans at a meeting of the Board for the Co-ordination of Malarial Studies during May 1944.[47] One of this group, diamadino stilbene, was contemplated for trial by Shannon as it had shown some activity against avian parasites. In his second report from Washington Ian Mackerras commented that these compounds were of interest as it was thought they may attack the undiscovered tissue stages of vivax.[48] It appears that these tests did not eventuate in America, but diamadino stilbene—together with another drug, neostam—was included in the instructions that Fairley gave for work to be done after his departure overseas in October 1944. There were two volunteers on each drug with four controls. Both drugs were administered intravenously daily for four days before exposure to infection, on the day of biting by 10 *Anopheles punctulatus* harbouring vivax sporozoites, and for four days afterwards. Neither drug prevented the onset of vivax malaria, but the infection in the two volunteers who had diamadino stilbene ran a very mild course. Parasites did not build up to the levels of the four controls and fever was not as marked. However, both drugs produced mild toxic symptoms.[49]

The report on sontochin incorporated the results summarised in Blackburn's progress reports of the short-term and long-term experiments. The experimental groups had started at various times during the preceding two months, and none of them had been carried through to completion. Nevertheless, sufficient data had already been accumulated to indicate the efficacy of sontochin against mosquito-transmitted vivax and falciparum malaria, and this was summarised and tabulated.

Fairley left Cairns on 5 October, and was due to leave for Washington during the following week. However, he had developed an upper respiratory tract infection while in Cairns, which caused ear trouble on the return flight to Melbourne.[50] The Director General of Medical Services would not agree to Fairley's flight overseas until he was quite well again, and this delayed his departure until 24 October. This extra time was not wasted, however, as it permitted a useful exchange of correspondence between Cairns and Melbourne to provide additional experimental results for the SN-6911 preliminary report. During this period Fairley sent a secret signal to Downie in Washington summarising the major findings for the Americans, and advising that a progress report was being sent by post.[51] Fairley's flight across the Pacific departed from Brisbane, and he arranged for the latest results and amended charts to be flown down from Cairns to connect with his US flight. Blackburn collated this additional data up to 20 October, and dispatched it to meet Fairley in Brisbane by direct air bag.[52]

By this time the first short-term vivax group on 200 mg daily (Experiment XXA) had virtually finished, except that the two volunteers on atebrin had not yet relapsed at 2/2 AGH. The second short-term vivax group were still on prophylactic dosage of 100 mg daily. It was then three weeks after their infective bites but none had yet broken through with malaria. The short-term falciparum group had ceased their drugs more than four weeks previously, and there had been no breakthroughs of men who had taken SN-6911 or atebrin. The report said: 'it is probable that cure has resulted'. This view was reinforced by the results of late subinoculations. There was as yet no evidence of malaria in recipients 11 days after receiving 200 ml of blood from donors who had ceased taking the drug three weeks previously. The long-term group had completed half of their three-month biting period. The report described the arduous conditions to which the volunteers were subjected in this 'field-type' experiment and indicated that at the time of writing they had received a total of 105 infective bites—from 80 falciparum and 25 vivax infected mosquitoes over a period of 40 days. None of the men on SN-6911 from this group had yet developed overt malaria. Subsequently, all of the test volunteers in the long-term (mixed infection) group broke through with vivax malaria between 19 and 33 days after ceasing the drug. None of them developed falciparum malaria.

Fairley submitted the report to the Board for the Co-ordination of Malarial Studies in Washington, where it was reproduced and circulated on 31 October 1944.[53] This was exactly five months after the initial request from the Board for the work to be done and only three months after the drug was actually received in Australia. This was an extraordinary achievement, particularly in view of problems encountered with mosquito collections in New Guinea, for not only did the results indicate the efficacy of the drug for prophylaxis against human malaria but they also indicated its mode of action, which was completely unknown at this time. The report stated:

> Subinoculation experiments in M.T. malaria were undertaken to determine whether asexual forms were appearing in the peripheral blood though they were not demonstrable microscopically in thick smears. Direct transfusion with 200 c.c. of blood obtained from the first four volunteers (SN-6911) on the 8th and 9th day induced malaria in the 8 volunteers injected. The findings . . . suggest that in M.T. infections SN-6911 does not act as a causal prophylactic but destroys the young asexual parasites . . . as they emerge . . . into the circulating blood from the 7th day onward.

The subinoculation technique made it possible for the Australians to relate the activity of the drug to the emergence of the parasites from the tissue phase thereby demonstrating that the drug did not destroy the tissue stages and was therefore not a causal prophylactic. The method suggested by the Americans—to administer the drug for five days after biting—would not have clarified this issue as SN-6911 persisted in the blood for considerably longer than this period. Consequently, as Blackburn pointed out in his comments on the original proposal, it would not have been possible to discriminate its action on the tissue stages from activity against the emerging blood forms.

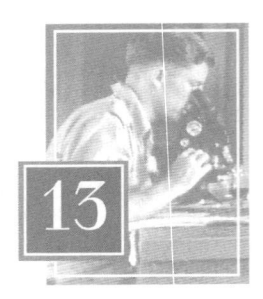

The Birth of Chloroquine

THE EVALUATION OF sontochin provided a promising new direction for the American malaria program during the first half of 1944 while, at the same time, synthesis and preliminary pharmacological investigations of other related 4-amino-quinoline compounds were undertaken in the hope of finding new drugs with even greater activity against human malaria. Colonel Downie wrote to Fairley on 7 June that 'a further point of interest is that Marshall considers that SN-6911 may not be the best of the series'.[1] He went on to say that one of the analogues, SN-7618, had already shown great promise in bird and animal tests.

The methods devised for experiments with avian malaria parasites compared the test drugs with quinine to arrive at the 'quinine equivalent' (the letter Q followed by a number). This was estimated from experimental data and was based on the minimum effective doses of the two drugs that caused a drop in parasitaemia relative to that of untreated control birds. Thus, a quinine equivalent of Q4 indicated that the test drug was four times more active than quinine under the conditions of the test and against the particular combination of host and parasite being tested. Tests of SN-7618 in ducks, conducted by Marshall at Johns Hopkins University, showed that it had quinine equivalents of Q32 against *Plasmodium lophurae* and Q8 against *P. cathemerium*.[2] Dr E. M. K. Geiling, at the University of Chicago showed that SN-7618 had an activity of Q8 against *P. gallinaceum* in chickens. These results were two to four times better than those obtained with atebrin against bird malaria. Even though it was realised by this time that there may not be a direct relationship between the action of a particular drug against human and avian parasites, this provided a positive indication that further development of this compound was warranted.

Experiments in animals were undertaken by Dr Leon Schmidt and his colleagues at the Institute for Medical Research, Cincinnati, Ohio, to compare the acute and chronic toxicity of SN-7618 with SN-6911 and atebrin.[3] Considerable species differences were noted. Experiments with rats showed that SN-7618 was more toxic than SN-6911, but slightly less toxic than atebrin. Tests in dogs showed that SN-7618 was more toxic than SN-6911. However, SN-7618 had the same or slightly less toxicity for monkeys than SN-6911, and it was definitely less toxic for monkeys than atebrin. This result was considered to be of more importance than the findings in other animals as it was felt that humans should react more like monkeys than rats or dogs. In view of these favourable results it was decided, at an executive session of the Board for the Co-ordination of Malarial Studies on 31 May, to assign SN-7618 to preliminary evaluation in humans.[4]

The first clinical tests, undertaken by Shannon's group in New York during early June, followed the usual experimental procedure of this laboratory in which the effects of the test drug were observed in blood-induced infections. This method bypassed the normal tissue development of the parasite following natural inoculation of sporozoites by mosquitoes. Nevertheless, it had the advantage that the results were obtained quickly, in two to three weeks, and they could be compared with those obtained with the standard drugs, quinine and atebrin, which had already been accurately characterised by this technique with a high degree of reproducibility.

Ian Mackerras remained in Washington during June 1944. He had fruitful discussions with US scientists, particularly with Dr Marshall, and subsequently prepared two reports (Recent Developments in Malarial Drug Research) for Australian Army medical authorities that were classified as secret. In his second report, of 19 June, he referred to the favourable results obtained with SN-7618 against bird malaria. He wrote: 'It is being screened in paretics by Dr Shannon at New York, and the few cases so far treated (including one very acute falciparum) have cleared up very promptly. This drug is to be regarded as decidedly promising'.[5] By the end of the month Shannon's experiments had confirmed that its high activity against animal parasites also carried over to human malaria and that, dose for dose, it was more active than atebrin and sontochin against the blood stages. It immediately became a priority compound for accelerated development and clinical evaluation.

At this time most members of the Board thought that SN-7618 was an entirely new drug that had not previously been synthesised and offered the prospect of a new lead in malaria chemotherapy for the USA. This is clear from the minutes of a Panel of Review meeting in June:

> In view of the fact that this compound was originally conceived by the Panel of Review and that as a result of this idea, Dr Blanchard was asked to request the Winthrop Chemical Company to synthesise this compound, it was recommended

that this information be brought to the attention of the Patent Division of OSRD [Office of Scientific Research and Development] for any action which is deemed necessary by that office.[6]

A month later, however, Dr Kenneth Blanchard wrote to the Secretary of the Board, Dr G. A. Carden:

> For the record, it should be pointed out that a gross error has crept into the minutes of the Panel of Review ... this compound (7618) was not conceived by the Panel of Review but was described in the patent ...which is the property of the Winthrop Chemical Co.[7]

A report prepared by US government patent lawyers was later considered at a closed session of the Board.[8] This document, classified under the *United States Espionage Act* and explicitly labelled 'Confidential—Special', considered the concerns of American commercial interests who were involved in the Wartime Cooperative Program and the patent aspects of the 4-amino-quinolines. It specified that both SN-6911 and SN-7618 were described as being new compounds and as being therapeutic agents for malaria in the original German patent so they could not be subject to further patents in the USA. This eliminated the possibility of patenting SN-7618 as a purely American discovery, but accelerated development of this drug continued. The co-operating scientists were told that 'any report dealing with or even mentioning the compound SN-7618 must be labelled confidential since this compound had been classified confidential by the Joint Security Control Board'.[9]

An important first step in development of the new drug was to ensure that adequate amounts were produced so that large-scale testing could proceed as rapidly as possible. It was unanimously agreed that arrangements should be made for a large-scale synthesis of SN-7618 and that, to this end, Winthrop be asked to produce 10 kg.[10] If the company could not comply with this request promptly then arrangements for its manufacture would be made elsewhere. Winthrop responded positively to the request from the Board, and agreed to deliver the requested amount as soon as possible.

In the meantime, the early promise of SN-7618 was reinforced as further data accumulated from the clinical trials conducted in New York. It was appreciated by senior members of the Board that the development of SN-7618 to the stage of operational use could not be undertaken without the support of the military authorities in the USA. Were the Army and Navy sufficiently interested to sponsor an 'all out' effort for its rapid evaluation as well as to lay plans for future production? Furthermore, if the promise of the new drug was confirmed by trials in military hospitals, would the Armed Services be prepared to use it in the field to replace atebrin? The answers to these questions were sought at a specially convened executive session in early August.[11] Dr Shannon reviewed the current data on SN-7618, and pointed out that it was at least twice as effective as atebrin and SN-6911 against the blood stages of vivax malaria. The chairman, Dr R. F. Loeb, then asked the Army and Navy representatives of the Board 'if their respective services would be interested in employing a compound which had this type of quantitative superiority'. Brigadier General Hugh Morgan replied that the US Army 'was interested in a compound which is distinctly superior to quinacrine . . . and is prepared to exploit in every possible way the development of any substantial improvement of antimalarial therapy'. These views were supported by Captain E. G. Hakansson on behalf of the US Navy. At the request of the chairman, Dr C. S. Marvel then explained the difficulties encountered in progressing 'from production on a small scale in glassware to large scale production in kettles and drums'. He pointed out that the solution to such engineering problems usually takes six months, so this would be how long it would take to produce sufficient drug for extensive field trials. Captain Hakansson said that he 'did not believe that CMR [Committee of Medical Research] could justify any position in which funds for large scale production of SN-7618 were withheld'. The Board then agreed that all available evidence of antimalarial activity and toxicity of the new drug would be prepared and circulated to members as soon as possible in anticipation of clinical trials in Army and Navy hospitals in the USA. If these studies 'do not disclose any unforeseen toxicity or other disadvantages, it was agreed that this drug will be required in increasingly large amounts for extended exploitation under field conditions'.

The Vichy French found no adverse symptoms during their field trials of SN-6911 in Tunisia during 1942, and this enabled the Americans to conduct clinical tests of this drug with some confidence that it would be safe. But there was no equivalent information on SN-7618 at the time that it was decided to actively promote its development. The data derived from the initial toxicity studies on the new drug in animals and preliminary trials in human subjects suggested that it was likely to be no more toxic than other existing antimalarial compounds. Nevertheless, it was appreciated by the Board that the entire program of clinical tests involving this compound would need to be reviewed if long-term use or the administration of higher doses produced adverse effects.

Concerns about toxicity of the new drug were raised in early September when tests of SN-7618 were temporarily discontinued at Atlanta Penitentiary by Dr W. H. Sebrell, Chief of the Division of Physiology, National Institutes of Health (NIH), who was the clinical investigator responsible for the Atlanta program. In a letter to Dr G. P. Carden, Sebrell explained that he had taken this action because the NIH pharmacologists were worried at the sharpness of the toxic range in experimental animals and the possibility that severe toxic reactions might occur in humans with little or no warning as the dose was increased.[12] He said that, on the basis of recently supplied information on toxicity, the NIH group were prepared to continue testing the drug at doses of 400 mg per day for six days and they would increase the test dosage above these levels if the pharmacologists considered that further toxicological evidence suggested that it was safe to do so.

All available data on the pharmacology, toxicology and antimalarial activity of SN-7618 were considered at a meeting of the Panel of Clinical Testing on 18 September.[13] Dr T. C. Butler, of Massachusetts General Hospital in Boston, explained the current status of tests to determine the maximum tolerated dose. A group of conscientious objectors took an initial dose of 900 mg, and had since been receiving the drug for 23 days at a daily dose of 400 mg without showing any adverse symptoms. A second group had taken 1000 mg on the first day and 500 mg for a week, and had also shown no toxic manifestations. It appears that this information alleviated the concerns raised by Dr Sebrell, as it was unanimously agreed to recommend to the Board that extensive clinical trials should be carried out in US Army and Navy installations in America and overseas. This resolution was formally accepted by the Board on 21 September.[14]

The decision to make a concerted and sustained effort to develop SN-7618 to the stage of operational use was based on the clinical experimental data obtained from Shannon's laboratory using blood-inoculated infections. This provided good evidence that the new drug was more effective against the blood stages of human malaria than other known antimalarial compounds, but there was no indication, one way or the other, whether SN-7618 could achieve the ultimate goal of the American program by acting as a causal prophylactic to prevent infection. The NIH group at Atlanta was the only clinical unit in the United States with the capability to undertake such experiments requiring the use of sporozoite-induced infections. On 11 August five prison volunteers received 400 mg of SN-7618 for four days before being bitten by mosquitoes infected with sporozoites of the St Elizabeth strain of vivax malaria, and for six days after being bitten.

The Americans were eager for tests on SN-7618 to be undertaken in Cairns as soon as sufficient drug was available. Close liaison with Fairley's group was maintained via Colonel Downie who was kept abreast of developments on the new drug by his attendance at Board meetings and in discussions and correspondence with the chairman of the Panel on Clinical Studies, Dr Shannon.

The enthusiasm for a trial at Cairns was reinforced by the views of Dr Robert B. Watson and Dr Fred C. Bishopp after their mission to Australia and New Guinea in July. On 10 August Shannon informed Downie that 'further work on SN-7618 continues to favour the view that it is not less than twice as active as atebrin'.[15] In a meeting with Downie on 7 September Shannon summarised the knowledge gained up to that time. The data implied that it was reasonably well tolerated at a dose 30 times greater than that required to terminate clinical attacks, and that it was less toxic and more effective against human malaria than atebrin.

On 14 September a signal was sent from the Australian Legation in Washington to Army Headquarters, Melbourne, formally advising that 'National Research Council desires Brig Fairley investigate SN-7618. Tablets available shortly will be forwarded with all information earliest opportunity'.[16] On the same date Downie wrote to Fairley that 'Winthrops have been rather tardy in producing tablets which are expected any day now', and he enclosed Shannon's estimation methods and 'a small quantity of SN-7618 powder in case you wish to commence work on estimation'.[17] Fairley notified Blackburn of the imminent arrival of the new drug and arrangements were made to have volunteers on stand-by in Cairns so that the experiments could start as soon as it was delivered. After further delays the tablets were finally brought to Jungara by safe hand of Major F. Ratcliffe on 21 October just before Fairley departed for America.[18] Blackburn held a staff meeting to initiate the work without delay. The test volunteers commenced their 'build-up' on 24 October and received their infected bites only a week after the drug arrived in Cairns.[19]

The experimental plan adopted for SN-7618 was virtually the same as that used for SN-6911. Atebrin was included for comparison purposes with both drugs administered under the same dosage schedules. There was to be a four-day build-up of 200 mg/day before biting, followed by the usual short-term period of 23 days on 100 mg/day. It was originally planned to conduct a long-term experiment on SN-7618, but this was stopped at the last moment. Fairley sent a signal from Washington in early November, which arrived in Cairns just seven hours before the men of this group were to receive their first infective bites.[20] He advised that, due to toxic symptoms encountered following administration of high doses in the United States, the drug was not to be administered for longer than one month and, consequently, the long-term experiment was not to proceed.

This decision arose from observations made in the previous month by Dr L. T. Coggleshall who was one of the more experienced clinical investigators associated with the American malaria program. In 1941 he played a pioneering role in the first field studies of the sulphonamides against human malaria while working for the Rockefeller Foundation in Panama. He later moved to the University of Michigan, where he was involved in the drug-screening program with avian malaria parasites. Coggleshall was called up for active duty in the US Navy in February 1944, and received a posting as medical officer in charge of a malaria unit at the US Marine Barracks, Klamath Falls, Oregon, where large numbers of marine personnel were subject to relapses of vivax malaria after returning from active duty in the South West Pacific Area. This facility provided a very useful opportunity to investigate therapy regimens with the objective of reducing the number of relapses, and both SN-6911 and SN-7618 were assigned to Coggleshall's group for this purpose.

Coggleshall advised Shannon of his experiences with SN-7618 in a letter of 7 October.[21] He said that he had treated a group of five vivax patients with an initial dose of 1200 mg, followed by 800 mg daily for five days. Toxic symptoms, including blurring of vision and general excitability, were observed in four of the patients, and drug administration was immediately discontinued. This dosage regimen exceeded the levels that had been tested for safety by Butler's group in Boston, and Shannon replied that he was surprised that such a high dosage schedule had been employed.[22] Coggleshall later wrote that that he administered this regimen in order to determine the highest tolerated dose in the belief that this was what Shannon himself had specifically mentioned at a recent Board meeting. His letter concluded: 'Even if there was a misunderstanding I am sure of one thing, that we have found what the maximum tolerated dose is'.[23] Shannon responded with a conciliatory 'Dear Coggy' letter on 1 November in which he expressed his regret at the misunderstanding that had arisen. He also said: 'I believe that the toxic reactions which you have uncovered, together with those which have apparently persisted in Atlanta, and those at Boston which, in retrospect, appear more important, will warrant a scaling down of the dosage recommended for trials of SN-7618'.[24]

The topic of human safety was discussed at considerable length in a closed session of the Board, convened specifically for this purpose on 6 November 1944 and limited to Board members and those actually working with SN-7618.[25] It was attended by Fairley who had recently arrived in Washington. The observations on toxic symptoms encountered in the participating laboratories were reviewed, and it was decided to investigate the possibility that there was a 'contaminating substance in certain batches' of the drug. Until this matter was resolved it was decided to cease studies at Army and Navy installations in the USA. Fairley asked whether this decision was also meant to apply to the studies in Australia already in progress. It was felt that 'Since the Australian volunteers are taking smaller doses of SN-7618 than did the subjects who have exhibited toxic symptoms, the studies at Cairns should continue at the present dosage unless information is forthcoming that the drug in use there contains a toxic contaminant'. Shannon and Marshall undertook to investigate the origin of the samples sent to Australia and communicate this to Fairley as a matter of urgency.

The proposed long-term experiment at Cairns was not undertaken. Presumably, Fairley felt that administration of the drug for three months, even at low doses, could not be justified until further data on toxicity had been accumulated. The Batches of SN-7618 that had previously produced toxic symptoms in human subjects at high doses were investigated by chronic feeding experiments in mice by the Americans. By mid-December 1944 these tests had shown no batch differences in toxicity, and it was concluded that toxic contaminants were not present.[26]

Meanwhile, the short-term experiments of SN-7618 in sporozoite-induced vivax and falciparum infections continued at Cairns. Experiment XXXA consisted of 12 volunteers (eight on SN-7618; two on atebrin and two controls) who received 20–22 infective bites of *Anopheles punctulatus* mosquitoes harbouring sporozoites of *P. vivax* on 28 October 1944.[27] Both controls developed overt vivax malaria after the normal incubation period. None of the men developed parasitaemia during the period that they were taking the drugs, but one of the two volunteers on atebrin and all of the eight volunteers on SN-7618 showed either minor clinical or laboratory features of suppressed malaria. Both men who were taking atebrin developed malaria after ceasing the drug, one after 25 days and the other after 40 days. All of the eight volunteers in whom major symptoms had been suppressed with SN-7618 had attacks of vivax malaria between 40 and 64 days after ceasing the drug.[28] Experiment XXXB was conducted under identical conditions except that there was only one control and the volunteers were exposed to 17–18 bites of falciparum-infected mosquitoes on 13 November 1944.[29] Most of the men had transient minor clinical symptoms but none showed any evidence of parasites while taking the drug, and none developed falciparum malaria after drug administration ceased.

Eighty-one days after they stopped taking the drug the volunteers in this group were bitten again by mosquitoes infected with the same strain of *P. falciparum* (New Guinea 'H' strain) to which they had originally been subjected. Subsequently, they all developed falciparum malaria within the usual incubation period, thereby confirming that they had no pre-existing immunity. In the vivax group (XXXA) 200 ml of blood was transfused from test volunteers to uninfected recipients. Subinoculations made on days Z+9 and Z+10 were positive in six out of six men taking SN-7618, even though their blood films were negative. Similarly, two volunteers receiving the new drug in Experiment XXXB were subinoculated on the eighth day after exposure to falciparum-infected mosquitoes. In both instances the recipients developed attacks of malaria. These subinoculation results indicated that asexual parasites of both species of human malaria were present, even though they were not observed during microscopic examination of the donor's blood.[30]

The results of the Cairns experiments showed conclusively that both SN-6911 and SN-7618 acted in an identical fashion to atebrin when administered for prophylaxis. Each of the drugs prevented the primary attacks of vivax and falciparum malaria by acting on the parasites soon after they appeared in the blood, before they multiplied to cause overt attacks of malaria. Falciparum malaria was cured after all of the parasites were eliminated from the bloodstream. In the case of vivax malaria, parasites emerged again from the tissue phase to cause relapses some weeks after drug administration ceased. This research had far-reaching implications for understanding the antimalarial activity of the 4-amino-quinoline compounds and played an important role in influencing the subsequent direction of the wartime malaria program in the United States. In 1946 SN-7618 was given the non-proprietary name of chloroquine.[31]

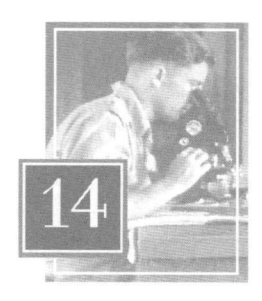

The Problem of Vivax

THE EXPERIMENTS AT Cairns demonstrated unequivocally that a daily tablet of atebrin suppressed malaria infections in men living under conditions of arduous physical stress similar to those encountered in jungle warfare. When this dose was taken with religious regularity on each day while in malarious areas and continued for a month afterwards, it provided complete protection against falciparum malaria by suppressing and then curing the infection. Atebrin was able to protect against vivax malaria, too, as long as prophylactic doses continued, but relapses occurred at irregular intervals for up to three years after drug administration ceased. The lack of a cure for vivax malaria had a direct effect on the manpower resources available to carry the fight against the Japanese. Men suffering relapses required hospital treatment. This placed a strain on medical facilities and also delayed the return to combat fitness of seasoned troops who were needed for later campaigns. These considerations were a powerful stimulus to develop compounds that might prevent vivax relapses, and the search for a drug that could achieve this goal became an important focus of the malaria research effort both in the United States and in Australia.

This issue was discussed at a conference convened in Washington to review the American malaria research program on 29 March 1944. Dr Shannon said '*P. falciparum* infections are not the problem. This main issue at stake is the discovery of a drug which will prevent or cure *P. vivax* infections'.[1] But the problem was how to undertake clinical experiments that would identify such a drug in a timely manner. Until then all of the clinical trials associated with the US malaria program were made with North American strains of vivax that were characterised by having a prolonged period of latency, usually six months or more, between the primary attack and the first relapse. This led to long delays in evaluation of drugs that might act against the stages of the parasite giving rise to such relapses. For example, the first report on the quinine experiments at Atlanta was prepared on 15 September 1944—five to six months after the volunteers were exposed to mosquitoes infected with the St Elizabeth strain of *P. vivax*. Data on primary attacks under the different dosage regimens were presented, but it was noted that 'a later report will be necessary to include the period of late primaries and late relapses, which usually occur 6–12 months after exposure'.[2] Similarly, experiments with SN-6911 against mosquito-transmitted vivax malaria commenced in Atlanta in June 1944, and a progress report was circulated in September with results showing that infection had been prevented for at least two to three months. It was stated 'from our previous experience it is expected that any infections will not now become evident until 6 to 10 months after exposure. Observations, for at least a year, therefore, will be necessary'.[3] This was a matter of considerable concern, and Shannon considered that it was unlikely that any promising new drugs 'will be forthcoming from the program within a period short enough to be of use in the present war unless more rapidly relapsing strains of [*P. vivax*] are put into use in the testing program'.[4]

The question of vivax relapses came up during a Board meeting on 31 May 1944, when Lieutenant Colonel Mackerras reviewed the experiments at Cairns. A discussion ensued regarding the difference between South West Pacific strains and those currently used in the United States. Mackerras pointed out that the Australian work had shown conclusively that, when atebrin was administered in doses of 100 mg daily for two weeks before and for 23 days after exposure to infected mosquitoes, vivax malaria was completely suppressed during drug therapy. When the drug was withdrawn, the vivax cases came down with a clinical infection within a three-week period. Mackerras said that this was an invariable phenomenon. Both Dr M. F. Boyd and Dr Coatney, the former working with the McCoy strain of vivax and the latter with the St Elizabeth strain, found that atebrin tends to delay the primary attack for long periods of time, sometimes for as long as nine months. The minutes of this meeting stated 'Dr Shannon believes that the apparent difference in characteristics of New Guinea versus North American strains may be explained by a difference in the size of inoculum utilized. Col. Mackerras was not inclined to agree'.[5]

Shannon's comments indicate that he thought that the difference between the Cairns relapses and American relapse patterns were because the former received a larger dose of sporozoites. However, the data at Cairns showed unequivocally that early relapses were the rule in South West Pacific strains of vivax malaria. Mackerras's comments to the Board were probably based on information in the fifth interim report submitted by Major Andrew on 26 November 1943, which stated that 'all [vivax] cases on atebrin or atebrin with A-S

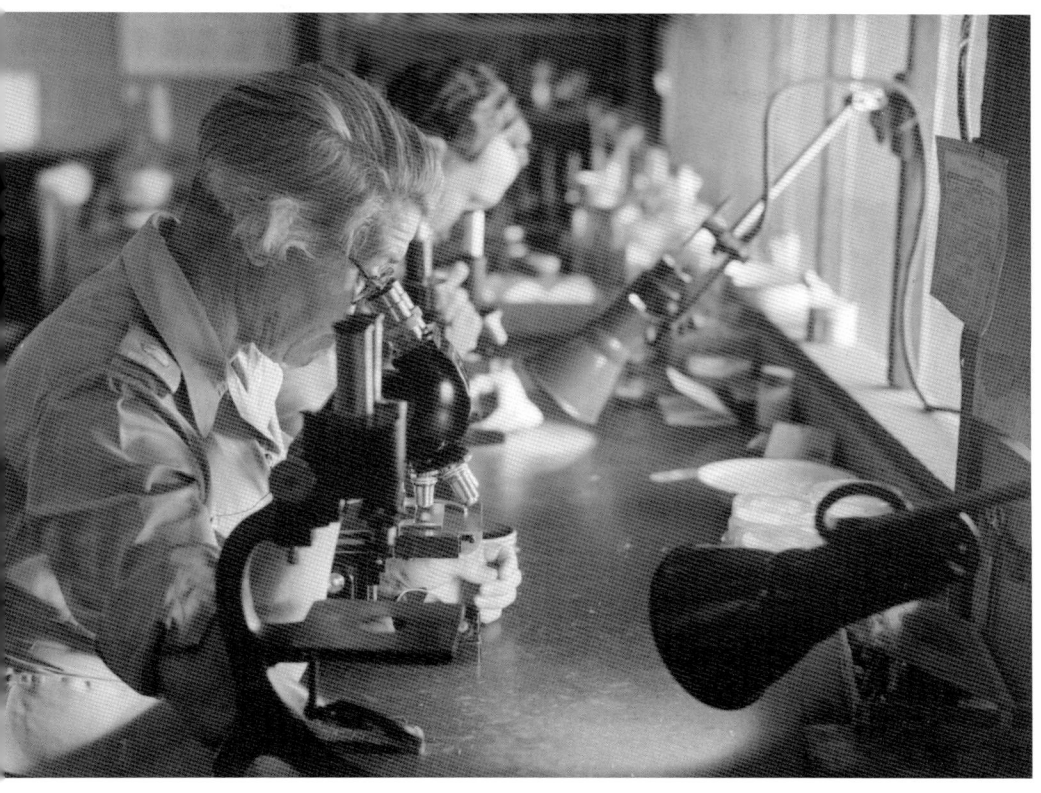

Major Jo Mackerras and entomology staff examining mosquito salivary glands under the compound microscope to determine whether they were infected with malaria sporozoites

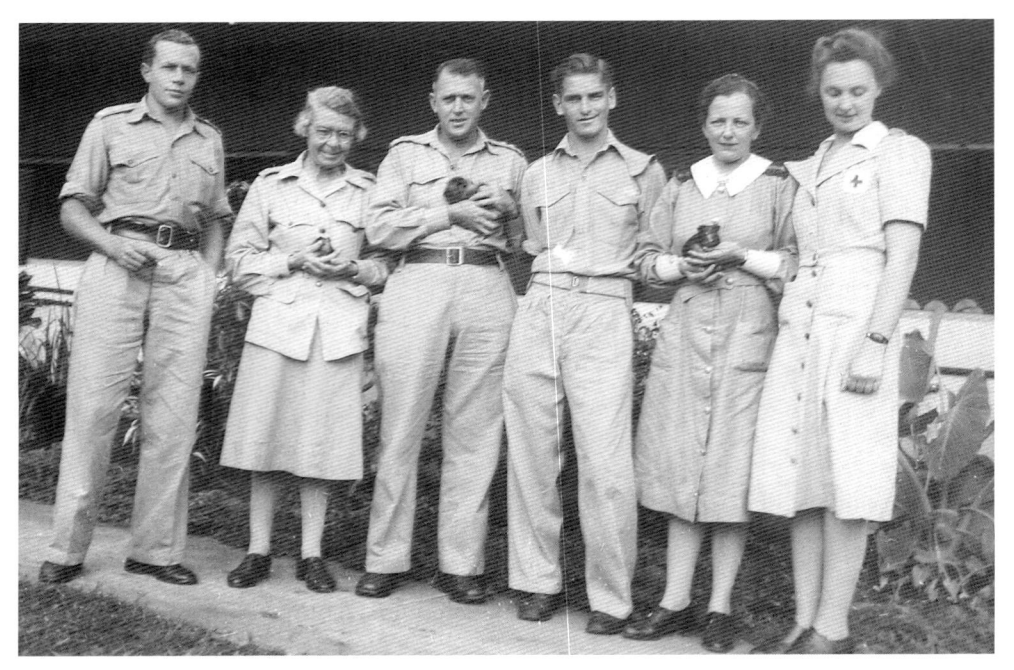

Entomology staff LHQ Medical Research Unit with guinea pigs used for mosquito feeding: (from left), Lieutenant Tom Lemerle, Major Jo Mackerras, Lieutenant Tony Ercole, Corporal George Merritt, Captain Bobbie Fenner, Private Patricia Johnson

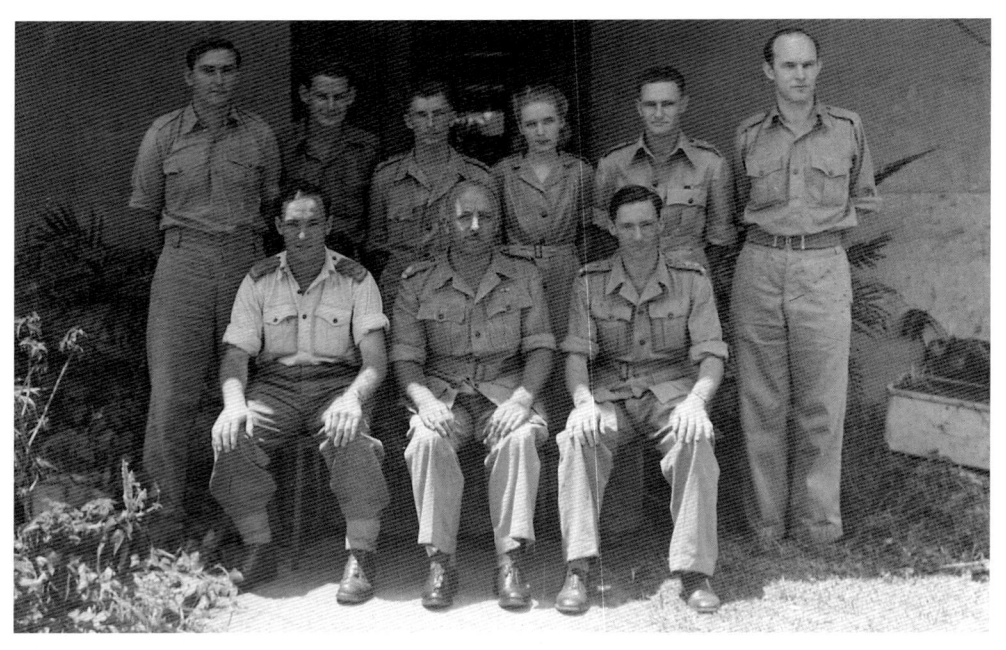

Pathology staff, LHQ Medical Research Unit: (standing, from left) Private Harry Harper, Private Ernest Challinor, Lieutenant Max Swan, Private Alexia Clarke, Lieutenant Tom Akhurst, Staff Sergeant James Findlayson; (seated, from left) Lieutenant Ken Pope, Major Tom Gregory, Lieutenant Ray Dunn

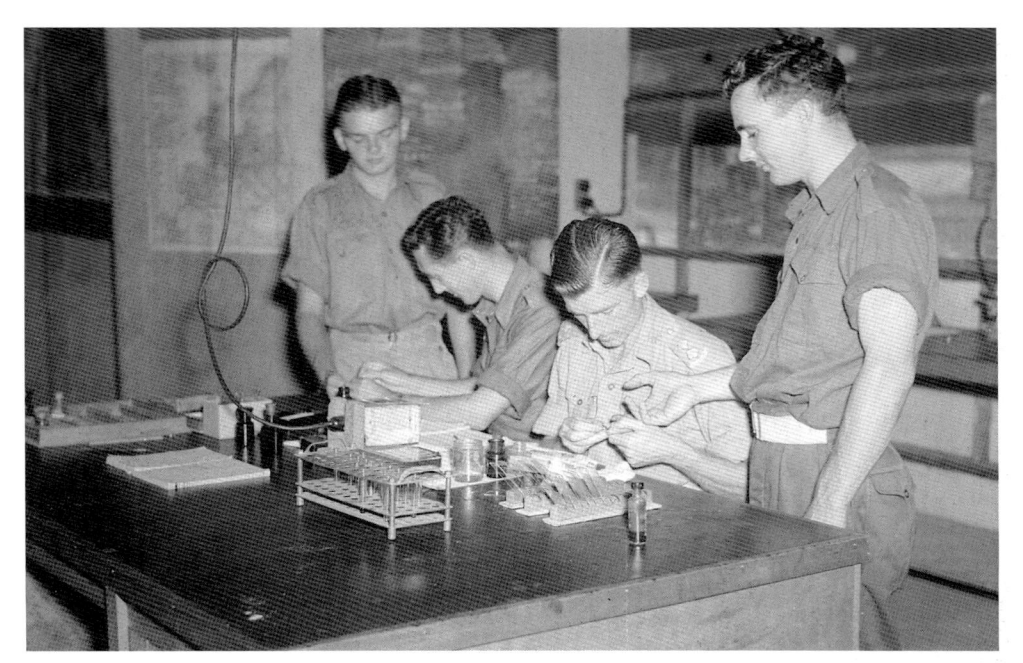

Routine blood collection from malaria-infected volunteers. A drop of blood was taken each day, smeared on a glass slide, stained and examined under the microscope for the presence of malaria parasites. Volunteers, standing from left: Private Hector Anderson, Private Gilbert Tuck; Staff, seated from left: Sergeant Howard Davies, Lieutenant Max Swan

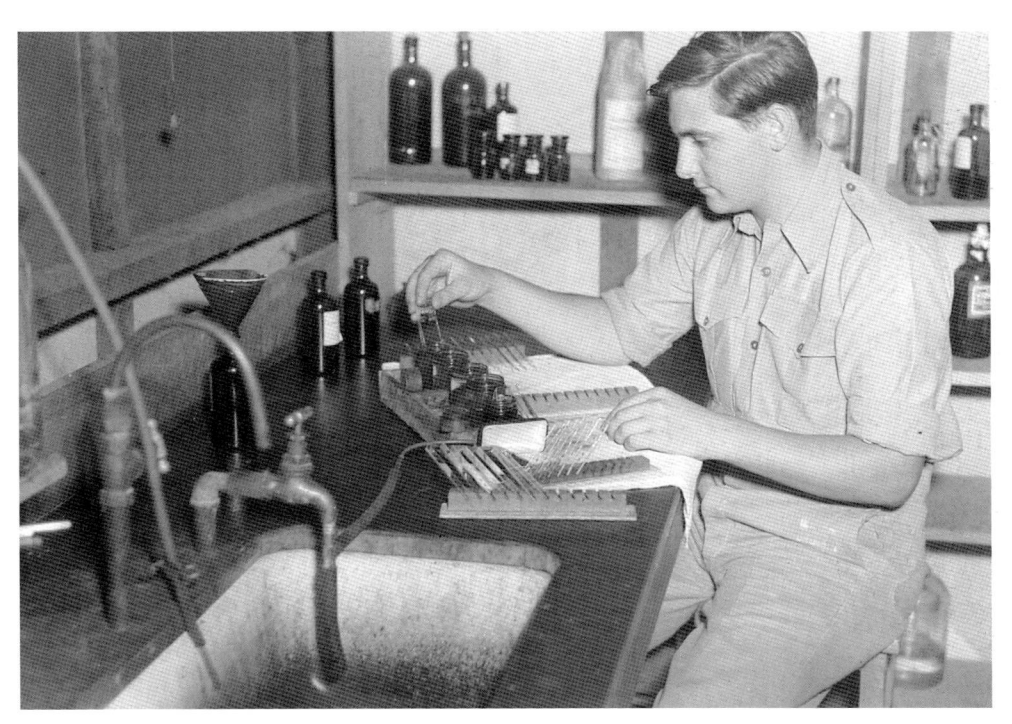

Private Harry Harper staining blood slides taken from volunteers before examination under the microscope

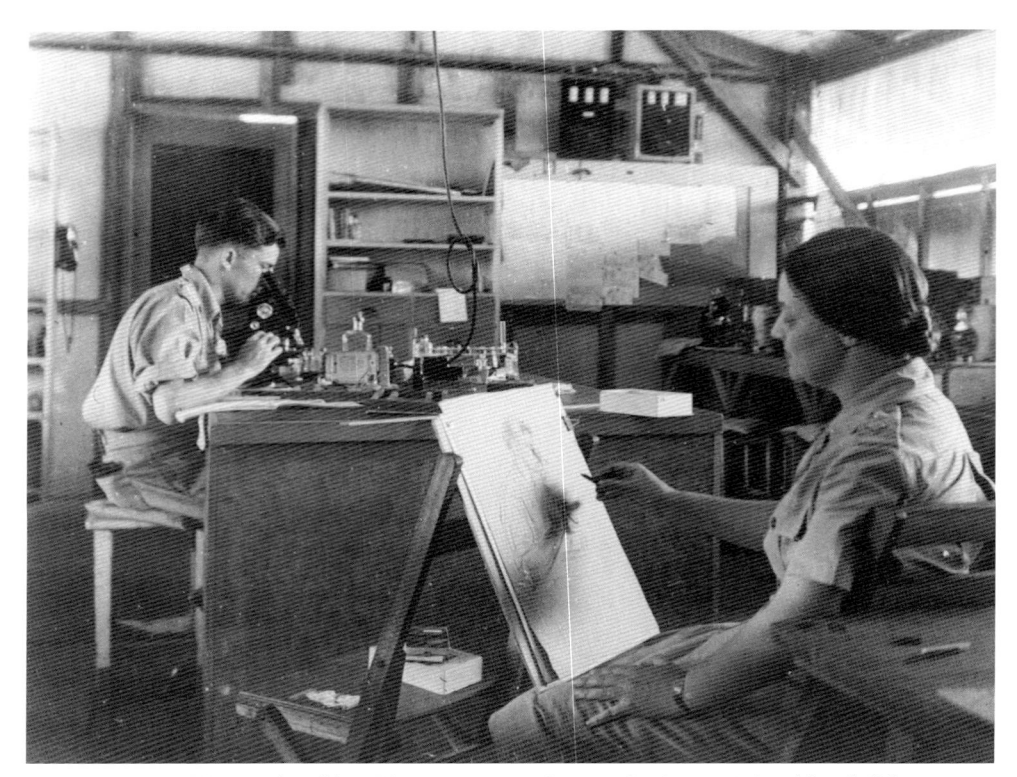

War artist Nora Heysen sketching Lieutenant Max Swan, who is examining blood slides under the microscope

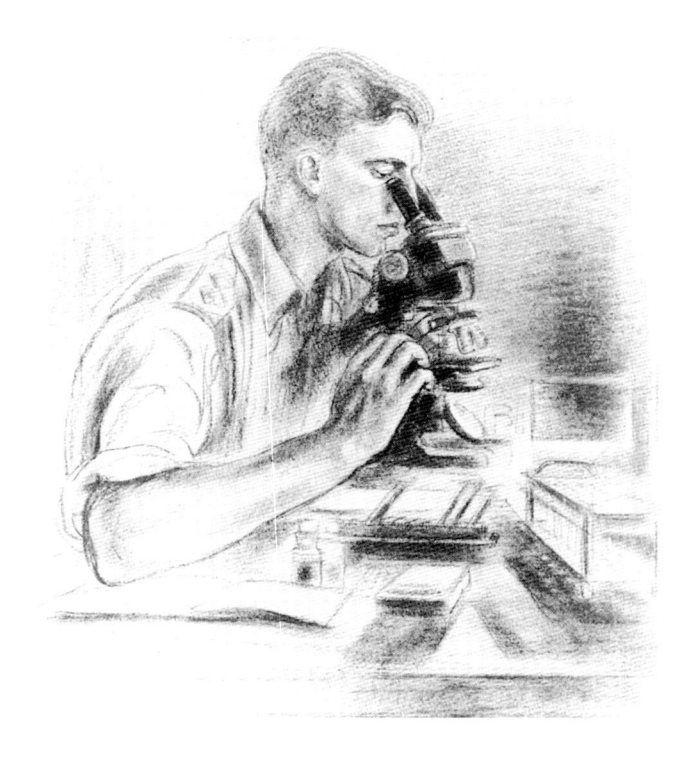

Lieutenant Max Swan examining blood slides under the microscope (sketch by Nora Heysen)

drugs have broken through 22 days after the drug has been stopped'.[6] Subsequent data indicated that the relapses were not quite this rapid, but, nevertheless, the timing of the first relapses were several months earlier that those observed with the North American strains. For example, progress notes prepared on 6 March 1944 indicated that 27 out of 32 vivax-infected volunteers (tests and controls in the sulphonamide experiments) had a mean relapse time of 43.5 days after ceasing the drug.[7] Data on relapses reported in volunteers exposed to mosquito-transmitted vivax malaria during the first year of the experimental work at Cairns were collated by Blackburn in September 1944.[8] The intervals between relapses were recorded as the time in days between occasions when the volunteers reported sick with overt malaria. Forty-four of the 49 volunteers had at least one relapse and two of them had as many as four relapses. After leaving Cairns none of the men resided in a malarious area where they may have been re-exposed to the parasite. Although the records were not complete they showed that there was no significant difference between the time intervals of the different relapses. Moreover, the relapse pattern of control volunteers who received no drugs was the same as that of the test volunteers whose first attacks were deferred by suppressive therapy with either atebrin or the sulphonamide drugs. These observations provided a good indication that the test drugs had no effect on the parasite stages responsible for relapses.

The Americans finally came to agree with Australian evidence that South West Pacific strains exhibited a different relapse pattern compared to those with which they had been working. They were probably influenced by a summary of the first year of the Cairns experiments received by the Board on 3 August 1944: 'Some 250 volunteers, being all "clean skins", have during this period been the subject of the most exhaustive and thorough experiment, unique in the history of malaria investigations'.[9] This provided a two-page outline of the work on the sulphonamides and atebrin, and discussed the implications of the results for troops engaged in jungle fighting in malarious areas: '3 to 4 weeks after such troops stop taking atebrin, attacks of benign tertian malaria will develop'. A letter Shannon received from Watson during his mission to Australia around this time probably contributed to his change of views on this subject. Watson wrote: 'In B.T. infections [on atebrin] there is universal suppression, and universal breakthrough when the drug is withdrawn, usually in about 28 days'.[10]

A more detailed account of the first year's work at Cairns was received on 20 August.[11] Data of the atebrin experiments were included in tables that showed that that sporozoite-induced vivax malaria was suppressed by 600 mg of atebrin per week, but 12 out of 12 men on this regimen relapsed within 19–26 days after they stopped taking the drug. Similarly, all 20 volunteers in the long-term field experiments receiving 100 mg of atebrin per day (with or without 1000 mg per day sulphamerazine) relapsed with vivax infections between 19 and 50 days after drug administration ceased. After seeing these detailed results, the American scientists would have had no option but to accept that New Guinea strains relapsed more rapidly than those of American origin, and this stimulated them to obtain such a strain for use in their clinical studies.

After a meeting in New York during the first week of September 1944, Colonel Downie wrote to Fairley:

> Dr Shannon raised the question of difference between the McCoy strain and the New Guinea Strain and expressed the hope that it might be possible to import into this country at some time some of the New Guinea Strain. He stated that it might be possible to send larvae of an. quadrimaculatus [*sic*] which travel well, infect the mosquitoes in Australia and return them to U.S.A. in order to compare the behaviour of the two strains under identical conditions.[12]

This was an unnecessarily complicated notion. A far simpler method would be to transport the parasites by air freight within a container of infected blood. If this failed, the strain could be imported in a suitable patient with gametocytes in his circulation. These possibilities were canvassed by Dr Loeb at a meeting of the Board on 21 September.[13] Colonel Downie, who attended this session along with Lieutenant Colonel Mackerras, said that he would respond to a formal request to import a suitable strain from Cairns and make every effort to facilitate this matter. The Board passed a resolution that the chairman should make such a request and, next day, Loeb wrote to Downie:

> Our program for the appraisal of the antimalarial activity of newly synthesised drugs in this country is seriously handicapped by the fact that the strain of malaria employed does not precipitate clinical activity for some 7 to 9 months following infection when atebrin or quinine is used as a suppressive drug. At the meeting of the Board for the Co-ordination of Malarial Studies held yesterday the fact was stressed that were it possible to obtain a strain of vivax malaria which would produce with regularity clinical activity in 3 to 4 weeks following the termination of a regime of suppressive atebrin therapy, our work would be greatly expedited and better direction could be given to both synthetic chemists and pharmacologists. The members of the Board are greatly impressed by the important contribution being made to the study of antimalarial drugs by Brigadier Fairley at Cairns and feel that it might prove mutually advantageous were it possible to carry on parallel studies with his strains of vivax malaria and strains now available here in relation to the response of infection to various antimalarial agents. The Board expressed the hope for these reasons that it might be possible to obtain one of Brigadier Fairley's strains which he finds regularly capable of producing clinical activity promptly following discontinuation of suppressive therapy ... Any suggestions which you and Brigadier Fairley may have concerning the possibility of solving the problem in this country will be deeply appreciated. May I take this

opportunity to express on behalf of the Board its gratitude for the fruitful cooperative effort which has been developed through the rapport established between the Australian and American groups interested in the problem of malaria.[14]

The strains used at Cairns were not specially selected for their capacity to relapse rapidly. Moreover, the Australian research had already demonstrated that this was a typical characteristic of vivax malaria originating from New Guinea. An even simpler method of obtaining such a strain for American studies would be to isolate one from among the many soldiers being treated in hospitals in the United States for relapses of vivax malaria acquired in the South West Pacific. It is interesting to note that this had already been done by scientists working under the auspices of the Board on two separate occasions in 1943. It seems that this work was undertaken to investigate the possibility that local North American mosquitoes might be able to transmit exotic strains of malaria, imported in returned soldiers, and start local epidemics of the disease. Dr R. L. Laird collected *Anopheles quadrimaculatus* larvae near Ann Arbor, Michigan, reared them to the adult stage, and then fed the females on soldiers with relapses of vivax malaria acquired in the South West Pacific Islands. Approximately a third of these mosquitoes developed oocysts on the stomach and sporozoites in the salivary glands.[15] Dr R. B. Watson, in Memphis, Tennessee, infected the same species via blood from soldiers suffering vivax relapses of South Pacific origin. He reported that 'Primary data indicate that *A. quadrimaculatus* can be infected about as easily with these strains as with the McCoy strain which was used as a standard of comparison; Also, that mosquitoes fed on patients with very low gametocyte levels may become infected'. An abstract of the interim report on this work, dated 1 November 1943, stated 'Salivary gland infections developed in mosquitoes applied to patients with three of the six strains studied, and sporozoite transmission of the strains was accomplished in these instances'.[16] Surprisingly, the subsequent course of these infections and their relapse patterns do not appear to have been studied and documented.

Thousands of cases of South West Pacific vivax malaria were treated in military installations in the United States during 1943 and 1944, and this was well known to the Board for the Co-ordination of Malarial Studies. However, systematic attempts to isolate such a strain for experimental purposes were not made until August 1944 when Board members became aware that *P. vivax* strains derived from soldiers who had acquired infections in the South West Pacific were being used at Harmon General Hospital in Longview, Texas, for malaria therapy of patients with syphilis. Dr Loeb sent a memorandum to Brigadier General Hugh J. Morgan, the US Army Chief Consultant in Medicine on 'the use of standard strains of vivax malaria versus exotic strains in the evaluation of prophylactic chemotherapy of malaria'.[17] Loeb pointed out that drug studies with the St Elizabeth strain at Atlanta were 'handicapped by the necessity to wait 5 months or more before knowing whether the drug in question has exhibited a prophylactic effect', whereas the experiments conducted by Brigadier Fairley in Australia had found that clinical activity of New Guinea strains occurred within three to four weeks after cessation of suppressive therapy. The memorandum asked whether a study could be undertaken to determine whether sporozoite-induced infections using the South West Pacific strains at Harmon were capable of producing early relapses similar to those observed at Cairns.

An accompanying protocol, which outlined the essential details of the proposed study, stressed the importance of using the most virulent strain available in consultation with Dr Martin D. Young of the NIH Malaria Research Laboratory at Columbia, South Carolina. *Anopheles quadrimaculatus* mosquitoes from this laboratory were used for the causal prophylactic studies in prison volunteers at Atlanta and it was suggested that mosquitoes from this source should be used at Harmon with the active involvement of either Dr Coatney or Dr Young to supervise the biting and dissection of infected specimens.

General Morgan wrote to Colonel G. V. Emerson, the Commanding Officer of Harmon General Hospital, requesting his co-operation 'in a study of the effect of atebrin in suppressive doses on the subsequent development of malaria inoculata when the latter is induced by mosquitoes infected with "Pacific strains" of *P. vivax*'.[18] A favourable response was received, and this was communicated to the Board on 31 August. By this time attempts to isolate a vivax strain had already commenced at Harmon under the supervision of Dr Young.

The report of the US Malaria Mission to the Southwest Pacific by Bishopp and Watson included an account of the experimental work at Cairns, which stated that 'all vivax infections develop clinical expression about 28 days following the discontinuation of atebrin'.[19] The report was critical of what the authors perceived to be deficiencies in strain standardisation: 'In all of these studies Brigadier Fairley has assumed that the strain of malaria parasites he has used, all from New Guinea are either identical or very closely related. In the absence of experimental evidence, this assumption does not seem justified'. Some of the strains used at Cairns were, in fact, studied at length and documented precisely.[20]

However, the significant advantage that the use of New Guinea strains could provide to the American research program was completely overlooked. This classic example of 'not seeing the wood for the trees' was due to Watson, who had the responsibility of representing the clinical and chemotherapeutic aspects of the mission. Watson himself had transmitted such strains via American mosquitoes to humans in Memphis the previous year. He did not study the relapses of these cases and, even when their early relapse patterns were explained to him, he did not appreciate the advantage of using these strains for experimental evaluation of drugs.

Further evidence of Watson's lack of critical insight on this subject was provided at a meeting of the Panel of Clinical Testing on 18 September. Dr Alving reported that they were ready to start sporozoite testing in the newly developed facility at Montano State Hospital, Illinois, as the insectary was completed and the only matter delaying the initiation of mosquito-induced infection was the decision as to which strain of vivax malaria should be employed. Watson said that 'there would be, from the standpoint of the overall program, some advantage of using the McCoy strain in that it would bring into the program another strain of vivax malaria for sporozoite testing since the Atlanta group is using the St Elizabeth strain'.[21] Chairman Shannon was quick to point out that 'if the studies at Harmon General Hospital uncover a New Guinea Strain with a short delay between termination of suppression and primary clinical activity it would be desirable for the Chicago group to use this strain'. In the meantime, it was decided to start experiments with the St Elizabeth strain 'pending receipt of information on characteristics of the exotic strain under study at the Harmon General Hospital'.[22]

The first indication of the results at Harmon were presented by Lieutenant Colonel Dieuaide at a Board meeting on 6 November:

> On 11 Sept 1944 under the supervision of Dr Martin Young, 12 patients were bitten by mosquitoes infected with a New Guinea strain of *vivax* malaria. Five of these patients received quinacrine from 7 to 30 September inclusive ... Four of the 5 patients who received quinacrine have developed positive smears and clinical malaria 25 to 32 days after cessation of quinacrine, and the 5th patient complains of malaise at this writing. The consistent results of this experiment indicate that a New Guinea strain will give much quicker information concerning the value of suppressive drugs than the St Elizabeth's strain previously used.[23]

These findings would not have been a surprise to Brigadier Fairley who attended this meeting in company with Colonel Downie.

Dr Coatney discussed the advantages of using the strain isolated at Harmon in future studies undertaken under the US malaria program at an executive session of the Board on 22 November. The chairman, Dr Loeb, emphasised that the strains already introduced into the United States by returning troops were presumably identical with, or closely related to, this new strain. It was therefore highly desirable to have available for experimental study a freshly isolated 'natural' strain rather than a domesticated variety that had been in laboratories and clinics for many years. The Board recommended that the new strain be introduced in the Atlanta, New York and Chicago units.[24] There were obvious advantages in using a strain that did not exhibit the delayed relapses characteristic of the McCoy and St Elizabeth strains, but it was also appreciated that the various strains could differ in other important characteristics. In his letter recommending the initial study at Harmon, Loeb mentioned to Brigadier General Morgan that 'there is a growing feeling of insecurity in relying upon the results of tests with a strain of vivax malaria which may differ markedly from the strains prevalent in the Southwest Pacific'.[25]

By a coincidence, similar studies recently completed in the USA and Australia had already shown important strain differences in drug activity, though the two groups of investigators were unaware of this at the time. The first experiments using prison volunteers in Atlanta were made by Coatney's group in March and April 1944 to provide baseline data on the protective effects of quinine against sporozoite-induced vivax malaria. The results showed that quinine, administered at a dose of 500 mg/day for 20 days, suppressed the primary attack of the St Elizabeth strain of vivax malaria.[26]

In contrast to the American results, the Australian tests showed that quinine did not suppress primary attacks of mosquito-transmitted strains of New Guinea vivax malaria. A summary of these experiments, conveyed to the American scientists in August 1944, concluded: 'It is evident from these observations that quinine given in doses of five or ten grains a day is inadequate to suppress the strains of *P. vivax* and *P. falciparum* found in Papua when inoculated by mosquitoes into healthy volunteers'.[27] One grain equals 65 mg, so the Australian dosage regimens (325 mg and 650 mg) straddled the dose used by the Americans. The differences between the American and Australian results were significant and underscore the fact that different strains of human malaria parasites may have different biological characteristics. The vivax strain employed by the Americans had been maintained for many years in therapeutic malaria patients at St Elizabeth's Hospital in Washington and at the South Carolina State Hospital. A comparison of the results from the two countries indicated that this strain was more susceptible to quinine than the strains used by the Australians. This was an important consideration, as the experiments at Cairns were made with vivax and falciparum malaria isolated from troops in New Guinea. The response of these parasites to drug therapy was more relevant to the malaria problem in the South West Pacific than the drug response of strains that originated in other parts of the world.

Graphic confirmation of the superiority of South West Pacific strains of vivax malaria for experimental purposes was provided by a comparison of the results of the SN-6911 and SN-7618 experiments at Cairns and Atlanta. There were five men in each test group for each drug in both places. The day of biting for the Atlanta experiment on SN-6911 was 9 June 1944, with relapses of the test subjects occurring between 12 March and 6 May 1945. The day of biting (Z day) for the Cairns SN-6911 experiments was 5 August 1944. All of the test volunteers relapsed between 20 and 27 September. Similarly, the day of biting

14 *The Problem of Vivax* 145

Atlanta SN-6911

Start 9 June

Relapses 12 March – 6 May

JUL 1944 — OCT — JAN 1945 — APR

Cairns SN-6911

Start 5 August

Relapses 20–27 September

JUL 1944 — OCT — JAN 1945 — APR

Atlanta SN-7618

Start 11 August

Relapses 21 April – 14 June

JUL 1944 — OCT — JAN 1945 — APR

Cairns SN-7618

Start 28 October

Relapses 31 December – 24 January

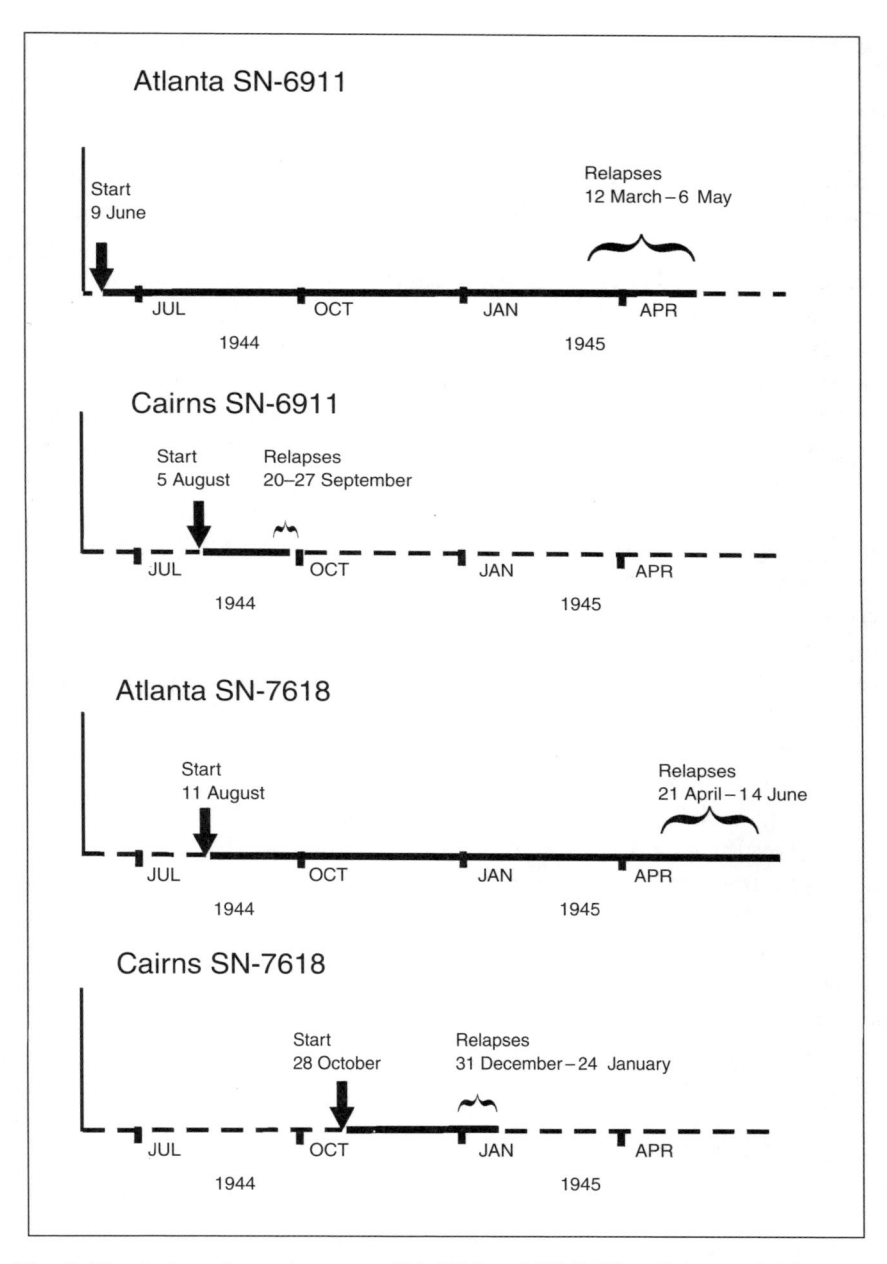

JUL 1944 — OCT — JAN 1945 — APR

Fig. 9 The timing of experiments on SN-6911 and SN-7618 at Cairns and Atlanta

The Atlanta experiment with SN-6911 commenced two months earlier than the equivalent experiment at Cairns, but the relapses in test subjects at Atlanta did not occur until five to six months later than those at Cairns. In the case of SN-7618, the Atlanta experiment commenced six weeks earlier than that at Cairns but the Atlanta relapses were three to five months later than the Cairns relapses.

for the SN-7618 experiment at Atlanta was 11 August, with relapses between 21 April and 14 June 1945. Z day at Cairns for SN-7618 was 28 October 1944 with relapses occurring between 31 December 1944 and 24 January 1945. Even though the experiments at Cairns commenced around two months after the Atlanta experiments, the relapses occurred between four and six months earlier than those at Atlanta (see Fig. 9). Thus, the prolonged latency period of the St Elizabeth strain between the primary attack and the first relapse was responsible for long delays in the American evaluation of these drugs for radical cure of vivax malaria.

A very brief report entitled '*Plasmodium vivax* Chesson Strain' was published in the American journal *Science* in April 1945.[28] It mentioned a vivax infection diagnosed in a soldier at Harmon General Hospital that had been contracted in New Guinea. The strain 'reacted differently to certain drugs than did the St Elizabeth Strain of *P. vivax* which has been extensively used for drug testing. This and other characteristics suggest that it might be a strain distinct from some of the American malarias'. The report concluded that, as there were 'indications that this new strain might be widely used for experimental procedures, it seems desirable to give it a definite designation', and it was designated Chesson—the name of the patient from whom it was obtained. Curiously, the article did not mention that this strain relapsed much more quickly than those of American origin. Nor did it mention that the stimulus to isolate such a strain was derived from the Australian work undertaken at Cairns under the direction of Fairley that had shown that this early relapsing tendency was a feature of South West Pacific strains of vivax malaria. The belated use of a South West Pacific strain by the Americans had a decisive impact on the significant progress achieved in their malaria research program in 1945 and in the years after the war. The so-called 'Chesson strain' has since become a standard strain for assessing drug effects on relapsing vivax infections. It is accepted in the scientific literature as the classic rapid-relapsing strain as compared with the slow-relapse pattern exhibited by American and European strains.

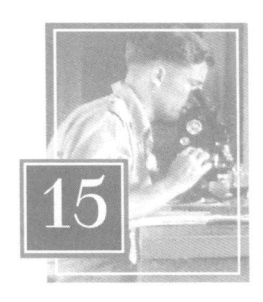

Reorientation of the US Program

FAIRLEY ARRIVED IN Washington during the last week of October 1944, where he remained for about a month. An important highlight was his review of the work at Cairns, which was presented at a meeting of the Board for the Co-ordination of Malarial Studies on 6 November.[1] The results of the experiments on sontochin were illustrated by a series of specially prepared charts that Fairley brought from Australia and a preliminary report that was circulated to the Board members.[2] The data obtained on the new drug were compared with those from the Cairns experiments on atebrin. Fairley pointed out that atebrin and sontochin appeared to be of equal value in suppressing vivax malaria and that both drugs were able to suppress and cure falciparum malaria, though the effect was not one of causal prophylaxis 'since it was possible to demonstrate the transient presence of [parasites] during the period of drug administration'.[3]

He also attended several other Board meetings, presented a paper at a joint meeting of the National Malaria Society and the American Society of Tropical Medicine at St Louis, Missouri (on 15 November[4]), and had ample opportunity for discussions with prominent scientists involved in malaria research. The far-reaching research developments in the USA and Australia since his last visit, two years previously, provided a fertile background for fruitful dialogue. Fairley's handwritten notes of important conversations provide interesting insights into his contemporary views and those of his American counterparts. His visit coincided with a period of intense soul-searching and re-evaluation by the Americans, and his opinions were eagerly sought by Shannon, Marshall, and Loeb—key members of the Panel of Review who had the responsibility of deciding on the entire direction of the American wartime program.

Fairley visited Shannon in his laboratory in New York on 4 November, and spent the morning and early afternoon of 8 November with Marshall at the School of Pharmacology and Experimental Therapeutics, Johns Hopkins Medical School, Baltimore.[5] Fairley's diary notes record that they both

> accept the view which I have strongly sponsored, ie, that in the absence of a true causal prophylactic what is required is a drug which would cure B.T. malaria in therapeutic dosage ... From a practical viewpoint if we possessed [such a drug] the whole malaria problem would be solved from the Army viewpoint.

He also wrote that they

> accept fully the findings in the Cairns report on SN-6911—and agree that this compound is not a true causal prophylactic and that the others [4-aminoquinolines] are not likely to be so. They have also experienced in patients tested with SN-7618 minor toxic features which are mainly subjective in nature and they are, consequently, somewhat depressed about the whole group—prematurely in my opinion.[6]

A major reason for their disappointment with the 4-amino-quinolines, a group of compounds on which they had pinned such high hopes, was the findings at Cairns that SN-6911 only acted on the blood stages of human malaria. In this respect it was similar to atebrin, and so was not able to prevent the disease. But they were particularly despondent with results just received from one of their collaborating institutions, which invalidated a key premise of American clinical evaluation of antimalarial compounds. It was thought that compounds that act upon the blood stages of human malaria might also have an effect on the tissue forms if they were administered in very high doses. This theory could not be tested with quinine and atebrin as there was only a relatively slim margin between therapeutically effective doses and toxic doses of these drugs. However, if a drug could be found that was very active against the parasites in the blood while also having a very low level of toxicity, it might be possible to destroy both the blood and tissue stages and eliminate the infection completely. This was the working hypothesis, advocated by Shannon, which underpinned the rationale for clinical evaluation of drugs against blood-inoculated infections in which effective therapeutic doses of different test compounds were compared in terms of plasma concentrations.

If this premise were correct, it followed that high doses of a very active drug administered for treatment of clinical attacks of vivax malaria should also prevent further relapses. As noted already (Chapter 13), Commander Coggleshall had administered very high doses of SN-7618 for treatment of vivax relapses in US Marines at Klamath Falls, Oregon.[7] These doses, which were higher than those approved by the Board, produced toxic symptoms in the patients.

During the first week of Fairley's visit to Washington a telegram sent to the Board from Klamath Falls stated 'Dr Coggleshall reports three parasite relapses on special drug [SN-7618]'.[8] These findings were discussed by the Panel of Clinical Testing on 20 November. This meeting, attended by Fairley, was convened to consider the orientation of the clinical program. Chairman Shannon said:

> The working premise has been accepted that a compound may be found to possess such high antimalarial activity of a conventional nature that, in addition to interrupting the asexual cycle, it would destroy the non-erythrocytic forms of the parasite and thus terminate relapsing *vivax* malaria ... Fortunately, SN-7618 has sufficiently high antimalarial activity of a conventional nature against *vivax* malaria to test this hypothesis. The preliminary data from Klamath Falls would appear to indicate that the working premise is incorrect.[9]

Shannon concluded from these results that 'a marked increase in antimalarial activity of a conventional nature does not necessarily alter the type of the antimalarial action to the point where it shows an effect on the underlying tissue phase of *vivax* malaria'.

Marshall and Shannon had frank discussions with Fairley about these discouraging developments, and they sought his views on the future orientation of their research program. His notes revealed that the Americans thought that 'causal prophylaxis has completely broken down as far as man is concerned ... Of the various compounds to date holding any prospect of success, no original ones appear to have been discovered in USA'.[10] Fairley felt that efforts to find a cure for relapsing vivax malaria should be given the highest priority in all therapeutic studies on new drugs but Marshall replied that he found it difficult to see how this could be done using bird malaria as an index. More than 11 000 new compounds had already been screened in bird malaria, but experience had shown that this was of doubtful value in identifying drugs that were active against human malaria. For example, a number of sulphonamides were true causal prophylactics of bird parasites but they did not act in this way against the malaria parasites of humans: 'If this be the case it follows that the only rational procedure is to extend human studies'. The discussion then focused on plasmoquine, as both Marshall and Shannon thought that analogues of this drug should be studied. Fairley wrote in his notebook that 'this would involve switching over practically the whole of the malarial drug research activities to this objective. The reason for this volte face was that of the known antimalarials so far explored, plasmoquine alone has been found to be a true causal prophylactic'.[11]

The use of this drug, the first synthetic antimalarial compound, had a mixed history since its synthesis and the discovery of its therapeutic action by the

Germans in the 1920s. Studies in India reported in 1930 by J. A. Sinton and his co-workers yielded 'a high proportion of permanent cures [of vivax malaria], with little toxic risk in a robust population, with even as small a dose as 0.04 gm plasmoquine, if this is combined with quinine'.[12] In the following year experiments conducted at St Mary's Hospital in England by S. P. James, W. D. Nicole and P. G. Shute showed that plasmoquine was able to prevent the primary attack of vivax malaria in 10 volunteers when it was administered at a daily dose of 60 mg, commencing on the day before biting with sporozoite-infected mosquitoes and continuing until the sixth day after infection. Five of the subjects subsequently came down with attacks of the disease during the following six to nine months but these findings implied that the drug exerted a prophylactic affect on the tissue stages to prevent the initial attack of the disease. James later found that, when the dose was increased to 80 mg per day for the first six days after biting, 'in no case did any manifestations of malaria (either early or late) occur in persons who underwent this prophylactic course'.[13] This dose was too near the level of human toxicity to be safely taken for more than a few days.

As time went on there were many independent reports that toxic reactions, ranging from mild to severe, were often produced—sometimes with startling suddenness. Gastrointestinal complaints were the most frequently reported symptoms (abdominal cramps, nausea, vomiting, or diarrhoea). Occasionally, sudden severe haemolytic reactions occurred, associated with shock and anaemia, which could prove fatal to the patient. It was observed that these severe toxic reactions were most often noted in black patients and rarely in Caucasians. Both mild and serious effects occurred at the original recommended doses, and it was realised that the drug was much more toxic than had been initially considered. These concerns were reflected by revised dosage schedules advocated by the League of Nations in 1933, in which the daily dose of plasmoquine was reduced to 27 mg and its administration with quinine for malaria therapy was limited to seven days.[14] At this lower dose plasmoquine did not prevent vivax relapses. It was not until after the war that studies in the USA confirmed that toxic symptoms due to plasmoquine and 8-amino-quinoline compounds occur in individuals who are deficient in the enzyme glucose-6-phosphate dehydrogenase (G-6-PD).[15]

Early in the war the Americans included plasmoquine in therapy for clinical attacks, though some members of the Board for the Co-ordination of Malarial Studies had doubts about its value. In July 1943 a joint meeting of the Sub-committees on Tropical Medicine and Co-ordination of Malarial Studies, which was convened to review drug regimes for suppression and treatment of malaria, recommended that its use be discontinued for routine therapy by the US Army and Navy.[16]

A regime of intensive treatment with atebrin was then adopted by the US Forces including those in the South West Pacific. The Australian malaria treatment regimen in the Pacific campaigns was a 13-day course of quinine, atebrin and plasmoquine known as 'QAP therapy'. This was a complicated treatment regimen comprising 2000 mg of quinine for three days, followed by a five-day course of atebrin (600 mg on the first day, and reduced by 100 mg on each of the following four days to 200 mg on the fifth day), and finally five daily doses of quinine (1000 mg) and plasmoquine (30 mg). It soon became apparent that it was ineffective in preventing vivax relapses. Nevertheless, plasmoquine destroyed the gametocytes of *Plasmodium falciparum*. These stages were able to persist in the circulation and infect mosquitoes for six weeks or more after patients were clinically cured. The gametocytes were not affected by quinine and atebrin, and could be an important source of infections if troops were only treated by the latter drugs and if they remained in a malarious area.

The Australians considered that this provided a positive argument in favour of the continued use of plasmoquine, but the Americans did not agree and they continued to have negative views about it. This was indicated at a meeting on 22 December 1943 when Lieutenant Colonel Dieuaide mentioned that studies were being conducted at Harmon General Hospital to evaluate the effect of plasmoquine in preventing relapses. Drs Shannon, Marshall and other members discussed the evidence regarding plasmoquine, and felt strongly that the studies 'could not be justified in the light of discouraging results which have been obtained with this drug in the past'.[17]

However, at a Panel of Review meeting on 28 April 1944 plasmoquine and its analogues were discussed again, and it was decided that 'the chemical panel should investigate the possibilities of nuclear substitution and evaluate these compounds pharmacologically as a basis of further synthesis'.[18] Shannon may have been responsible for this renewed interest as he suggested that synthesis of related compounds should 'go hand in hand with quantitative pharmacological studies'. This work was not accorded a very high priority, and it appears to have been proposed in the hope that some other derivatives of plasmoquine may be less toxic and more active, even though Shannon believed at this time that plasmoquine itself 'is of little value as an anti-relapse factor in *P. vivax* infections'.[19]

Several months later, the Panel of Review requested Dr Hamilton Southworth, of the London Mission of the Office of Scientific Research and Development, to forward an enquiry to Colonel James seeking information of the present status of the prophylactic use of plasmoquine in vivax malaria. James replied on 11 August that, in his opinion, the state of knowledge of the drug was the same as that stated in the report by the League of Nations in 1933. He added 'no additional experiments of that kind have since been made at Horton or elsewhere in England'.[20]

On 9 August 1944 Shannon wrote a letter to Dr Henry Packer, who worked with Watson at Memphis, Tennessee, in which he mentioned that the first of the plasmoquine analogues was available for clinical trial, and suggested that they be studied at Memphis.[21] The Panel of Review thought that it would be advisable to obtain some background information on plasmoquine itself before proceeding with tests on the new series of compounds. He referred to details of S. P. James's original reports in which 40 to 80 mg per day were administered during the incubation period, with the highest dose providing complete protection from vivax malaria. Accordingly, the first experiments with plasmoquine, using James's high-dose regimes during the incubation period, commenced at Memphis during the last week of September 1944. Daily doses of either 40 mg or 60 mg during the incubation period did not prevent the primary attack of sporozoite-induced infections of the McCoy strain of vivax malaria. However, one vivax patient who had been treated with 80 mg remained free of malaria for 30 days, as did two others on the same drug regimen but infected with sporozoite-induced falciparum malaria.[22] These experimental results were the reason for the American interest in plasmoquine and its analogues at the time of Fairley's visit to the United States in November 1944.

In his talks with Marshall and Shannon, Fairley said that, as the strains used by James and the group at Memphis were characterised by having delayed relapses, they were not comparable to New Guinea strains. Also, subinoculations had not been done. He suggested that 'before such a drastic step was taken [ie to change the direction of the entire program], it would be wise to repeat this experiment at Cairns, with subinoculations on the 7th, 8th and 9th days to see whether the action was being exerted on the sporozoites or tissue forms'.[23] The Americans thought that this was a good idea, and it was brought up again at a meeting of the Panel of Clinical Testing on 20 November after a report on the results at Memphis was presented. The minutes for this meeting state:

> In the discussion which followed ... Brigadier Fairley pointed out that a study could be designed to test the prophylactic action of plasmoquine very precisely by administering the drug in one experiment for 6 days after exposure and a second experiment during days 7 to 12 after exposure to infected mosquitoes. This would accurately characterise the type of effect: ie, whether on the pre-erythrocytic forms of the disease or whether upon the trophozoite and the non-erythrocytic forms which are presumed to exist between attacks and are thought to play a part in the production of the relapsing character of the disease. The panel agreed that the study outlined by Brig. Fairley would yield particularly useful information in the reorientation of the clinical program and recommended to the Board that it communicate to Brig. Fairley an expression of its keen interest in the conduct of such studies.[24]

These recommendations were accepted at an executive session of the Board on 22 November, and Loeb made a formal request through Colonel Downie for the continuation of these studies in Australia:

15 Reorientation of the US Program 153

> The Board expressed the hope that it might be possible for Brigadier Fairley to undertake such studies at Cairns [to extend the observations of Watson's group at Memphis]. Should a further confirmation of James's work ensue from these studies, information of the greatest value would accrue to those charged with the direction of the chemical synthesis of anti-malarial drugs in this country.[25]

Fairley had already left for London by the time this letter arrived, but Downie replied that

> I can, however, assure you that before he left Washington, Brigadier Fairley drafted a critical series of experiments which should settle the problem you mention. These directions have already been sent to Australia with the highest priority. Therefore, it should not be too long before he will be in a position to provide you with an answer.[26]

Blackburn received Fairley's instructions about the plasmoquine experiments on 18 December 1944, and made preparations to start the vivax group before the New Year.[27] The question of toxicity was an important consideration that had been recently highlighted in a patient at the unit. Ten days later Blackburn wrote to Fairley:

> I enclose a brief history of a patient with haemoglobinuria resulting from the administration of plasmoquine, whom you saw at 2/6 AGH in August before you left. I had him transferred to me and the notes enclosed shew that he had a very severe reaction to plasmoquine ... For a while I thought he was going to die. He has been sent south and his papers clearly indicate that he is not to be given plasmoquine again under any circumstances.[28]

In order to prevent a recurrence of this experience it was decided to undertake a preliminary drug sensitivity test so that any volunteer with an idiosyncrasy to plasmoquine could be excluded. This involved the administration of 30 mg of the drug on three consecutive days to each test volunteer, the last dose of which was given not less than seven days before starting the experiment.

The objectives of this series were to observe the activity of plasmoquine against mosquito-transmitted vivax and falciparum malaria when it was administered, either during the incubation period of the infection, or when trophozoites were first expected to appear in the peripheral circulation. There were two groups of ten volunteers comprising two controls and eight test cases. Both groups were to be subjected to 20 bites at one session—one group with mosquitoes infected with *P. vivax* and the other with *P. falciparum*. Each was divided into two subgroups, the first of which closely followed the test procedure used by James: four men received 80 mg of plasmoquine, commencing one day before biting, on the day of biting, and for the next five days. The other subgroup received the same daily dose of the drug commencing on the sixth day after biting, and continuing until the tenth day.

The vivax subgroups were bitten by infected *Anopheles punctulatus* mosquitoes on 15 January 1945.[29] All four volunteers who had plasmoquine from Z–1 to Z+5 subsequently developed attacks of malaria. However, the observation of parasites in their peripheral circulation and the development of clinical attacks of the disease occurred several days later than normal. For example, the controls had parasites in their blood on the 12th day, and required therapy 17–19 days after biting. On the other hand, microscopic densities of parasites were not seen in the test volunteers until 17–23 days after biting, and the average date on which treatment commenced was 27–29 days after their infective bites. Subinoculations to uninfected recipients were made by direct transfusion, following the normal procedures developed at Cairns, on the 9th and 10th days after biting. Recipients of blood from the controls and the test volunteers receiving plasmoquine from days Z+6 to Z+10 developed malaria, thereby demonstrating the presence of submicroscopic parasites in the donors. However, in contrast to all other subinoculation experiments conducted to that time, the recipients from test donors who had taken plasmoquine from days Z–1 to Z+5 did not develop vivax malaria.[30] These findings indicated that plasmoquine was unable to prevent infections of New Guinea strains of vivax malaria if it was administered during the first five days after sporozoite inoculation. However, there was clear evidence that it prolonged the incubation period.

The falciparum group were bitten on 8 February, around the time that the first group of vivax test volunteers on plasmoquine were having their primary attacks. All four volunteers who received plasmoquine from the 6th to the 10th days after biting developed malaria, and were treated for overt attacks within a week of ceasing the drug. Unlike the vivax group, three out of four men who received plasmoquine from days Z–1 to Z+5 failed to develop attacks of falciparum malaria. Negative subinoculations showed that these men did not have circulating parasites on Z+9 and Z+10. The other man had parasites at microscopic levels on Z+14, and commenced treatment therapy on Z+17. Positive subinoculations from this man and from the four volunteers who received plasmoquine between Z+6 to Z+10 showed that they had parasites in their blood at submicroscopic levels after the usual incubation period.[31]

The results of the plasmoquine experiments at Cairns implied that there was an essential difference between the action of the drug in the two species of human malaria. It acted as a partial causal prophylactic of *P. vivax* by delaying the primary attack when administered at a daily dosage of 80 mg/day during the incubation period, or during the time when the blood stages first appear. With falciparum malaria, on the other hand, this dose of the drug acted as a true causal prophylactic in three out of four volunteers when given during the incubation period, but it did not prevent or delay the development of the disease when administered during the period that the blood stages first appear in the circulation. Serious toxic features were not encountered in any of the volunteers in the plasmoquine series though some of the men had minor side effects.

A signal was passed on from the Australian Legation in Washington to the Board during the second week of February 1945 advising that 'Brigadier Fairley reports in plasmoquine vivax experiments Cairns no evidence causal prophylaxis as all 4 volunteers had demonstrable parasites by 20th day following exposure'.[32] Information on the negative subinoculation results were not included, so the Americans were not aware from this that the Cairns work showed that the drug, in fact, did exert some effect on the tissue stages by delaying the development of the primary attack. However, by this time another five patients at Memphis had been infected with sporozoite-induced vivax malaria (McCoy strain) and subjected to James's high-dose plasmoquine regimen during the incubation period. There had been no breakthroughs more than 50 days after stopping therapy, though observations were still continuing.[33]

The Americans also became aware of British work at Colchester and other military hospitals in England, which commenced in 1944 to compare 10-day intensive courses of either atebrin or plasmoquine, combined with quinine, for treatment of naturally acquired vivax malaria in soldiers returned from malarious areas. It was shown that 34 per cent of more than 600 cases treated with atebrin had relapses, whereas only 10 per cent of relapses were recorded in a similar number of men treated with the quinine and plasmoquine combination.[34]

Shannon reviewed again all of the earlier British work on plasmoquine.[35] He was particularly impressed with Sinton's work from India, which showed a significant reduction in vivax relapses if plasmoquine administration was continued for 10 days or more in contrast to conventional therapy of less than a week as recommended by the League of Nations. He resolved to undertake an experiment in New York to see whether such long-term administration of plasmoquine could prevent relapses of vivax. In March 1945 nine conscientious objectors at Goldwater Memorial Hospital were infected with the mosquito-induced 'Chesson' strain of vivax from Harmon Hospital. The primary attacks of these men were treated with 90 mg of plasmoquine, together with 2 gm of quinine per day for 14 days. None of them had relapses.[36] These results, together with the findings from Memphis, convinced the Americans that plasmoquine was active against the tissue forms of vivax malaria. This provided the rationale for an extensive exploration of other 8-amino-quinoline compounds that dominated the American malaria research effort in 1945.

Further collaborative work between the Australian and American groups was not undertaken, though cordial relations continued and research reports were exchanged on a regular basis. The Australian research effort changed direction in 1945 to focus on evaluation of an entirely new group of antimalarial compounds discovered by British scientists.

16

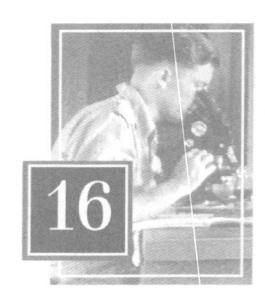

The Answer to the Maiden's Prayer

FAIRLEY ARRIVED IN England from America on 26 November 1944. British malaria research had expanded in the two years since his previous visit, albeit on a smaller scale than the malaria program in the USA. The entry of Imperial Chemical Industries (ICI) into this field was encouraged by a leading British malaria researcher, Professor Warrington Yorke, of the Liverpool School of Tropical Medicine. At Yorke's suggestion a co-operative arrangement was initiated, in early 1943, between the ICI laboratories at Blackley, North Manchester, and the British Medical Research Council for testing and evaluating new antimalarial compounds.[1] They adopted an approach similar to that used by the Americans, in which the drugs were screened for activity against avian malaria parasites. Most of the test compounds came from their own research program, though some came from other sources. The initial thought was to concentrate on seeking a causal prophylactic, but in view of perceived problems associated with atebrin (including skin yellowing) and the Japanese capture of Java, which jeopardised future supplies of quinine, they decided to look for better suppressive drugs as well.

The first priority facing Drs D. G. Davey, F. H. S. Curd and F. L. Rose, the key scientists at Manchester, was to decide on a screening system to identify promising compounds that would then be evaluated further. The work commenced using W. Roehl's test involving intramuscular injection of test compounds to canaries infected with *Plasmodium relictum*. They appreciated that the logic of this approach was contingent on the assumption that the activity of the test compounds against avian parasites was similar to their action against human malaria. They also realised that it was questionable whether the chemotherapeutic index of a drug determined for bird malaria was of any value in assessing the drug for clinical use against human malaria. For example, none of the sulphonamide drugs, which had already been shown to have activity against the human malarias, exhibited any antimalarial activity using Roehl's procedure. Consequently, there was a distinct possibility that other promising compounds might be overlooked if they were screened only in this system. In a contemporary review describing the rationale for the ICI malaria program, Curd argued that such exploratory investigations should include more than one avian parasite.[2] Curd and Davey decided to abandon Roehl's test and to set up a *P. gallinaceum*/chick system under standardised experimental conditions in which the test drugs were compared with atebrin. The activity of promising compounds was also assessed against other avian parasites, including *P. lophurae* and *P. cathemerium*, and chronic toxicity was investigated in mice.

After the discovery of plasmoquine and atebrin, most of the chemical work undertaken in various parts of the world had been concerned with derivatives of acridine or quinoline that were chemically related to the new synthetic antimalarials. The British group at Manchester decided to break away from investigations of these structures and to investigate some other systems in the hope of finding new antimalarial compounds that might be easily synthesised. They explored derivatives of pyrimidine, as it was known that these compounds play an important role in cell metabolism. It was thought that 'pyrimidine would possess important intrinsic chemotherapeutic properties and these would include activity against malaria parasites'.[3]

The ICI chemists synthesised a large series of related substances and subjected them to their systematic screening program. The first one to show a definite action against *P. gallinaceum*, code-named M.2666, was five to six times less active than atebrin; it was also two to three times more toxic than atebrin in mice. However, it was an entirely new type of antimalarial drug, so they decided to give it a preliminary clinical trial in humans. Therapeutic tests conducted by Dr A. R. D. Adams at the Liverpool School of Tropical Medicine against five cases (two of falciparum; two of vivax and one of quartan malaria) produced negative results at a dose of 40 mg three times a day. Even at this small dose toxic symptoms were encountered and further work on this compound was abandoned.[4]

The first drug to show promise against human malaria was a methylpyrimidine compound with a guanidine component code-named M.3349. This was selected for clinical tests after it had shown activity equal to atebrin against *P. gallinaceum* in chickens. More than 200 cases of vivax and 80 attacks of falciparum malaria were treated at Liverpool with this drug.[5] The attacks were arrested with doses of 600 mg/day for a week, but there was a high incidence of recrudescences after treatment ceased. It was found that this drug was less effective than atebrin against West African strains of falciparum malaria.

The chemists then followed the avenue of synthesis suggested by M.3349 to investigate related compounds, including several biguanide derivatives. One of the latter group, M.4430, had a broader spectrum of activity against avian parasites than the other compounds previously tested. It had a pronounced action against the blood forms of *P. gallinaceum* in chickens and *P. lophurae* in ducks. More significantly, it acted as a causal prophylactic against the former parasite by affecting the primary tissue forms, as well as the sporozoites. On the other hand, it had no causal prophylactic action against *P. lophurae*, *P. cathemerium* or *P. relictum*. Investigations of the toxicity of M.4430 indicated that its adverse effects in laboratory animals were much less severe than those associated with atebrin. Observations in humans suggested that toxic effects did not occur in daily doses of less than 1000 mg.

Preliminary therapeutic trials were in progress when Fairley arrived in England. These involved tests conducted at Liverpool against naturally acquired clinical cases of human malaria. The initial results were encouraging, as good clinical responses occurred in all treated test cases.[6]

In early 1945 another biguanide, closely related to M.4430, was shown to have an even greater range of activity against bird parasites by acting as a causal prophylactic against *P. gallinaceum*, *P. relictum* and *P. cathemerium*. This drug, designated M.4888, had not yet been subjected to clinical trials, but its promising activity against avian malaria implied that it might be the best of the group.

At the end of 1944 the British workers found themselves in a situation analogous to that of the Americans six months previously. They had identified compounds with very promising antimalarial activity but, although they were able to proceed with limited clinical testing, they lacked the capacity to undertake large-scale clinical trials that would clearly define the mode of action and practical value of these drugs against human malaria. They were aware of the Australian investigations at Cairns, as Fairley had been in regular correspondence with Major General A. G. Biggam, Chairman of the Malaria Committee of the Medical Research Council, but they did not know the full scope of the work, even though some of the progress reports had been seen by members of the British Medical Research Council.

Soon after arriving in London Fairley was invited by Biggam to present an account of the Cairns experiments at a meeting of the Malaria Committee.[7] Among those present were the most prominent British authorities in tropical medicine and malaria, including the eminent malariologist Colonel S. P. James (co-discoverer of the tissue stages of bird malaria), Brigadier J. A. Sinton VC (who, as a Major in India, demonstrated the value of plasmoquine against vivax relapses), and the distinguished mosquito entomologist Sir (Samuel) Rickard Christophers, formerly of the Indian Medical Service. Two senior members of the Liverpool School of Tropical Medicine, Professor T. H. Davey and Lieutenant Colonel B. Maegraith, were also present. Both were involved in testing the new compounds synthesised by ICI. Fairley summarised the events leading to the formation of the malaria experimental group at Cairns, and then outlined the results of the experiments with the sulphonamides, atebrin, quinine and sontochin that had been undertaken during the previous 18 months. The minutes of the meeting state that, 'after various questions had been asked and answered, the chairman thanked Brigadier Fairley for this account of the valuable work, and the committee expressed appreciation of the great importance of the investigations he had described'.[8]

The members of the Malaria Committee immediately realised that the Cairns unit was the only facility in the world that could test their new drugs on a sufficiently large scale to provide a rapid and thorough evaluation of their efficacy. This view was reinforced by the first formal scientific presentation of the work that was made by Fairley in a paper presented at a meeting of the Royal Society of Tropical Medicine and Hygiene held in Manson House (the Society headquarters) on 18 January 1945. The format was similar to his presentation at the Atherton Conference in June 1944, but the experimental results were rigorously described and documented with graphs and tables arranged for a scientific audience. Fairley outlined the organisation of the laboratories and wards at Cairns and Rocky Creek, indicated the names and areas of responsibility of the senior staff members, and described the methods used in the entomology, pathology and clinical sections. He related the organisational set-up to the overall plan of the investigations, and then went on to provide a chronological narrative of the experiments on sulphonamides and atebrin. The short-term experiments induced by infected mosquito bites or by inoculation of infected blood were described, as well as the conditions of extreme physical stress and other methods employed in the long-term 'field type of experiments' to investigate the possibility of breakthroughs while on atebrin. The results were discussed in relation to plasma atebrin levels and the findings of subinoculation experiments. The quinine experiments, which demonstrated that this drug was not able to prevent overt attacks of South West Pacific strains of falciparum or vivax malaria, were also described. Fairley concluded by indicating that the military implications of the work were that 'granted infallible atebrin discipline, it should be possible to fight a non-immune force for many months in hyperendemic areas of malaria without significant malaria casualties'.[9]

Some of the most significant findings at Cairns were made by following leads originating from the work of James, and it was particularly fitting that he opened the discussion. He said: 'Brigadier Fairley is to be congratulated sincerely on his successful accomplishment and on obtaining results which permit no doubt of the efficacy and practicability in the field of the protective measures tested'.[10] After further discussion and comments by various speakers Brigadier Sinton 'congratulated Brigadier Fairley and his team upon the conclusive results obtained by experiments so clearly planned and brilliantly executed. He also desired to thank him on behalf of the [British] army for the irrefutable evidence produced as to the outstanding value of atebrin suppression during military operations in the tropics'.[11] In addition to these meetings Fairley talked on numerous occasions to different groups, including combatant staff, the Inter-Allied Military Conference, the Epidemiological Section of the Royal Society of Medicine, and the Royal Society of Tropical Medicine and Hygiene.[12] In a letter to Burston he wrote: 'For the most part it has either been an "atebrin crusade" based on our Cairns findings and the field results in New Guinea, or a review of medical achievements in jungle warfare'.[13]

The Australian Army Medical Services had two very competent medical officers among the military staff at Australia House in London: Colonel J. H. (Jock) Anderson, the Medical Liaison Officer, and Major S. J. M. (Stan) Goulston. Goulston was responsible for the staff work associated with Fairley's mission in London. He accompanied the brigadier on official visits, including an important trip to Liverpool and Manchester between 10 and 14 February 1945 to see the progress of research on the new ICI compounds.[14] Fairley visited the Liverpool School of Tropical Medicine and the Tropical Diseases Centre at Smithdown Road Hospital, where he met Dr A. R. D. Adams, who was overseeing the administration and clinical evaluation of the new drugs in malaria patients. He gave a lecture at the University of Liverpool to a large audience on 'Medicine in Tropical Warfare'. In Manchester he went to see the malaria research work at the ICI laboratories, and had long discussions with Dr D. G. Davey, the senior scientist involved in the malaria drug program.

The workers at Cairns had exhaustively tested all the known antimalarial drugs, including the most promising new drugs identified by the Americans. In spite of the demonstrated value of atebrin for prophylaxis they appeared to have come no closer to finding a causal prophylactic drug that would prevent infection with human malaria. This was the ultimate goal of the research, but they had also reached a dead end in their efforts to eliminate relapses of vivax malaria. Fairley was excited by the possibilities offered by the new British compounds to solve these problems—particularly M.4888 the first compound shown to destroy the tissue forms of all the avian parasites against which it had been tested. He considered this to be the most promising drug discovered since plasmoquine and atebrin, and resolved to have it tested at Cairns as a matter of urgency and with the utmost priority. Before departing from Manchester Fairley and Davey discussed the experiments that could be conducted in Australia.

During the next two weeks Fairley was preoccupied with setting up all the necessary preparations so that the Australian experiments could proceed as soon as possible. On the one hand, the administrative arrangements needed to be formalised with the British authorities and Australian Army Headquarters. At the same time, a detailed experimental plan of the work had to be prepared and sent to Cairns. On 17 February he had a meeting with Sir Edward Mellanby, Chairman of the Medical Research Council, to arrange for the drugs to be sent to Australia through the auspices of the council.[15] A signal marked Top Secret was sent from Australian Army Staff, London, to AHQ Melbourne on 20 February stating that: 'the British Medical Research Council urgently desires two recently discovered drugs to be tested at Cairns. Brig Hamilton Fairley advises one hundred volunteers be collected Cairns and highest priority given this investigation. Drugs and detailed instructions follow by air. Information regarded as most secret'.[16]

Fairley then wrote to Major General Burston to explain the background and importance of the proposed experiments.

> As indicated by cable, Sir Edward Mellanby has asked if we will test out two remarkable anti-malarial drugs discovered by I.C.I. at Manchester ... M.4888 is the first drug to be discovered acting as a *general* causal prophylactic for bird malaria; it acts on the early tissue stage of the parasite in all the different species of bird malaria parasites so far tested. It may well act as a causal prophylactic in benign tertian malaria and or cure B.T. infections in man. From a theoretical viewpoint it looks like the answer to the maiden's prayer and is what all the malaria research workers have been looking for both in U.S.A. and U.K. ... We will be the first to work with M.4888 on experimentally infected volunteers and on our results will largely depend any decision made in regard to future mass production.[17]

Fairley also sent a letter to Colonel Keogh on the same date that he wrote to Burston (24 February) outlining the status of the new drugs and emphasising that they should be tested experimentally at Cairns with a minimum of delay. He told Keogh that he was sending initial batches of each drug (500 tablets) by air at the same time as the letter, and later batches were to be sent within a few days.[18]

On 20 February Davey sent to Fairley a report of all the work that had been done on M.4888, together with a draft outline of the proposed experiments he had prepared from notes of their meeting in Manchester.[19] This formed the starting point for discussions held in London on 23 February between Fairley, Davey and a senior executive from ICI, Dr C. M. Scott, to finalise the Australian experimental program. Davey had also brought summaries of the latest information on M.4430 and M.4888. This was supplemented by a letter from Dr Adams to Fairley providing a synopsis of clinical test data of the two drugs in patients at Liverpool. By that time more than 50 cases had been treated at Liverpool with doses of M.4430 ranging from 20 to 500 mg (three times daily) for a week. Most patients were suffering from vivax malaria, although some were falciparum cases and there were two cases of quartan malaria.[20] Parasites disappeared from the blood of all the test cases in three to four days, but approximately half of them relapsed within one to two months afterwards.[21]

An experiment with M.4430 had been completed on British Army volunteers by Major J. Reid, Flight Lieutenant M. Joekes, and P. G. Shute at the Royal Army Medical College, Millbank. Five men receiving 1200 mg of the drug for three successive days were injected with sporozoites of *P. falciparum* on the second day. The results indicated a causal prophylactic action, as none of them became infected, whereas an untreated control and another volunteer on atebrin for the same period subsequently developed falciparum malaria. Trials of the suppressive action of M.4430 against vivax malaria were about to commence at Millbank, and investigations were in progress at Colchester by Major R. D. P. Johnstone to determine the effect of this drug on relapses.

The first therapeutic tests of M.4888 started in January 1945 at the Liverpool School of Tropical Medicine to provide a preliminary indication of effective dose regimens for therapy of clinical attacks. In laboratory animals it appeared to be absorbed more rapidly and was more persistent than M.4430, so it was decided to administer the new drug twice (rather than three times) a day for 14 days.[22] By the end of February 29 cases of vivax malaria, mostly relapses in military personnel from the Burma campaign, as well as two falciparum cases, had been treated with twice daily doses that varied from 10 mg to 150 mg. In every case fever and asexual parasites disappeared from the blood within two or three days. At the completion of treatment microscopic examination of blood was made at least twice weekly in all cases. The longest period of observation was only three weeks at this time but so far none had relapsed, nor had parasites yet been observed in any blood slides examined.[23] After their treatment was finished, the Liverpool patients were discharged from hospital to local convalescent homes, where they were accessible to the clinical staff. In spite of this arrangement Adams had difficulty keeping patients under observation long enough to follow up possible vivax relapses.[24]

Blackburn had been sending regular letters and reports to Fairley to keep him abreast of the experimental work at Cairns. These included monthly progress reports with updated results and tabulated data on the experiments in progress. Fairley replied at length in a long letter on 16 February 1945, in which he gave the first hint of the new British drugs: 'I am hoping to arrange for testing at LHQ Medical Research Unit in the immediate future [of] two ... recently discovered compounds (secret). If so, this investigation must be given A1 priority. Its importance needs no emphasis'.[25] He probably considered it premature to provide more information to Blackburn at this point, as the administrative formalities had not been completed. He then went on to outline his current views on the most appropriate experimental approach to evaluate newly discovered antimalarial compounds. He wrote: 'owing to the light it throws on tissue forms [subinoculation] is of considerable practical importance as it is almost now certain that the cure for B.T. malaria will come from drugs which act on known tissue forms in bird malaria'.[26] Fairley asserted that the data collected at Cairns showed that the action of drugs on the parasite could be investigated by administering the test compounds for precise periods corresponding to the different stages of the life cycle in the experimentally infected volunteer. Thus, drug administration on the day before biting and the day of biting would investigate drug action on the sporozoites. Administration of the test compound in the first five days after biting in falciparum infections and the first seven days in vivax infections could be employed to study the effects of drugs on the primary tissue stages. Action against the blood stages could be assessed by administering the drug from the sixth day after biting in falciparum infections and the eighth day after biting in vivax infections. Finally, he postulated that drugs that acted against the secondary tissue forms (presumed responsible for vivax relapses) could be investigated by administration during the latent phase, and preferably at a time when subinoculation is negative. This approach was well suited for determining the mode of action of a drug like M.4888 that does not persist in the blood at active levels for more than a day after administration. Co-ordination of drug administration with different phases of the parasite cycle would yield ambiguous results in longer-acting drugs like chloroquine or atebrin that remain in the circulation for much longer periods.

Such considerations influenced Fairley's choice of the experimental protocol. The overriding hope was that the latest ICI drug would act as a causal prophylactic in vivax infections as this was the most important practical need. The plasmoquine experiments were still in progress in Cairns, but he was aware that initial results had already shown that, even though the incubation period of vivax malaria was prolonged, this drug failed to eradicate the infection. This news, together with the early indications that vivax relapses still occurred after therapy with M.4430, stimulated enthusiasm for M.4888 as the last hope for finding a practical and effective causal prophylactic of both falciparum and vivax malaria before the end of the war.

The original plan, which was sent to Australia during the last week of February, was based on three groups of experiments. Each group was to consist of two vivax experiments, one with M.4888 and the other with M.4430, and a similar pair of falciparum experiments. The first group was to follow the usual scheme of short-term experiments with test cases receiving the test drug each day from Z–1 to Z+23. Drug administration in the second group was to be restricted to the incubation period (Z–1 to Z+7 for vivax, and Z–1 to Z+5 for falciparum) to investigate causal prophylactic ability. The final group, in which the two drugs were to be administered for two weeks, commencing on Z+8 for vivax and Z+6 for falciparum, was designed to test their action on the blood stages.[27]

The experimental team at Cairns had been alerted to the impending experiments on the new drugs by Fairley's letter to Blackburn in mid-February. On receipt of the detailed instructions all available resources were immediately allocated to the new project. The first experiment commenced just over a month after the first drug samples were dispatched to Australia. This was a repetition of the rapid response to the American request in the previous year, and was a further dramatic indication of the ability of the group at Cairns to undertake large-scale clinical evaluation of an entirely new compound at very short notice. The new series of experiments proposed by Fairley would require 80 men. Unfortunately, the number of volunteers was very low at this time, as only 26 were available in April 1945.[28] It was proposed to issue a further routine order calling for additional volunteers, but any large increase was not anticipated. It was suggested by Land Headquarters in Melbourne that nothing further be done about this matter until Brigadier Fairley returned to Australia.[29]

Fairley indicated that, if volunteers were scarce, M.4888 should be given first priority over M.4430, so the work was scaled down according to these guidelines and it was decided to defer experiments with M.4430 until more volunteers were available. Four experiments with M.4888 (one with falciparum and three with vivax malaria) commenced in early April[30] (see Table 2). Six test volunteers commenced a daily dose of 100 mg of M.4888 on 1 April 1945. Those in the first falciparum subgroup (named CIII), which also included a man on atebrin and an untreated control, were bitten by 20 mosquitoes infected with sporozoites on the following day, and continued to receive the drug for the subsequent 23 days. Three vivax experiments, each involving administration of M.4888 to four volunteers, commenced on 9 April. The first, designated CI, followed the same plan as falciparum subgroup CIII. The second vivax subgroup (CV) was subjected to the procedure laid down for the causal prophylactic experiments with 300 mg/day administered during the incubation period. The third concurrent vivax experiment (CIX) investigated the effects of M.4888 on the blood stages by administration of 200 mg for two weeks from the ninth day after biting. Subinoculations of 200 ml of blood were made from the subjects in the falciparum experiment, using the usual procedures, on the seventh and twelfth days after biting.

By the end of April it was apparent that all subinoculations had yielded negative results (as none of the recipients went down with malaria) and all of the test volunteers in this experiment remained in good health. This was an exciting outcome and a clear indication that M.4888 acted as a true causal prophylactic against falciparum malaria by preventing the infection from invading the blood. Plasmoquine was the only other drug to demonstrate this ability during previous studies at Cairns but, unlike the new drug, it was much too toxic for general use in the field as it could only be administered for a limited period under strict medical supervision. Subinoculations were made in the first two vivax experiments on the ninth and fourteenth days after biting. These also proved negative in all recipients, providing another demonstration that the normal development of the blood stages in the primary attack of vivax had been delayed.

Fairley left Britain on 5 March in company with Brigadier Sinton to visit India and Burma to advise on tropical disease problems in the South East Asia theatre of operations at the request of the British Director General of Army Medical Services. Consequently, he was absent from Australia when the first series of experiments on M.4888 were carried out, and he did not arrive in Melbourne until late May 1945 after the initial results had confirmed the early hopes for the new drug. It was already clear that this compound acted on the human malaria parasites in a different way to previously known antimalarials. None of the test volunteers broke through while on the drug, but it was still too early to know whether the drug was able to prevent vivax relapses. By the end of the month all of the test cases in Experiment CV had attacks of vivax malaria and so had one man from Experiment CIX. However, none of the test

Table 2 Cairns experiments with M.4888 First Series

Experiment	*Procedure*	*Results*
CIII falciparum	Short-term; drug from Z–1 to Z+23; 20 bites; Z = 2 Apr 1945; 6 men on M.4888; 100 mg/day.	No breakthroughs; negative subinoculations Z+7 and Z+12; first evidence of causal prophylaxis.
CI vivax	Short-term; drug from Z–1 to Z+23; 20 bites; Z = 9 Apr 1945; 4 men on M.4888; 100 mg/day.	No primary attacks; negative subinoculations Z+9 and Z+14; all had relapses 7 Jun–3 Sept 1945.
CV vivax	Causal prophylactic drug from Z–1 to Z+7; Z = 9 Apr 1945; 4 men on M.4888; 300 mg/day.	Negative subinoculation on Z+9; all broke through 10–29 May 1945.
CIX vivax	Against blood stages; drug from Z+8 to Z+21; Z = 9 Apr 1945; 4 men on M.4888; 200 mg/day.	No primary attacks; all broke through 21 May– 11 Jul 1945.

volunteers in Experiment CI had yet developed any indications of overt vivax infections.

On 5 June a signal was drafted for transmission to London summarising these first encouraging findings. It concluded that 'subinoculations indicate drug has inhibitory or curative action on tissue stage of human malaria parasites and preliminary results indicate superiority to atebrin. Several types of experiments being repeated with higher dosage designed to ascertain cure of vivax infection. Additional supplies urgently needed'.[31]

During the first few months of 1945, while Fairley was overseas and the work at Cairns was devoted to the first series of experiments with the new British drug, there was a major resurgence of malaria amongst Australian troops engaged in operations against the Japanese on the northern coast of New Guinea. This was an entirely unexpected development, given the excellent results of the Cairns experiments that showed that atebrin was able to completely suppress the disease under operational conditions, provided that there was strict malaria discipline as endorsed by the Atherton Conference in June 1944. Fairley was alerted to this situation immediately on his return to Australia. The resolution of this problem, as well as further comprehensive experiments on M.4888, occupied his full attention (and the work of the Cairns unit) for the closing months of the war.

17

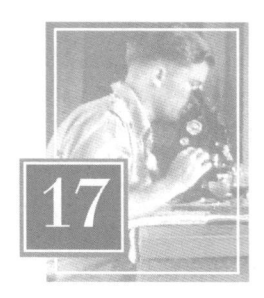

The Possibility of an 'X' Factor

DURING THE LAST year of the war the character of the South West Pacific campaigns changed from a series of bitterly contested strategic struggles of uncertain outcome to mopping up operations against isolated enemy forces. Allied operations in the previous two years had effectively reduced Japanese aircraft and ships to the point at which they could not effectively support their land-based troops. The major enemy-occupied areas were the west Sepik region, on the north coast of New Guinea, as well as the islands of Bougainville and New Britain. The Americans landed at Hollandia and Aitape, on the New Guinea north coast, in April 1944. The port and airfields in these bases were developed as staging points to support the advance to the Philippines. US Army troops repulsed a strong enemy attack at Aitape in August but did not engage in offensive activities to eliminate the enemy from the surrounding area. This responsibility was relegated to 6th Australian Division, comprising 17 500 men of 16th, 17th and 19th Infantry Brigades, under the command of Major General J. E. Stevens. The first elements of the division arrived in September 1944, but lack of shipping delayed the arrival of the full complement of the three brigades until the end of the year.

The area of operations covered 160 km from Aitape to Wewak and inland across the adjacent mountains (see Fig. 10). The flat coastal plain is relatively narrow, ranging from 6 to 20 km wide, and it rises abruptly to the rugged features of the Torricelli and Alexander Ranges, which extend in an east–west direction parallel to the coast, with peaks of the range averaging 1200–1500 metres. In some places rainforest-covered spurs, with steep ridges and deep gorges, extend right down to the sea. The terrain near the shore is often swampy and interspersed with many streams subject to rapid flooding. The

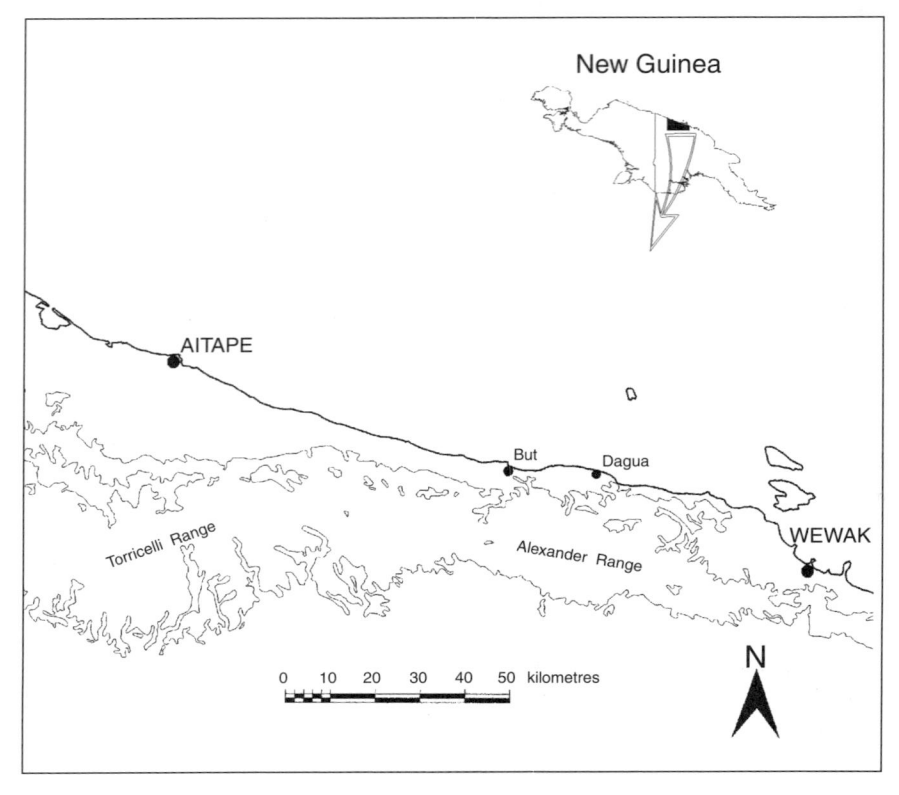

Fig. 10 Area of operations during the Aitape–Wewak campaign, November 1944 to August 1945

whole area, like virtually all of the coastal areas of the island of New Guinea, is highly malarious.

In November 1944 units of the 19th Brigade began a series of active patrols around Aitape to establish the disposition and strength of the enemy forces. The first cases of malaria in the campaign were reported from among these men. Unlike some of the earlier operations in New Guinea, during which malaria rates soared to alarming levels before effective counter measures were instituted, the situation was immediately taken seriously and dealt with promptly. This reflected the dramatic change in attitude of the Australian Army to malaria since the Atherton Conference.

In early December cases rose to around 10–14 per 1000 men per week, and Major G. Read, the Deputy Assistant Director of Health of 6th Division, prepared a report on the status of the disease. Information provided by the malariologist of 43rd US Division indicated that the malaria incidence in

American forces increased from 25 cases per 1000 men per year in June to 125 cases per 1000 men per year in November. Major Read's report concluded: 'The formation is occupying a highly endemic area with the conditions of transmission so well established that the present status approximates to an artificially suppressed epidemic. The slightest laxity in malarial precautions will take its inevitable toll of casualties'.[1]

Major General Stevens held a conference to discuss what should be done. The actual numbers of cases were still relatively few, but boards of investigation were appointed to enquire into possible administrative failures and weaknesses of preventive measures. The commander ordered that every case was to be investigated and, if necessary, disciplinary action was to be taken. He invoked the special provisions of the routine orders on malaria to increase atebrin to two tablets daily, as an emergency measure, and he put the whole of 19th Brigade on this higher dose from 13 December until the end of the month. This measure appeared to be successful, as the malaria cases declined dramatically.

Just before Christmas 1944 the 19th Brigade began to advance along the coast towards Wewak. In late January 1945 the malaria incidence rose again to more than 40 cases per 1000 men per week. Major Read prepared a report that provided a detailed analysis of the malaria cases occurring up to the week ending 26 January. The division had suffered 348 malarial casualties, while the base troops at Aitape had 47. Most cases (71 per cent) proved to be of falciparum malaria; 23 per cent were vivax malaria; and in 6 per cent of cases the parasite species was not determined. Read wrote:

> The conviction is held that there has been an earnest endeavour to ensure thorough atebrin administration. A small proportion of units ... have been found wanting ... There are also units, in which an investigating officer has failed to detect imperfections in administration of atebrin; as a result of this, the officers and men of these units are not only bewildered but fearful of the mounting toll of malaria and the consequences of this—in their minds has arisen some doubt as to the efficiency of the suppressive action of atebrin ... This attitude has been fostered by some medical officers casting around to find alternative solutions.[2]

Read investigated possible reasons for the increase in malaria cases. He found that there was no apparent relationship between conditions of fatigue, exposure, or diet hardship and the incidence of proven malaria because some units enjoying the most favourable circumstances had significant malaria rates, whereas other units who were operating under more trying conditions and in contact with the enemy had few malaria cases. Read reasoned that 'If there were a bulk failure [due to inferior supplies of the drug], a large number of cases of reasonably equal distribution would be expected. With a faulty batch, a reasonably equal distribution for a few days or an increase in malarial casualties, would result. Neither of these conditions has obtained'.[3] However, he noted that there were marked differences in malaria rates between units. Even within a particular battalion the rate of infection in one company was often significantly different from the rate in another company. Read concluded that failure of atebrin administration was the only explanation left that could account for the varying incidence and distribution of malaria cases in the division. Investigations had shown deficiencies in some units but not in others that recorded significantly high malaria rates. In the latter instances it was concluded that

> The nature of the investigation [was] such that minor failures [were] not detected ... The inherent difficulties in proving or disproving perfect atebrin discipline have produced a deadlock. The determining stage is the link between the junior leader and the individual soldier and it is felt that the failure has occurred here.[4]

The senior medical officer of 6th Division, Colonel H. M. Fisher, agreed with Read's assessment.

On 29 January Major General Stevens ordered that the atebrin dose should again be increased to two tablets per day for the whole division. Two days later he convened a conference of commanding officers at divisional headquarters to discuss the alarming increase in malaria in the current campaign, and to consider what could be done to prevent it. Investigations of 150 cases of malaria indicated that in almost all instances there was evidence that atebrin had been taken and that protective measures had been observed, but some lapses were discovered. Disciplinary action was taken against officers where deficiencies were found, and in one case a platoon commander was removed from his post. Stevens said:

> Brigadier Fairley ... is the most eminent malariologist in the world. He has devoted his whole life to this disease. He carried out the most extensive investigations and experiments made in the history of mankind and from that made a definite pronouncement that one tablet of atebrin per day will suppress malaria. It would be presumptuous for us to suggest this authority is not absolutely correct. There must be no weakening of our faith in his doctrine, otherwise the whole structure of anti-malarial measures will collapse.[5]

The order on atebrin administration emphasised that, whenever possible, it was to be given on a formal parade under the command of an officer whose responsibility was to ensure that the tablet was placed in the recipient's mouth after which he was to swallow a drink of water and call his name in a loud voice. Stevens directed that these stringent regulations were to be further tightened. He ordered that the drug was always to be administered on a parade. After taking their tablets the men were to open their mouths so that the inspecting officer could see that they had been swallowed. The new instructions specified that this 'is not a suggested method of ensuring the taking of atebrin, but is the *actual method* which they are ORDERED TO FOLLOW'.[6]

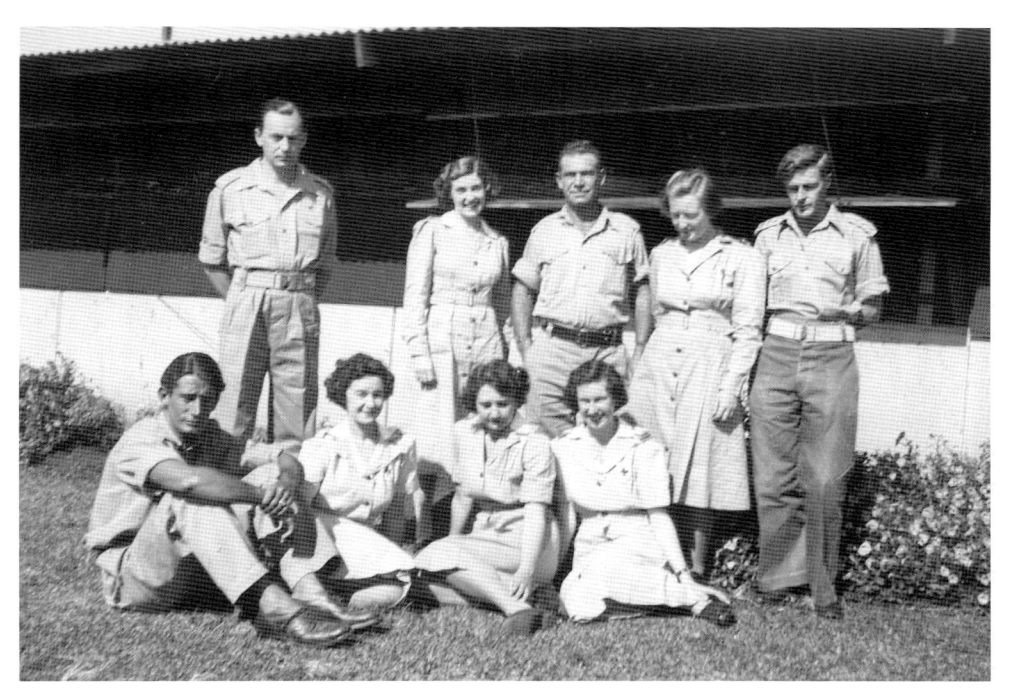

Headquarters staff, LHQ Medical Research Unit: (standing, from left) Lieutenant Colonel Ruthven Blackburn, Corporal Rosemary Gore, Warrant Officer Bill Winterbottom, Private Lorna Hunter, Captain Robert Black; (sitting, from left) Corporal Patrick Fitzherbert, Private Betty Wild, Private Margary Dymock, Private J. A. Birt

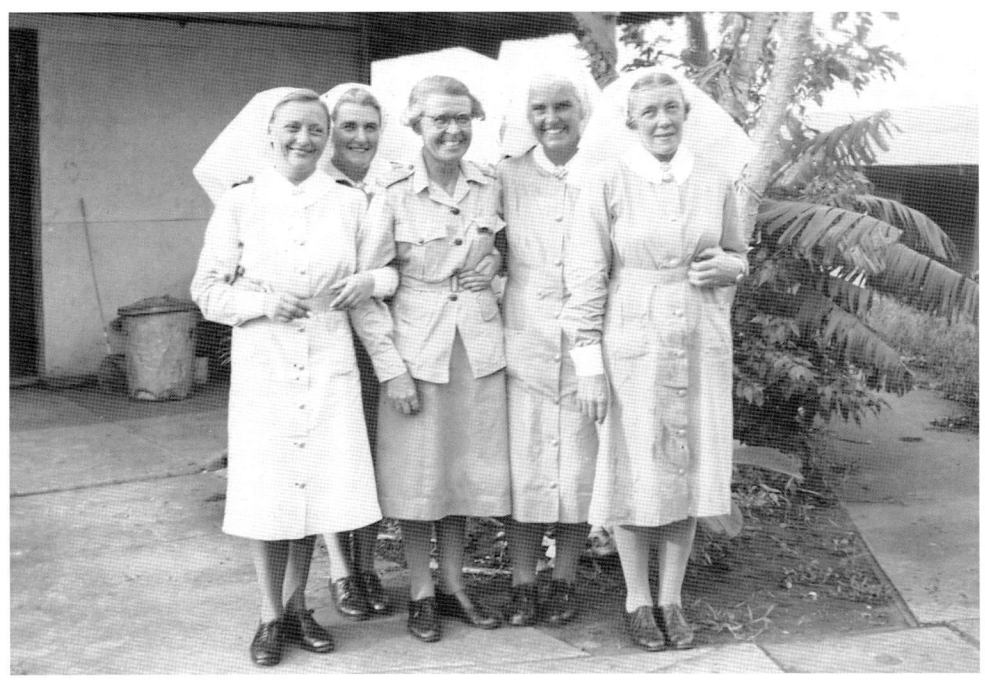

Nursing staff, LHQ Medical Research Unit: (from left) Lieutenant Margaret Stretch, Lieutenant Gladys Goodger, Major Jo Mackerras, Captain Beryl Burbidge (matron), Lieutenant Grace Banks

Lieutenant Colonel Ruthven Blackburn, Major Jo Mackerras, Brigadier Neil Hamilton Fairley

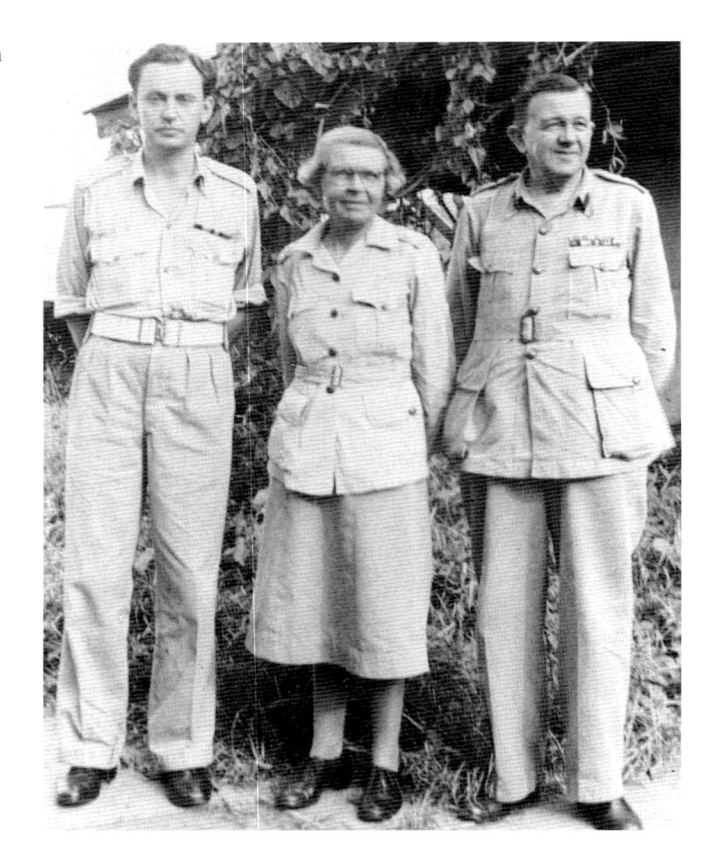

American malaria scientists attached to US 42 General Hospital, Brisbane: (from left) Lieutenant William Trager, Lieutenant Fred Bang, Lieutenant M. Ferguson

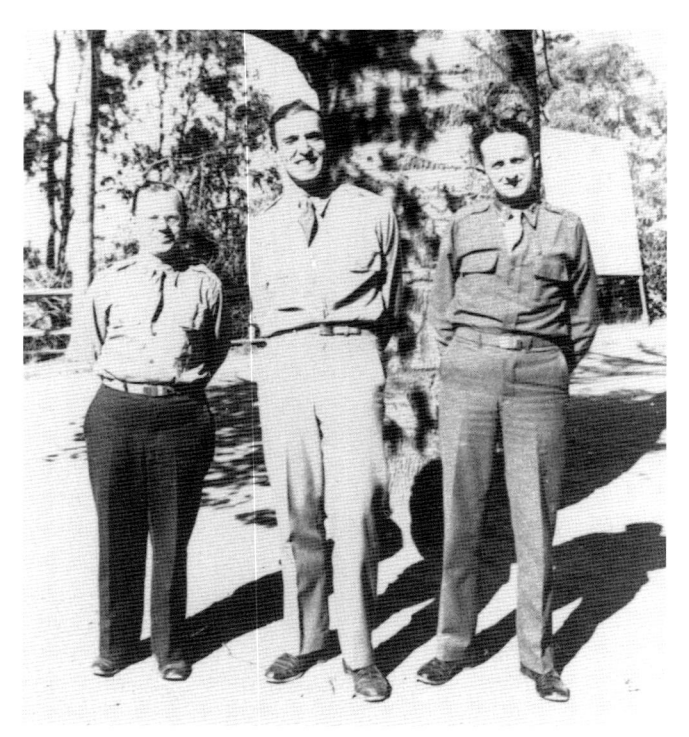

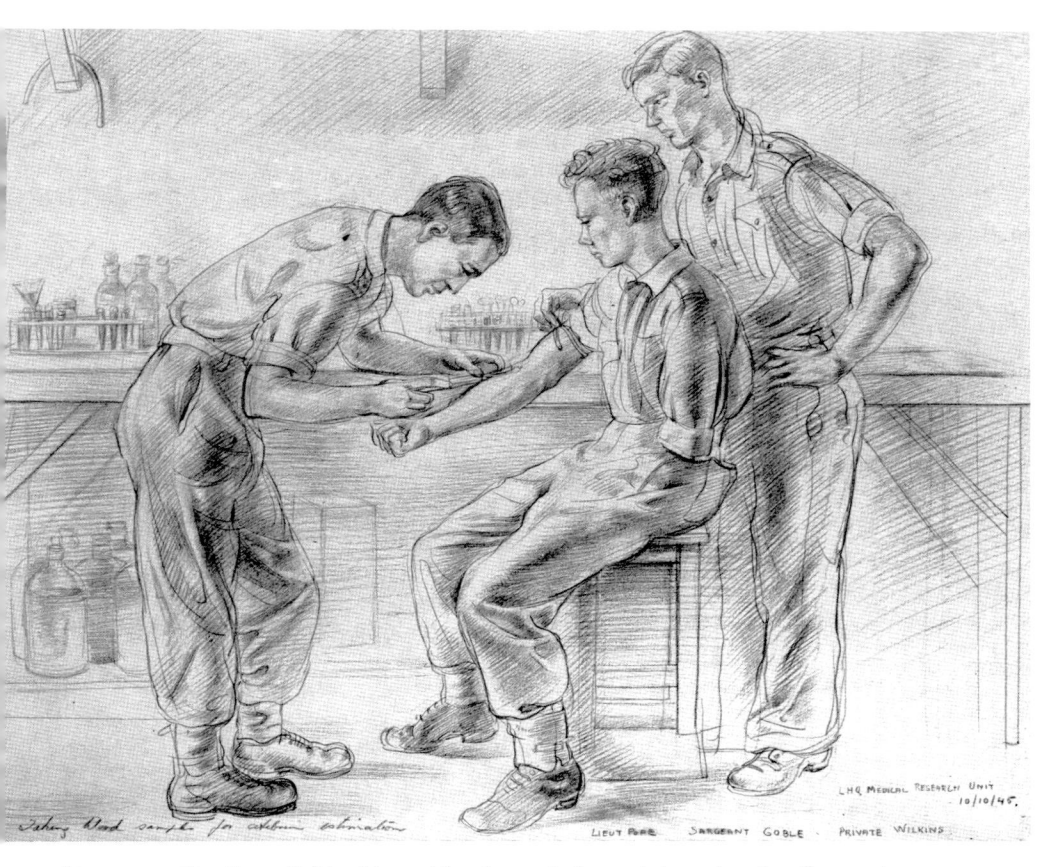

Lieutenant Ken Pope (left) taking a blood sample for atebrin estimation from volunteer Sergeant L. T. Goble. Another volunteer, Private B. Wilkins (right), is assisting by holding the tourniquet (sketch by Nora Heysen).

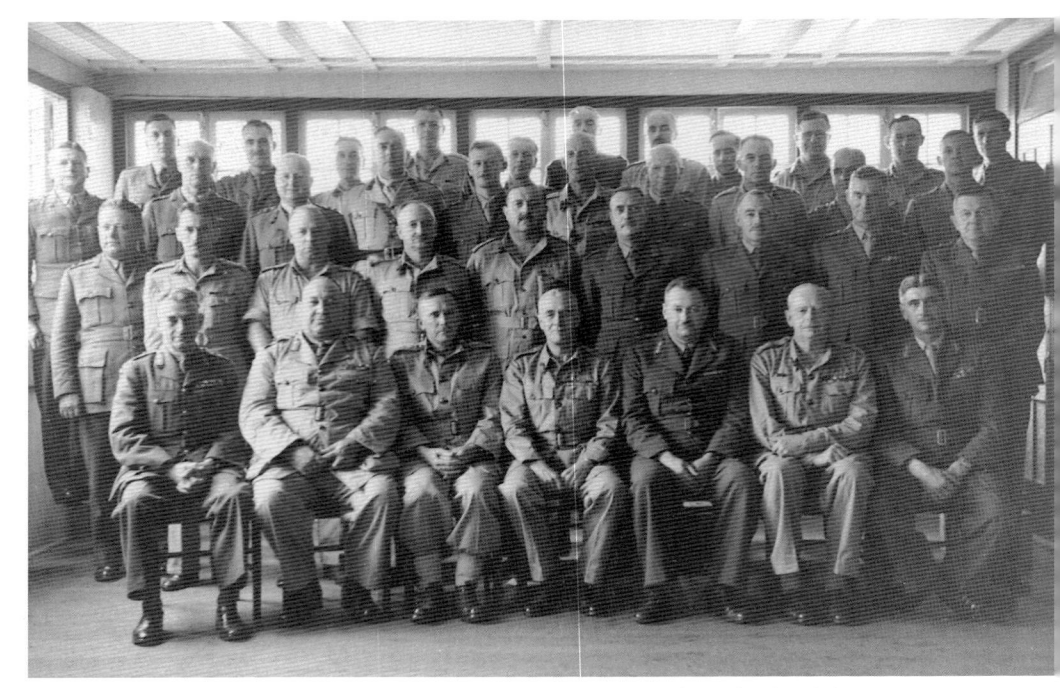

Participants in the conference 'Prevention of Disease in Tropical Warfare' at Atherton, Queensland, 12–13 June 1944. Front row: Major General J. E. Stevens, Commander, 6th Australian Division (extreme left); Lieutenant General V. A. H. Sturdee, General Officer Commanding 1st Australian Army (centre); and Major General S. R. Burston, Director General of Australian Army Medical Services (second from right). Brigadier Neil Hamilton Fairley is on extreme right of the second row

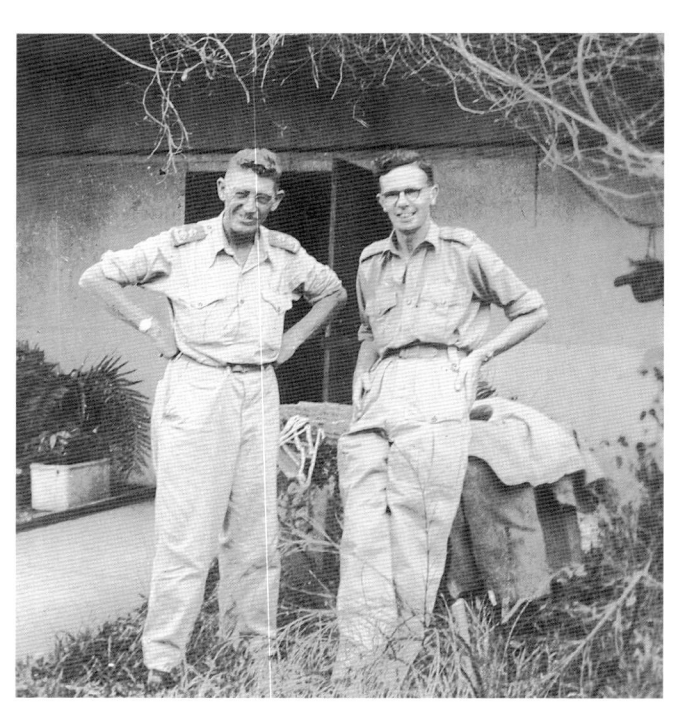

Lieutenant Colonel Ian Mackerras and Major John Tonge

These changes were not well received and some voiced their objections, including the commanding officers of 2/1 Field Ambulance and 2/7 Infantry Battalion, as well as the Division Legal Officer. The Commanding Officer of 2/2 Field Ambulance, Lieutenant Colonel R. S. Smibert, expressed the opinion that the order was wrong in principle, and that the rigid new measures should only be adopted in cases where a soldier had previously contracted malaria. In a formal letter submitted through the chain of command Smibert wrote that if he were in the soldiers' place he would resent the order and the implication that he was not capable of being trusted to carry out a simple instruction. He pressed these arguments strongly in two interviews with Stevens, and requested permission for his views to be passed on to higher authority. Stevens overruled these objections, and directed that the new instructions were to stand.[7]

There is little doubt that an additional underlying reason for the objections to the new order was that many combatant and medical officers of the division firmly believed that the men were already taking their atebrin religiously but that the drug did not always prevent attacks of malaria. In his report of an investigation of cases in 2/7 Battalion Smibert wrote: 'It is felt by some that those who have had repeated attacks of malaria, may not have it suppressed on 1 tablet of atebrin per day'.[8] Smibert thought that one of the cases he investigated was of interest in this respect. This man had had five previous attacks, and was being treated for his second attack in the Aitape area. His brother had died of malaria at Milne Bay in 1943, and his fear of the disease was such that he had been taking two atebrin tablets a day for some considerable time. He was willing to have a blood atebrin test done, and Smibert thought that he should be sent to the LHQ Medical Research Unit at Cairns for further study. Smibert's report was not appreciated by Colonel H. M. Fisher, and it appears that his suggestion to send this patient to Cairns was not followed up.

Brigadier G. B. G. Maitland, the Director of Medical Services of Australian Army forces in New Guinea, visited Aitape at this time for discussions on the malaria problem. Maitland agreed with the decision to place the division on two tablets of atebrin daily as a temporary measure but, in his view, the necessity for doing so was an admission of an administrative failure to ensure that atebrin was being taken by the troops as laid down by Army orders. Maitland was particularly concerned that some unit medical officers had questioned the ability of atebrin to completely suppress every case of malaria. 'The odd spoken word by a unit RMO [regimental medical officer] may undermine all our efforts as regards our inherent belief in the efficacy of our methods ... A case of malaria among medical personnel is a major disaster'.[9] He acknowledged that the medical officers of the division had received no information on the experiments carried out by the LHQ Medical Research Unit. The proceedings of the Atherton Conference had a very limited distribution, and Maitland requested that further copies should be made available to all medical officers, and that they should also be provided with additional details of the studies at Cairns. A special technical instruction on the efficacy of atebrin was subsequently issued from Army Headquarters. This concluded with the statement that 'review of the experimental data and careful analysis of Australian Military Forces malarial statistics make it possible to state with certainty that malarial rates consistently in excess of the minimum must be attributed to some breakdown in administration of suppressive atebrin'.[10]

But there had been attacks of malaria among men of the highest reliability, and this fuelled the misgivings of many members of the division. For example, a private of 3/14 Field Ambulance contracted vivax malaria in December 1944. The Commanding Officer, Lieutenant Colonel R. F. K. West, wrote that he 'has been most thorough in all aspects of malaria precautions. Question arises as to possible necessity of increasing dosage of atebrin in this area'.[11] The following week Lieutenant Colonel West was paraded before the Area Commander and questioned about the case of malaria in his unit. The Standing Orders for malaria prevention of the unit were inspected and found to be satisfactory. In fact, these orders, like all those of the division, were particularly thorough. In addition to the atebrin regulations, the men were given precise and comprehensive orders to prevent themselves from being bitten by mosquitoes. The vectors of malaria bite at night, so personnel were ordered to remain fully dressed with long trousers, long-sleeved shirts rolled down, and wearing boots and gaiters from dusk to dawn except when inside their mosquito nets. Mosquito repellent was applied to all exposed skin before the evening meal, and clothing was not permitted to be removed for purposes of ablutions. A whistle was blown at two-hourly intervals from dusk until 'lights out', as a signal for more repellent to be applied. Before retiring at night and on rising in the morning, the men were instructed to spray the inside of their nets and tents with 'flit guns' containing pyrethrum insecticide to kill adult mosquitoes. On 27 January, the day before Brigadier Maitland arrived in the area, Lieutenant Colonel West himself was diagnosed with falciparum malaria and was evacuated to hospital.[12] This clearly came under the category of 'major disaster' as defined by the brigadier and it must have been the source of lively discussion among West's fellow medical officers. Under these circumstances one can understand the origin of the 'odd spoken word' that Maitland feared would undermine the antimalarial efforts of the division.

Cases of malaria subsided to very low levels throughout 6th Division during February 1945 while the men remained on two tablets of atebrin each day. The 19th Brigade at Aitape went back to one daily tablet at the end of February, but the other two brigades on active operations continued with the higher dose until 22 March. During this period the 16th Brigade continued the coastal advance and cleared the enemy from the airfields at But and Dagua. In mid-April malaria flared up in the units of 16th Brigade, and developed into a sustained epidemic, with weekly incidences of more than 70 cases per 1000 men persisting for the next two months. A reappearance of malaria in 19th Brigade occurred earlier than this, during March, but remained at relatively lower levels of 10–20 cases per 1000 men per week until May.

Wewak was captured on 10 May but the enemy continued to put up a stiff resistance in the adjacent inland hills. There was a sharp rise of malaria amongst 19th Brigade units at the end of May. This could have been partly influenced by increased exposure to infected mosquitoes, as the upsurge occurred two to three weeks after the brigade took over the lead on the coast in the final advance towards Wewak. Cases in 17th Brigade, which was engaged in operations inland from the coast, also increased, but they remained at lower levels than the other two brigades. The epidemic peaked in June with an incidence rate of more than 1200 cases per 1000 men per year.[13] This outbreak, in which more than 80 per cent of confirmed cases were falciparum malaria, caused consternation at all levels of command (see Fig. 11).

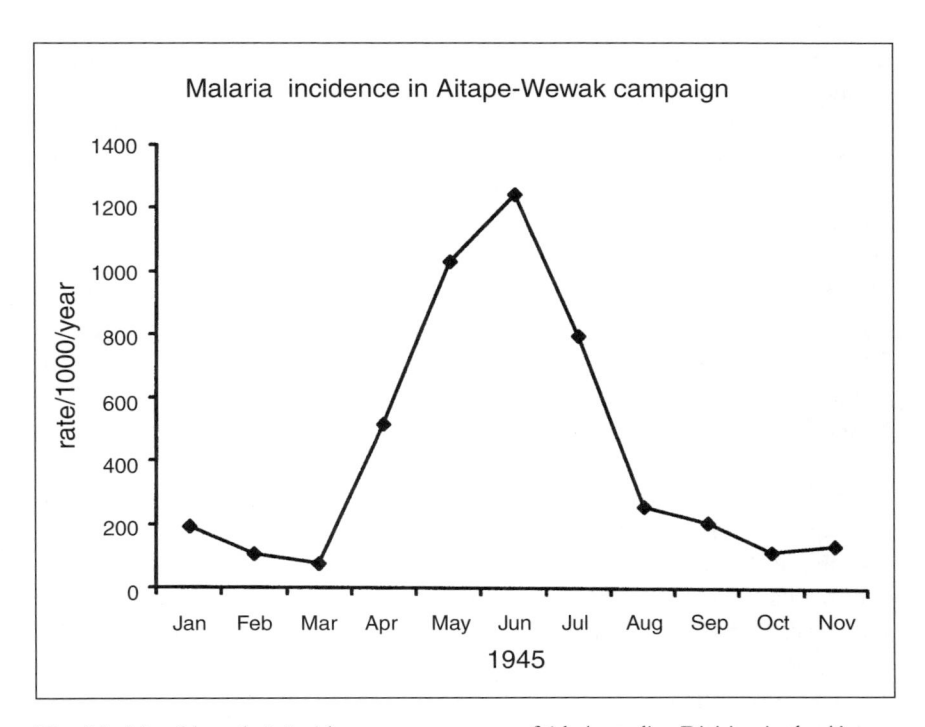

Fig. 11 Monthly malaria incidence among troops of 6th Australian Division in the Aitape–Wewak area during 1945

The high incidence of malaria in the Aitape–Wewak area was in marked contrast to the very low rates prevailing elsewhere in the South West Pacific Area at that time. At the peak of the epidemic, in mid-June, Major General Stevens ordered two experienced unit commanders, Lieutenant Colonel C. H. Selby of 2/7 Field Ambulance, and Lieutenant Colonel R. F. Jaboor of 2/2 Field Regiment, to visit 3rd Division on Bougainville and 5th Division in New Britain. They were instructed to find out the details of all measures adopted in these areas for prevention of malaria in order to investigate whether any additional precautions could be employed by 6th Division. The investigating officers found that in many cases the actual amount of atebrin taken was more than the regulation dose of one tablet a day. Some units were put on two tablets a day when the malaria incidence seemed to be rising, and other units were put on this increased dose when engaged in strenuous marches or patrols. One combatant officer said the troops preferred atebrin to aspirin for headaches. Selby and Jaboor visited 15 units and Headquarters in Bougainville, and estimated they were taking 12–14 atebrin a week. After returning to his unit in Wewak, Selby wrote that, in his opinion, 'Brigadier Fairley is absolutely wrong in saying 1 atebrin a day in a highly malarious area under fighting conditions will control malaria'.[14]

Lieutenant Colonel Blackburn often received correspondence from individual medical officers requesting advice on malaria treatment and prophylaxis. He heard of the worrying malaria situation at Aitape from similar sources as the problem developed. For example, Major Frank Fenner, malariologist of 1 Australian Corps, wrote in early May 1945: 'I suppose you know that 6 Div figures are up again—300 a week'.[15] He requested details of the Cairns results on atebrin, and asked how many cases had been on weekly atebrin regimens of 600 mg or more without any failures of suppression. Some other comments Blackburn received around this time suggested that there appeared to be breakdowns in the ability of atebrin to prevent attacks of malaria in the Aitape area. His response was to urge that examples of falciparum malaria cases demonstrating this phenomenon should be immediately transported by air to LHQ Medical Research Unit so that their parasites could be studied.[16] The mechanism for evacuating malaria-infected soldiers was well established by the practice of obtaining gametocyte carriers from New Guinea for the Cairns experiments. Lieutenant Colonel Smibert's suggestion, in January 1945, that an interesting case should be sent from Aitape to Cairns was not heeded, but ultimately, a man with a history of relapsing falciparum malaria was evacuated from Aitape and admitted to LHQ Medical Research Unit (as case 620) on 11 May.[17] He was reported as having six attacks in 14 weeks.

This soldier had been off atebrin for two weeks before his arrival in Cairns and he exhibited blood stages of falciparum malaria within several days. His plasma atebrin levels were around 2–5 µg per litre, and it was known from previous results that this was insufficient to suppress *Plasmodium falciparum*. His parasitaemia rapidly increased into a full-blown attack with high fever (39.8°C) on 19 May. He was then given 2000 mg quinine (in divided doses over two days), and supervised administration of 100 mg atebrin per day was commenced. His parasitaemia declined initially after drug therapy commenced, but blood stages persisted at moderately high levels for the next two weeks despite his daily atebrin intake. Blood atebrin levels were monitored closely during this period, and were in the range 14–27 µg per litre. Previous work at Cairns had shown that atebrin levels consistently higher than 12 µg per litre were sufficient to suppress falciparum malaria. So the persistence of parasites in this man, despite an adequate amount of the drug in his circulation, was unique, as such a phenomenon had not previously been observed. However, 'one swallow does not make a summer', and this observation, while of consuming interest, did not constitute sufficient evidence to demonstrate a general breakdown in the ability of atebrin to suppress malaria in the Aitape–Wewak area.

Fairley was absent from Australia when these events were unfolding. He remained in England until the first week of March 1945, and then left for a tour of Burma, India and Sri Lanka to advise on malaria and other tropical disease problems in South East Asia Command. He made this trip in company with his friend and colleague Brigadier Sinton. While in Burma, Fairley heard that there had been a serious malaria breakdown among 19th Brigade in January–February 1945. During April he met Major General S. R. Burston in India, who advised that the rate had fallen following the institution of increased atebrin dosage to two tablets a day.[18] Fairley and Sinton travelled together until the final leg of their trip, which ended in Colombo. Sinton left for Australia by air on 6 May and later in the month he visited New Guinea, accompanied by Ian Mackerras. On 30 and 31 May Sinton attended conferences of medical officers and unit commanding officers in Wewak convened to solicit his opinion on the serious malaria problem. He heard first-hand accounts of the epidemic from those who were actually involved in dealing with the situation. In the course of an informal chat with Lieutenant Colonels Smibert and Selby, both Sinton and Mackerras conceded 'that there might possibly be some factor not found elsewhere which is preventing atebrin from suppressing malaria'.[19]

Fairley returned to Australia on 21 May, and received orders from General Thomas Blamey to proceed to Wewak to personally investigate the situation.[20] He had addressed similar issues several times already during the present war. While in London during January 1945 he expressed his current thoughts on the possibility of malaria breaking through standard atebrin prophylaxis. During the Burma campaign several medical officers in a field ambulance developed attacks of malaria, despite the fact that they were reputed to have been conscientiously taking atebrin. But there was no evidence of the drug in their urine. In response to a written request from Sinton for his opinion on this matter, Fairley replied:

> In the past year I have been led up the garden path myself by similar stories. Since the Cairns experiments I no longer believe them ... I do not believe that the majority of Burmese strains are likely to be so atebrin-resistant that 1 tablet taken every day will not result in clinical suppression in the majority of cases. Nor do I know of any scientific evidence that such atebrin-resistant strains do in fact exist.[21]

Fairley's initial thoughts on the Aitape–Wewak epidemic have not been recorded, but there is little doubt that he considered it in the same light. This view would have been reinforced by the fact that there were extremely low rates among all other Australian units operating in highly malarious areas at that time. The most likely explanation was that the malaria problem in 6th Division was due to failures of atebrin discipline. Fairley, Blackburn and others at the Cairns unit certainly subscribed to this opinion when first hearing of the problem, and they had extensive and impeccable experimental results to back it up. There had been no failures of atebrin prophylaxis in 113 experimentally infected volunteers, despite massive mosquito infections involving South West Pacific isolates of both falciparum and vivax malaria and exposure to the most arduous conditions of physical stress. On the other hand, some medical personnel and combatant officers who were in the Wewak area and saw the situation at close quarters entertained serious doubts as to the consistent efficacy of the drug. They felt sure that the vast majority of troops were complying with the extremely rigid atebrin regulations, and this belief was strengthened by attacks of malaria that occurred in some senior men of the highest integrity and reliability. For example, Brigadier J. E. G. Martin, the commander of 19th Brigade, was admitted to hospital with malaria on 25 May.[22] This event must have been very unsettling for his headquarters staff and the officers in his brigade who were personally responsible for implementing the regulations on atebrin. From such incidents there developed a strong suspicion that, for some unknown reason, atebrin was not always doing its job as a suppressive. Thus, the idea arose that this unknown 'X factor' was responsible for the epidemic.

By the end of May Blackburn had confirmed the persistence of *P. falciparum* in case 620, despite what should have been adequate atebrin levels to suppress the blood stages. But this was only one case that had not been exhaustively studied according to the meticulous experimental procedures followed at the Medical Research Unit. Blackburn knew that Fairley would soon return to Cairns, so he decided not to commence any experiments with parasites from this case before Fairley's arrival.[23] In the meantime, the administration of suppressive atebrin was continued, and the patient's parasitaemia persisted at moderate levels. Fairley flew up from Melbourne during the first week of June and remained at the unit for 10 days before departing for New Guinea to personally investigate the epidemic. Blackburn told Fairley about case no. 620, who still had parasites in his blood despite taking atebrin each day for three weeks, and they discussed what should be done.

Sinton and Ian Mackerras arrived in Cairns from New Guinea on 6 June and participated in the discussions. It was important that this case, with parasites refractory to atebrin, should be followed up with observations of other cases contracted in the Aitape–Wewak area. Fairley resolved that, on his impending visit to New Guinea, he would personally arrange for other men from 6th Division to be flown to Cairns so that their response to atebrin could be studied. The men would be specially selected on the basis of having recurring attacks of malaria contracted in the present campaign. In discussions with Blackburn, Jo Mackerras and other members of the research group, a detailed protocol was devised so that the individual isolates could be maintained either by directly feeding mosquitoes on the Aitape–Wewak cases (if gametocytes were present in their circulation) or by blood inoculation to volunteers who would later be subjected to mosquito feeding. The ultimate objective was to maintain a number of separate parasite isolates at Cairns, each derived from a different field-infected patient, which could then be subjected to drug sensitivity experiments in volunteers. In the meantime this procedure was commenced with the first Wewak patient already there. On 11 June 1 ml of blood from case 620 was subinoculated into an uninfected volunteer for further studies with his parasites.

Fairley flew to Port Moresby by Sunderland flying boat on 12 June, and left for First Australian Army Headquarters in Lae on the following morning. Over the next four days he had discussions on the malaria situation with the senior combatant and medical officers in the area, including the Commander-in-Chief of Australian Ground Forces General Blamey, the Commander of First Army Lieutenant General V. A. H. Sturdee, the Director of Medical Services Brigadier Maitland, and malariologist Lieutenant Colonel J. English. He flew to Wewak on 16 June, where he met Major General Stevens and Colonel D. M. Salter, the senior medical officer, and toured local medical units. On 18 June, before departing for Aitape, Fairley gave a talk on malaria to the medical officers of the division. Lieutenant Colonel West, who had already been hospitalised with malaria in the present campaign, recorded that this was 'a magnificent lecture . . . This was the outstanding lecture we have had since arriving in the area'.[24]

After inspecting the situation in the field and discussing the malaria problem with the local authorities Fairley decided that the factors that should be considered were:

> (a) Was 'Atebrin' being supplied in the correct dosage and was it being taken daily with unvarying regularity . . . (b) Was 'Atebrin' being absorbed normally and were adequate blood concentrations being built up in troops taking 'Atebrin' in the

Wewak area? (c) Were 'Atebrin'-resistant strains of *Plasmodium falciparum* and *Plasmodium vivax* affecting troops in the Aitape–Wewak area and if so to what extent were they responsible for the epidemic?[25]

Even though the atebrin tablets used by 6th Division were similar to those supplied to other Australian troops, it was decided to submit samples of various batches for analysis by Dr Adrien Albert of the Department of Organic Chemistry, University of Sydney. Albert's observations subsequently showed that the actual dosages and disintegration times of these tablets were within satisfactory limits.

Fairley decided that a field section of the LHQ Medical Research Unit should be formed and based at Wewak. In the third week of June Major I. C. Macdonald, malariologist of II Australian Corps, took up the appointment of Officer Commanding this section, which was attached to 104 Casualty Clearing Station, with Major J. I. Tonge as pathologist. Fairley returned to Wewak from Manila on 27 June where he met Major Macdonald, and next day laid down a program of work to be carried out by the field detachment. He instructed that an extensive clinical and parasitological survey should be made of troops in the area. Large numbers of blood samples were to be collected and flown to Cairns for plasma atebrin estimations. Lieutenant Colonel Ian Mackerras was appointed Malariologist, 1st Australian Army, and was sent to Wewak to study the entomological aspects of the epidemic. Mackerras conducted a survey of the area with Major J. E. C. Aberdeen to provide an epidemiological background to the investigation. During his visits to medical units in Lae, Wewak and Aitape, Fairley earmarked selected cases with a history of recurrent malaria attacks for evacuation to the Medical Research Unit at Cairns and arranged for further similar cases to be sent there after his departure. He flew from Lae to Cairns on 1 July by air ambulance, accompanied by five of these special cases.

The malaria epidemic peaked in 6th Division just before Fairley's arrival in Wewak. There was a decline in the number of cases in 16th Brigade during the second week of June. Atebrin dosage was increased to two tablets on 22 June, and the rate in the brigade declined further to around 10 cases per 1000 men per week by mid-July. Malaria figures in 19th Brigade followed the same trend by decreasing in mid-June, even though these troops remained on one tablet a day throughout this period. This reduction may have been partly due to the mosquito control commenced in the Wewak area during May with aerial application of DDT. From June until the end of the campaign 25 square km of the surrounding area were regularly subjected to spraying by aircraft, as well as by intensive control measures on the ground.[26]

The first group of five patients selected by Fairley from 16th Brigade units were admitted to the Medical Research Unit on 16 June. Three of these men had negative blood films at the time of admission but had a history of falciparum malaria characterised by one to three recrudescences within a short period after completing their initial treatment. All were immediately placed on the standard prophylactic dose of 100 mg atebrin daily. One man had low plasma atebrin on admission, but his levels increased gradually during the next two weeks; he was subsequently discharged without developing an attack of malaria. Another patient had satisfactory plasma atebrin levels when he arrived, but these declined during the next two weeks, even though the drug was administered under supervision. He was later observed to be chewing gum on atebrin parade. A well-known method to avoid swallowing atebrin was to secrete it inside the mouth within the gum. He was then told that he had little chance of obtaining leave, and would remain indefinitely in the north while his attacks of malaria continued. Subsequently, his plasma atebrin returned to satisfactory levels, though his blood films remained negative and he was discharged from the unit.

The third patient with negative blood films (case 2) had low atebrin levels when he was admitted on 16 June, and his drug level remained low despite daily atebrin administration. Blood stages of falciparum malaria appeared on 22 June, and his parasite levels rose during the following week while, at the same time, his atebrin levels declined. He was then informed that there was little chance that he would be able to proceed south on leave while his malaria attacks persisted. Thereafter his atebrin levels returned to normal, but falciparum stages remained at microscopic levels, even though the amount of atebrin in his circulation should then have been sufficient to destroy them. The failure of the drug to rapidly eliminate the parasites in this man was similar to the lack of atebrin response in case 620 during the previous month. Blood from case 2 was subinoculated into a volunteer on 26 June for further study of these parasites. The other two patients (case 4 and case 6) were both suffering from overt attacks of falciparum malaria when admitted to the Medical Research Unit. Their attacks were stabilised with quinine, and they were subinoculated into uninfected volunteers.

So, by the end of June the workers at Cairns had obtained tantalising preliminary evidence for two radically different explanations for the epidemic. Two of the patients evacuated to Cairns had been avoiding atebrin, so this supported the arguments of those who said that the malaria problem was due to deficiencies in atebrin discipline. Conversely, another two men had been shown to have sufficient atebrin in their circulation to eliminate the blood stages of falciparum malaria, but their parasites still persisted. This suggested that there was truth in the assertion that atebrin in the standard daily dose did not always prevent malaria in the Wewak area, and pointed to the possibility of resistance. Of course, this information was not released outside the unit at that time. This would have been premature as the investigation was far from complete.

It was initially hoped that mosquitoes could be infected from the first patients admitted to the unit from Wewak. This proved impractical due to pressure of work relating to other experiments on M.4888 in progress at the time. Also, some of the original cases had few gametocytes. However, the recipients of subinoculated blood from cases 620, 2, 4 and 6 all developed satisfactory numbers of gametocytes, and mosquitoes were infected from them.

During the next two months more than 40 selected patients were evacuated from Wewak to Cairns. Five of these (cases 7, 8, 19, 22, and 30) developed good numbers of *P. falciparum* gametocytes in their peripheral blood, and separate batches of mosquitoes were infected from each of them. Parasites persisted in the original patient (case 620) for more than a month despite his daily atebrin dosage that was confirmed by adequate blood levels of the drug. On 17 June he commenced a daily dose of 100 mg of M.4888 for a week. His blood films were negative within two days, and parasites did not return after drug treatment ceased. This suggested that, even if some of the parasites from the Wewak area proved to be atebrin-resistant, they might respond to the new drug.

A normal experimental approach to investigate the epidemic would have been to undertake preliminary clinical observations of the selected patients from Wewak, and then to progressively extend the work in order to systematically study the susceptibility of their parasites to the drug. However, those responsible for the health of the troops in the field needed the issue to be resolved as rapidly as possible, and the realisation that the war would soon end provided additional urgency towards finding a solution. A most elegant series of experiments was designed to unambiguously assess the atebrin sensitivity of the individual parasite isolates from the Wewak area in the shortest possible time. The strategy involved maintaining the parasites from each donor separately by feeding different batches of mosquitoes either on the recipients of infected blood from evacuated patients (isolates from cases 620, 2, 4 and 6) or directly on the patients evacuated from Wewak (isolates from cases 7, 8, 19, 22 and 30). These mosquitoes were used to infect volunteers in two experiments (AW-I and AW-II) conducted concurrently.[27]

In experiment AW-I the atebrin response of each of the nine parasite isolates was investigated separately in nine separate pairs of volunteers (see Table 3). One man from each pair took 200 mg of atebrin per day for a week before being bitten by infected mosquitoes and continued to take 100 mg per day for 28 days afterwards. The other man did not take the drug and acted as a control. Each pair was allocated a single parasite isolate from Wewak, and the two men received 10 infective bites from mosquitoes infected with that isolate. The mosquito batches were fed on donors at different times (to coincide with the presence of gametocytes in their circulation), so the actual day of biting varied accordingly, with the first pair of volunteers being bitten on 10 August and the

Table 3 Experiment AW-1: First documented evidence of drug-resistant malaria. Chronology of clinical experiments of nine isolates of *Plasmodium falciparum* from Aitape–Wewak area

Isolate[a]	Arrival at Cairns[b]	Z day[c]	Results
620[d]	11 May 1945	13 Aug 1945	Broke through on drug 26 Aug 1945.
4[d]	16 June 1945	10 Aug 1945	Broke through on drug 22 Aug 1945.
6[d]	16 June 1945	13 Aug 1945	Broke through on drug 22 Aug 1945.
2[d]	16 June 1945	10 Aug 1945	Broke through off drug 11 Sept 1945.
8[e]	1 July 1945	20 Aug 1945	Broke through on drug 1 Sept 1945.
7[e]	1 July 1945	22 Aug 1945	Did not break through.
19[e]	18 July 1945	22 Aug 1945	Broke through on drug 27 Sept 1945.
22[e]	26 July 1945	28 Aug 1945	Did not break through.
30[e]	5 Aug 1945	30 Aug 1945	Broke through off drug 8 Oct 1945.

[a] Isolate numbers correspond with those in the published report of the Aitape–Wewak investigation (Fairley et al., 'Atebrin susceptibility of the Aitape–Wewak strains . . .', pp. 229–73).
[b] Date of arrival at LHQ Medical Research Unit, Cairns of soldier from Aitape–Wewak area with history of recurrent falciparum malaria.
[c] Day of biting of 10 infected mosquitoes on volunteer test case at Cairns. Test case commenced 100 mg/day of atebrin seven days before biting, and continued for 28 days afterwards.
[d] Isolate subinoculated from Aitape–Wewak soldier to uninfected recipient volunteer. Mosquitoes fed on the recipient were used to infect a volunteer test case taking atebrin.
[e] Isolate transmitted experimentally by direct feeding of mosquitoes on Aitape–Wewak soldier. These mosquitoes were used to infect a volunteer test case taking atebrin.

last on 30 August. The volunteers were examined daily using the usual comprehensive clinical, parasitological and biochemical methods adopted for the Cairns experiments. After each control broke through, his parasites were maintained by subinoculation to an uninfected recipient.

One of the test volunteers in AW-I (isolate 4) broke through with blood stages of falciparum malaria on 22 August, 12 days after biting, while he was still taking 100 mg of atebrin per day. His parasitaemia increased during the next week into a full-blown attack. The atebrin dose in this man was increased to 200 mg per day on 30 August, but parasites persisted until his attack was terminated with M.4888. During the last few days of August three other test cases in this experiment broke through while taking atebrin (isolates 620, 6, and 8), and another three broke through within one to two weeks after they ceased taking the drug (isolates 2, 19 and 30). Only two isolates (7 and 22) did not break through in the test volunteers during the period of observations. The men in this experiment were subjected to the same drug-testing procedures as the atebrin groups at Cairns in early 1944. In the earlier experiments none of more than 100 test cases infected with falciparum malaria broke through, provided that they had a build-up before biting and maintained an adequate atebrin concentration by taking at least 600 mg of the drug each week throughout the period of exposure and for one month afterwards.

This result was the cornerstone of the rationale for drug prevention of malaria expounded by Fairley at the Atherton Conference, and subsequently promulgated with the full weight of the disciplinary provisions of General Routine Orders. Yet seven out of nine men infected with *P. falciparum* from Wewak developed overt attacks of the disease, despite the fact that they had been taking what should have been adequate prophylactic doses of atebrin. These breakthroughs provided unequivocal evidence that atebrin-resistant parasites were present in the Wewak area. This finding was without precedent in the history of the fight against malaria. There had been reports of suspected cases of resistance to quinine in several parts of the world, including Brazil in 1910, and in Macedonia during World War I. However, a review of these early reports suggested that they may have been due to strain differences of parasites in different areas.[28] Moreover, these previous observations had not been subjected to the painstaking experimental verification of the studies at Cairns.

The second experiment, AW-II, compared the activity of atebrin and M.4888 against simultaneous infections with all nine isolates from Wewak. This experiment was started shortly after AW-I, using batches of mosquitoes infected from the same nine donors. It included a subgroup of four volunteers on the same atebrin regimen as the first experiment, as well as another subgroup on 100 mg of M.4888 per day from the first day of biting until 28 days after the last bite. Each man in each of the two subgroups received a total of 41–3 bites (2–11 bites from different batches of mosquitoes infected with each of the nine parasite isolates) between 20 August and 3 September. All four men in the atebrin subgroup broke through with microscopic levels of parasites 7–12 days after the onset of biting while they were still taking the drug. None of the men on M.4888 developed malaria while they were taking the drug, nor was there any evidence of parasitaemia after drug administration ceased, thereby indicating that all were cured of their infections. Thus, these first two experiments not only confirmed the existence of parasites refractory to atebrin but also suggested that these resistant parasites could be dealt with by the new British drug.

During this period the field section of the Medical Research Unit collected many blood samples from 6th Division troops at Wewak. Fairley attempted to obtain representative samples by directing that surprise visits were to be made to units immediately before their daily atebrin parade, and groups of 10 men at a time were to be taken to the field section under close supervision for blood collection.[29] The plasma was separated by centrifugation in the field laboratory, and packed on ice for dispatch by aircraft to Cairns where the atebrin content was analysed by B. B. Brodie and S. J. Udenfriend's method. The results showed that the atebrin levels of most samples were within the range of values that should have been sufficient to prevent the development of malaria. The results of parasitological surveys among the troops showed that 14 out of 155 men had microscopic levels of *P. falciparum* parasites in their blood without suffering any symptoms of malaria, and atebrin estimations indicated that their drug levels were satisfactory. A result such as this had never been observed previously, even in heavily infected volunteers at Cairns. This provided direct evidence from the field that atebrin-resistant parasites were present in the Wewak area. It was also noted that the clinical attacks of malaria in the epidemic were unusually mild, with a very low incidence of the severe symptoms often associated with falciparum malaria. This indicated that, even when overt attacks developed, the clinical manifestations of the disease were ameliorated by atebrin.

Ian Mackerras directed his efforts towards investigating the source of the malaria infecting the Australian troops. During July he and Major J. E. C. Aberdeen made a malaria survey among New Guineans living in the coastal village of Hawain, about 16 km west of Wewak. Dissections of anopheline mosquitoes collected in the area showed that around 2 per cent were infected with sporozoites. Immediately after the end of hostilities on 15 August Mackerras and Aberdeen carried out a survey that showed that more than 50 per cent of Japanese soldiers had malaria parasites in their blood. This was done on the day that the enemy troops came in from their positions before their malaria rates had time to change. A summary of the survey results showed that the highest parasite and gametocyte rates in the area occurred in New Guinea infants, followed by older New Guinea children and the Japanese. The Australians were not near local children except for brief periods when they moved through villages, but the men in the forward units were often within mosquito flight-range of the enemy. The published report of the survey concluded that 'our troops acquired an overwhelming proportion of their infections in the coastal area from the Japanese'.[30]

Fairley was in Cairns when the war ended, and he returned to Wewak several days later where he addressed a conference on malaria. Those present included the 6th Division brigade commanders: Brigadiers R. King (16th Brigade), M. J. Moten (17th Brigade) and J. E. Martin (19th Brigade) (who had already contracted malaria in the present campaign). Unit commanders and local heads of services were also present. Brigadier King opened the meeting by outlining the purpose of the conference. He said 'Investigations had been made and were being made into the unusual incidence of malaria in this area. We have all been waiting with great interest to see what conclusions have been made. Brigadier Fairley asked that you come here today to hear his preliminary report and discuss such conclusions as had already been reached'.[31] Fairley then described the steps that were being taken to investigate the problem in the Aitape–Wewak campaign and the results obtained to date. Parasite rates in New Guinea villagers and mosquito surveys conducted by Mackerras suggested that the risk of infection in the Wewak area was no higher than in other coastal areas of New Guinea. This implied that the local malaria hazard must be regarded as similar to that of the other areas of current operations in Bougainville and New Britain. The higher incidence of the disease in the present campaign was discussed at length, and the data on cases in the different brigades of 6th Division were analysed.

In describing the current investigations at Cairns, Fairley related the observations of the specially selected cases evacuated by plane from Wewak. On the day that he was giving this talk the first test volunteer on atebrin in experiment A-W I broke through while still taking the drug. Fairley could not have known this at that time but, in any case, it would have been premature to promote the idea of resistance until the experiments were completed and all the data had been analysed. He emphasised the positive aspects of the present situation by pointing out that most men in the division had not contracted malaria. Moreover, the symptoms in those who had broken through were milder than expected, which he had no doubt was due to the suppressive effect of atebrin. However, he did say that a parasite survey had shown that 'a certain proportion of troops in the Wewak area [around 9 per cent] actually have malaria of a type that, though not at the time sufficiently severe for admission to hospital, may later produce symptoms necessitating this being done'. He concluded: 'If atebrin-resistant strains from Wewak are not discovered at Cairns no conclusion can be made from this investigation except that the vast majority of malaria attacks in the 6th Division had resulted from irregular atebrin intake'.

Within a month after the end of the war, the field investigations at Wewak were completed, and the final results of the two experiments on the Aitape–Wewak strains at Cairns were analysed. The findings showed: (1) evidence that some cases were due to failures of atebrin discipline and (2) unequivocal confirmation that some of the parasite isolates were resistant to atebrin. Two obvious questions arose from these results. First, what proportion of cases in the epidemic was due to failure to take the drug with unvarying regularity and what proportion was due to drug resistance? Second, what was the origin of the resistant parasites?

Seven of the nine strains investigated at Cairns were atebrin-resistant but these were isolated from specially selected cases characterised by having a history of multiple attacks of falciparum malaria. Also, some men flown down from Wewak were shown to be avoiding atebrin but, again, these were among the specially selected group. Consequently, these observations were of little value in answering the first question as they were not derived from a representative sample of the malaria-infected troops in Wewak.

However, other data were analysed by Fairley to address this question. Even though almost 90 per cent of confirmed cases in the epidemic were due to *P. falciparum*, there were four times as many *P. vivax* cases in the Aitape–Wewak campaign than in Bougainville and New Britain during late 1944–45.[32] Experimental work at Cairns demonstrated that the blood stages of *P. vivax* were more susceptible to atebrin than those of *P. falciparum*. Vivax malaria was invariably suppressed by weekly doses of 400 mg, whereas breakthroughs of falciparum malaria had occurred at this dose. Only one strain of *P. vivax* was isolated from the Aitape–Wewak area during the epidemic. It showed normal susceptibility to atebrin, and there was no indication that any *P. vivax* cases in the Wewak area failed to respond to the drug. Thus, as few as four tablets per week should have been enough to prevent clinical attacks of vivax malaria, yet more than 700 cases were recorded among 6th Division and base support troops who were supposed to be taking seven tablets per week (and for part of the time 14 tablets per week) throughout the campaign. Fairley concluded that these overt vivax attacks must have been attributable to defective atebrin intake.

The published account of the investigation noted that the incidence of malaria attacks in officers of the 6th Division was only half that of non-commissioned officers and privates.[33] The significance of this was not discussed, but readers might have inferred that officers had fewer attacks because they were more conscientious in complying with atebrin regulations than the other ranks. Another point raised in this article was that medical opinion in the Aitape–Wewak campaign considered that the epidemic was characterised by a high incidence of *P. falciparum* recrudescences. But this was not borne out by the overall multiple attack rate that indicated only 1.3 attacks for each infected case. This rate was about the same as in 7th and 9th Divisions in the Ramu campaign of the previous year, and was considered to have a direct bearing on the proportion of atebrin-resistant cases. Fairley pointed out that the Cairns experiments on the *P. falciparum* cases evacuated from Wewak had shown that they were not cured by routine quinine, atebrin and plasmoquine (QAP) treatment. Such a result had rarely been observed previously and was most unusual. He argued that, if atebrin-resistant parasites were responsible for most cases in the Wewak epidemic, there should have been many secondary attacks in the infected men, but this was not the case. Thus, the small number of subsequent attacks that were recorded at Wewak following treatment indicated that the common strain producing malaria was sensitive to atebrin. So, in reviewing all the available evidence, he clearly inclined to the view that, even though some *P. falciparum* parasites were atebrin-resistant, most cases that occurred in the Aitape–Wewak epidemic were due to failures of atebrin discipline.

But this was a matter of considerable controversy and there were some dissenting voices. Lieutenant Colonels Selby and Mackerras wrote separate letters to the editor of the *Medical Journal of Australia* shortly after Fairley's paper was published. Both agreed wholeheartedly with the major thrust of the article, but each raised concerns about this issue. Selby wrote:

> It was extremely difficult for a man to avoid taking the official dosage of atebrin, though no doubt a few possibly feeble-minded persons did so ... Brigadier Fairley's table wisely shows officers and other ranks separately. It is quite a fact and possibly an indication of bad discipline that many officers in the 6th Division were taking more than 1 atebrin tablet per day, as they should have been threatened with courts martial and disgrace should they contract malaria. This table is valuable, therefore, provided one does not assume that officers took only 1 atebrin tablet per day. One officer (evacuated through medical channels!) was taking 12 tablets a day.[34]

Fairley's point about failure of QAP treatment to cure cases of atebrin resistance was supported by the data generated at Cairns, but the evidence was not entirely clear cut. In experiment AW-II this treatment failed to cure three out of three test cases who broke through while receiving atebrin. Each of these men was infected with all of the nine isolates derived from Wewak patients. However, one man in experiment AW-I, who had been exposed to a single isolate of falciparum malaria derived from a Wewak patient, broke though five days after ceasing his daily atebrin dosage, and his infection was subsequently cured by QAP. None of the other resistant isolates was treated individually with this regimen, so it is not possible to know the proportion that it would have failed to cure. Nevertheless, one resistant isolate was cured by QAP. This weakens the argument that the lack of secondary attacks in the epidemic implied that most parasites were atebrin-sensitive.

The field investigation showed that around 9 per cent of the troops surveyed at Wewak had *P. falciparum* parasites in their blood, even though they had adequate atebrin levels and exhibited no symptoms of the disease. Fairley noted that 'it is evident from these observations that the degree of infection in the division exceeded the reported malaria rate, since such individuals were not admitted to hospital for treatment'.[35] It is probable that some of these cases were unreported recrudescences. There is also another possibility, which is purely speculative, but which might have some bearing on this issue. The men serving in this campaign had a powerful incentive not to report sick with malaria after being the object of official scrutiny following their first attack. Some may have resorted to self-medication with extra atebrin tablets on developing the premonitory symptoms of a second attack, rather than face the prospect of possible disciplinary action, and this may have resulted in under-reporting of recrudescences. Consequently, there may have been deficiencies in the figures quoted by Fairley to indicate that there were few secondary attacks following treatment and to support the argument that the majority of cases were due to atebrin-susceptible parasites. On the other hand, there has never been any indication that *P. vivax* parasites developed resistance to atebrin, so the vivax malaria cases recorded during the epidemic provided unequivocal evidence that some men avoided the drug. This must have been a significant factor affecting the number of *P. falciparum* cases that occurred. But what proportion fell into this category, and did it exceed the proportion of cases due to resistant parasites? These are vexed questions since there is insufficient information to provide accurate answers.

Fairley also considered the source of the resistant parasites. In the concluding remarks he wrote: 'The origin of the Aitape–Wewak relatively atebrin-resistant strain is a matter of conjecture. The fact that it was first found in an individual who had purposely been avoiding atebrin suggested that it might be arising like strains of bacteria resistant to sulphonamides . . . as a result of sub-optimal dosage'.[36] In a subsequent article he elaborated on this point:

> The quality of relative atebrin resistance may have arisen suddenly as a mutation in soldiers taking atebrin, or constituted an inherent biological characteristic of a geographically limited strain. On the other hand, the fact that it was first demonstrated in an individual who was purposely avoiding taking atebrin, suggested that it might be originating as a result of prolonged sub-optimal dosage.[37]

Mackerras disagreed strongly with the suggestion that inadequate atebrin dosages among 6th Division troops stimulated the development of resistant parasites: 'Whatever their sins of omission in taking their atebrin, one feels that they must be acquitted of the suggestion that they added to their woes by breeding atebrin resistance in their parasites'.[38] He believed that the development of such a phenomenon would have required many parasite generations through humans, as well as through the complete sexual cycle in mosquitoes. Mackerras felt that there was insufficient time for this to have occurred in the Australian troops who had only arrived in the area several months previously. He thought that the resistance may have been naturally present in a local strain of the parasite, or that it may have been selected by irregular atebrin intake by Japanese troops. Captured wartime documents revealed that the Japanese used atebrin for prophylaxis and treatment in New Guinea. Acute shortages of supplies in the latter half of the war probably led to administration of inadequate doses of the drug, and this could have contributed to the emergence of atebrin-resistant parasites.[39]

In the years since World War II many experiments with animal malaria parasites have demonstrated that drug resistance can develop rapidly following the administration of suboptimal levels of antimalarial compounds. It is now commonly believed that drug resistance to human malaria parasites can develop in a similar way, but it is difficult to pinpoint the origin of such occurrences in the field. The Aitape–Wewak epidemic is the only 'report of a reduction in the sensitivity of any human malaria parasite [to atebrin] that may be directly related to the use of the compound itself'.[40] It is not known why atebrin resistance did not develop in other areas of New Guinea and elsewhere. As Ian Mackerras pointed out:

> The greatest difficulty, however, in accepting atebrin resistance as a new character developed during the war was its complete failure to appear anywhere else in the field, although it had boundless opportunities to do so throughout 1943 and the first quarter of 1944. Nor did it appear in any strains previously isolated at Cairns, although many of these originated from men taking inadequate atebrin, for example, in areas where the official dosage was then 300 mg per week.[41]

This enduring puzzle has often been noted since then. Why has resistance developed in some areas against a particular drug but not in others? In most instances there are no clear answers to such questions.

A small proportion of *P. falciparum* parasites in the human population around Aitape may have already been naturally resistant to atebrin, and this proportion might have increased by genetic selection after the drug was introduced into the area. Alternatively, resistance may have evolved as a result of inadequate atebrin doses taken by some of the Australian force. The occurrence of a significant number of vivax malaria cases is a clear indication that some of the men were not meticulously following the atebrin instructions, and they might have formed a pool of inadequately suppressed hosts in which resistant *P. falciparum* developed.

There is another possible scenario that does not appear to have been canvassed previously. The Americans landed at Aitape in April 1944, more than six months before the Australians. The incidence of malaria in these troops increased from 25 cases per 1000 per year in August to more than 125 cases per 1000 per year in November, with most cases being due to *P. falciparum*.[42] The report of an American Malaria Mission to the South West Pacific in July 1944 noted that 'there was evidence [among American troops in New Guinea] of very extensive deviation from the recommended regime of 100 mg [of atebrin] per day . . . in some instances it appeared to be a matter of self discipline by enlisted personnel'.[43] Thus, it is possible that resistant parasites first appeared among troops of the original invasion force who were lax in taking atebrin, and that it spread to the Australians after their arrival in the area, some of whom were also neglecting to take the prescribed dose of the drug with scrupulous regularity.

During the latter part of 1945 and in early 1946 the atebrin-resistant parasites were maintained in volunteers at Cairns for further experiments using various drug regimens. It was confirmed that daily doses of M.4888 as low as 25 mg per day were able to suppress the atebrin-resistant isolates. It was also shown that the atebrin-resistant isolates were susceptible to the new drugs

SN-6911 and SN-7618, developed by the Americans.[44] The last experiment (AW-VI) was of particular interest. A volunteer taking 100 mg atebrin per day was bitten by mosquitoes infected with sporozoites of isolate number 8, but did not develop malaria while taking the drug or after drug administration ceased. This result was surprising because the original volunteer in experiment AW-I who was exposed to mosquitoes infected with this isolate broke through with an attack of malaria while he was taking this dose of atebrin. This highlighted the issue of differences in susceptibility to atebrin of the parasites isolated from the different cases infected in the field and the stability of this characteristic after the isolates were maintained at Cairns by cyclical transmission between human volunteers and mosquitoes.

The Atherton Conference in June 1944 was a turning point in the attitude of the Australian Army to the malaria problem. After Fairley's description of the experiments at Cairns, the ability of one tablet of atebrin per day to invariably suppress attacks of malaria was accepted with religious fervour, and the quest to achieve zero malaria cases throughout the various formations of the Army was pursued with missionary zeal. This attitude clearly influenced the extraordinary reduction in malaria casualties in the South West Pacific campaigns during 1945, and it had a direct impact on how the 6th Division dealt with the epidemic in the Aitape–Wewak area. On the one hand, senior officers, including Major General Stevens and Brigadier Maitland, were convinced that some men were lax in taking atebrin because, if they took the drug without fail every day, they could not have attacks of malaria. This argument was certainly valid as far as vivax malaria was concerned, and the *P. vivax* cases diagnosed in the campaign (as well as some of the *P. falciparum* cases) were almost certainly due to failures of compliance with the atebrin regulations. On the other hand, many commanding officers, including commanders of medical units, were convinced that virtually everyone in the division was complying strictly with the orders on atebrin, which indicated (to the exponents of this opinion) that the drug was not always effective in providing complete protection from malaria. The experimental evidence accumulated at Cairns confirmed the validity of this argument in a certain proportion of falciparum cases. So, in the final analysis, there was truth and error in both of the opposing schools of thought.

There was, however, one aspect of 6th Division's response to the epidemic as it developed in 1945 that, in retrospect, seems curiously flawed. The provision in the Army instructions for atebrin prophylaxis to be increased to two tablets daily was implemented for a limited period in December 1944 and again during February–March 1945. In both instances the malaria rate fell after its introduction, but rose again when the formation reverted to one tablet a day. It might have been prudent to continue the two-tablet regimen since field experience had demonstrated its efficacy in reducing the malaria rate in the present campaign. However, the command hierarchy of the formation seemed to place more importance on slavishly following the standard suppressive measures because Brigadier Fairley said that one tablet per day was sufficient to prevent malaria, even though experience had shown that the higher dose was necessary to achieve this goal.

It may be of interest to speculate on what might have happened if Fairley had been in Australia when the first cases of malaria appeared at Aitape. There is little doubt that he would have arranged for evacuation of selected cases to Cairns for investigation at the Medical Research Unit in January 1945. This should have resulted in early confirmation of atebrin-resistant falciparum malaria and would have led to a more accurate analysis of the proportion of cases infected with resistant parasites and the proportion caused by failures of drug compliance. It is important to appreciate, however, that no effective substitute was then available to replace atebrin, and Fairley's actions and those of the commanders in the field must be viewed against this background. The newly developed American and British drugs were still in the early stages of development, and only small quantities were available for experimental purposes. The only other drug which available for operational use in 1945 was quinine, and experiments at Cairns had already shown that it was not an effective suppressive of South West Pacific strains of malaria. It was important that the troops maintain faith in atebrin and continue to take the prescribed dose each day as they had nothing else to replace it. If there had been widespread failures of compliance, the malaria incidence would have been disastrously high and significant numbers of deaths from cerebral malaria could have ensued. The drug continued to provide suppression of vivax malaria and, even though there were confirmed instances of *P. falciparum* resistance, the symptoms were milder in those cases than in patients who were not taking atebrin at all. In his analysis of the situation at Wewak in August 1945 Fairley emphasised the fact that most of the men in 6th Division did not contract malaria and were protected by the suppressive effect of atebrin.

18

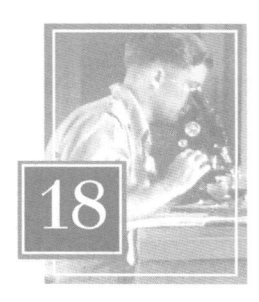

Paludrine

THE RESOURCES OF the Medical Research Unit were stretched to the limit in mid-1945. The operational situation demanded that the Aitape–Wewak problem be faced as a matter of urgency while, at the same time, there was a burning scientific imperative to evaluate the new British drug M. 4888. Both developed into major research activities that continued in parallel at Cairns during the closing months of the war.

An important question concerning the latter project was whether M.4888 could prevent relapses of vivax malaria. Consequently, the four test volunteers in the first short-term vivax experiment with M.4888 at Cairns (CI) were observed with particular interest after they had completed their 23 daily doses of the drug after being bitten by infected mosquitoes (see Table 2 in Chapter 16). The first man broke through with an overt attack on 7 June (Day Z+59)—36 days after the last dose—and this was recorded in the first preliminary report of the experiments sent under a covering letter to Colonel Anderson in London on 10 June.[1] When discussing the mode of action of the drug, the report noted:

> The results of these experiments, with particular reference to the subinoculations, indicate that administration of M.4888 (a) delayed the initial appearance of trophozoites in volunteers exposed to *P. vivax* sporozoites and (b) prevented the appearance of trophozoites in volunteers exposed to *P. falciparum* sporozoites. No evidence of a curative action has been obtained in the volunteers exposed to *P. vivax*.[2]

In the ensuing weeks this latter comment was reinforced as the other test cases in Experiment CI broke through with vivax malaria: one on 28 June; another in August; and the final case in the first week of September.[3]

But there was still the possibility that a higher dose might prevent the appearance of vivax relapses. This raised the question of the dosage range over which the new British drug was safe. During the earlier trials on the American-produced drugs SN-6911 and SN-7618 Fairley insisted that there was adequate data to confirm that they were safe for humans at the proposed dosage regimens before the experiments at Cairns commenced. The experiments on M.4888 were undertaken before complete toxicology data were obtained, but Fairley applied the same criteria by asserting that the test dosages to be used at Cairns would first need to be confirmed as being safe for humans. This was an important objective of the British testing program in which the drug was administered to different human subjects for varying periods and dose regimens. As the safety of lower doses was established the dosage was increased by small increments in successive tests during which the subjects were carefully monitored for toxicological manifestations. During February 1945 test cases of vivax malaria had been treated at the Liverpool School of Tropical Medicine with doses as high as 150 mg twice a day for 14 days without exhibiting any toxic signs or symptoms. So this was the highest dose regimen adopted for the first series of experiments at Cairns.

Sometime after Fairley's departure for Australia via India and Ceylon in March 1945 he received a signal from Major S. J. Goulston in London:

> Following impression gained during recent visit ICP [*sic*] Manchester and Tropical Medicine Liverpool. First. High dosage necessary [to] destroy all tissue forms in bird malaria. Second, Liverpool dosage now up to 350 mg twice daily for 14 days with no repeat no toxic symptoms ... Dr G. Davey recommends you run 23 day experiment on the lines of experiment one [i.e. CI of the first series] using 300 mg once daily and will provide further supplies of drug for this purpose.[4]

Goulston subsequently reported to AHQ Melbourne on a meeting of the Therapeutic Sub-committee, held in London on 27 April, at which it was mentioned that the dosage in experimental work at Liverpool was up to 550 mg twice daily for 14 days without any evidence of toxicity.[5]

These reports influenced the plan for the second series of experiments at Cairns, which was prepared and sent to London at the same time as the preliminary report.[6] The aims, as stated in the protocol, were:

(1) To observe whether malaria could be prevented or cure could be obtained by increasing the dosage of M.4888 used in earlier experiments.
(2) To determine the mode of action of M.4888.
(3) To observe the efficacy of 100 mg daily administered over a period of three months during intensive repeated infections.

The first objective was addressed by three experiments with vivax malaria, each with six test volunteers on M.4888, using the same format as those of the first series. The numerical designation was also the same, followed by the letter 'B'. Thus, CIB involved administration of 300 mg daily from the day before exposure to the 23rd day afterwards; the test cases on CVB took 1000 mg daily during the incubation period; and those of CIXB took 1000 mg daily for two weeks commencing on the ninth day after biting. The three groups each received 20 infective bites on 16 June 1945.[7] As with the first experiments none of the men broke through with parasites while taking M.4888. Only one man in CIB broke through during the observation period at Cairns, 19 days after ceasing the drug, but three of the remaining five men in this group subsequently had vivax relapses. Four of the six volunteers in each of the other two experimental groups developed malaria between three weeks and two months after the last dose. Drug administration in Experiment CVB was restricted to the period before the parasite entered the circulation so, even though the initial attack was delayed, the subsequent development of overt malaria showed that the drug was not acting as a causal prophylactic of *Plasmodium vivax*, even at a dose of 1000 mg per day.

The third objective in the protocol followed the scheme developed at Cairns for the long-term field-type experiments first used with atebrin. This involved a group of 10 volunteers who each received 100 mg of the test drug daily: eight with M.4888; the other two received the same dose of atebrin and acted as controls. This experiment, designated CXX, commenced on 9 June.

During the next two months each volunteer received a total of 250 bites from infected mosquitoes (130 with *P. falciparum* and 120 with *P. vivax*). The men were subjected to similar stresses as those of the earlier long-term groups: heavy exercise involving marching for long periods in mountainous tropical conditions, exposure to cold temperature in the Cairns meatworks, and adrenalin injections. For the last two biting sessions on 6 and 10 August each man received 10 infective bites from one of the atebrin-resistant strains isolated from the Aitape–Wewak area, after which they remained on the drug for a further 28 days. None of the men taking M.4888 had breakthroughs with *P. falciparum* either during or after the period of drug administration. Similarly, none had vivax malaria while taking M.4888, but all eight volunteers in this group had *P. vivax* parasites in the peripheral blood between 15 and 23 days after the last dose. All developed into clinical attacks of vivax malaria. The two men on atebrin remained free of the disease during the period of biting, but both came down with falciparum malaria while still on the drug within four weeks of the last infective bites. It is probable that the latter result was due to inadequate suppression of the 'relatively atebrin-resistant' strain. Both cases were cured by a course of treatment with M.4888.

The results of the first experiment with M.4888 (CIII—conducted in April 1945) showed that falciparum malaria was prevented by daily administration of

100 mg of the drug for 23 days after biting. This group followed the usual scheme developed for short-term experiments at Cairns, and the negative subinoculations from test cases on the seventh day after biting suggested that the drug may prevent the development of the disease before it entered the circulation.

During early September 1945 an experiment was undertaken in which M.4888 was administered during the incubation period of mosquito-induced falciparum malaria. There were two groups of three volunteers (one group receiving 100 mg per day and the other group on 300 mg per day) from the day before until six days after being bitten by 20 infected mosquitoes. Two other similar groups of volunteers were bitten at the same time, and received the same dose regimens for two weeks from the seventh day after biting. Subinoculations from all six volunteers receiving the drug in the first week after biting were negative, and none of these men developed malaria. On the other hand, all test cases in the other groups who received the drug in the second week after biting had positive subinoculations on Z+7, but none developed overt attacks after ceasing the drug. This implied that M.4888 was a true causal prophylactic of falciparum malaria if administered during the incubation period, and that it was also able to eliminate the blood stages if administration was delayed until the parasites entered the circulation.

These latter results were augmented by observations at Cairns in which the drug was administered for therapy of overt malaria in experimentally infected volunteers and in patients with naturally acquired infections. It was found that even a single dose of 100 mg given to volunteers with falciparum malaria eliminated their blood parasites and improved their clinical condition until they felt well. However, this result was only temporary, as parasites later reappeared and they developed another attack.

Several different therapeutic regimes were tested at Cairns, but the most common course adopted for falciparum malaria was 300 mg daily for 10 days. This treatment cured all but one of 88 sporozoite-induced infections.[8] More than 50 attacks of vivax malaria were cleared of parasites and clinical symptoms after treatment with 1000 mg daily for 14 days. For both kinds of malaria the clinical response was not rapid and symptoms persisted longer than did trophozoites in the peripheral circulation. It was hoped that the higher dose regimen might prevent relapses of vivax, but a number of subsequent attacks were recorded in the months following this treatment.

An experiment was conducted at Cairns with the other British drug, M.4430, during July 1945. This followed the usual short-term experimental procedure in which six volunteers were given daily doses of 200 mg from the day before being bitten with 20 vivax-infected mosquitoes until Z+23. Subinoculations indicated that the normal invasion of the circulation did not occur on the ninth day after biting, but all test cases developed overt attacks between 16 and 60 days after the last dose.[9] These results implied that the action of M.4430 against vivax malaria was similar to that of M.4888, as both drugs acted as partial causal prophylactics by delaying the primary attacks, but they were not able to prevent later attacks of the disease. No further work was done on M.4430 in Australia as preliminary work in England had suggested that it may be less effective than M.4888 and the potential of the latter had already been amply confirmed by the trials at Cairns.

The work on the British drugs conducted between June and September 1945 was the last large-scale experimental series carried out at Cairns. By that time the M.4888 experiments had involved more than 180 volunteers, and Fairley was tremendously impressed with the outcome. In a letter to Colonel Anderson in London he said:

> I have no doubt whatever regarding the unique position of this drug in malaria therapy. Provided it does not manifest unsuspected toxicity when given over prolonged periods of time, it will onset [*sic*] all other suppressive drugs not excluding atebrin and sontoquine and its modifications. When taking this drug, parasites are not liberated from tissue cells into the circulation. This holds for vivax as well as falciparum infections, though in vivax infections asexual parasites appear some time after ceasing the drug, whereas in falciparum infections they do not.[10]

However, a deficiency which hampered a complete understanding of the results was the lack of a method for measuring levels of the drug in the test subjects. This was clearly realised at the time that the first experiments were subjected to preliminary analysis, as indicated in a letter from Blackburn to Colonel Keogh (who by then had replaced Downie as senior medical officer at the Australian Legation in Washington) on 1 June 1945:

> The action of the drug appears to resemble plasmoquine in that we get negative subinoculations at the end of the sporozoite-schizont phase. Results of vivax malaria suggest that the drug may have a persistent effect not unlike that of atebrin as well. We have no clear information on this as we are not doing drug estimations.[11]

It was important to know for how long the drug remained in the body after administration and what plasma concentrations were required to kill the parasites or to prevent their multiplication. The amount required for suppression of the disease or for therapy of clinical attacks could not be determined without a method for measuring quantities of the drug in body fluids. Such a method would permit analysis of the rates of absorption into the blood after ingestion, as well as subsequent excretion in the urine. By this means it would be possible to establish the time required for equilibrium levels to be achieved in humans on a particular constant dose regimen and to determine the time for individual doses to attain peak blood levels, as well as to estimate the rates of 'die away' due to metabolism and excretion. The individual variability of drug levels between different people on the same dose regimen could also be investigated. These kinds of data formed an important part of the atebrin research at Cairns. At the time that the M.4888 studies were in progress, plasma atebrin estimations played a crucial role in analysing the factors responsible for the Aitape–Wewak epidemic, and helped confirm the presence of atebrin-resistant parasites. The lack of a similar method to estimate blood levels of the new drug must have been felt very keenly.

Confirmation of this was provided in a signal sent from AHQ Melbourne to Colonel J. H. Anderson in London:

> Fairley reports investigation being handicapped by lack of technical information re plasma estimations. Arrange through medical research council that details of any method available be supplied immediately. Also cable list of chemical reagents and special apparatus required so that these can be sent fastest from London if not available here.[12]

Professor Brian Maegraith of the Liverpool School of Tropical Medicine wrote a letter to Fairley in response to this signal on 24 September.[13] He said that a preliminary report of the Liverpool work with M.4888 was being forwarded via Anderson. This included a description of a method that was a modification of the analytical procedure developed by Spinks for the estimation of M.4430. They had found it 'workable and accurate' for estimations of M.4888 in whole blood, plasma and urine. The plasma build-up during 14-day courses of 50 or 500 mg at 12-hourly intervals rose to a plateau after four to five days, and the urinary excretion followed the same trend. It was observed that 'die away' in both plasma and urine concentrations was considerably faster than that of atebrin. In his reply of 5 December Fairley said the information 'in regard to the rate of disappearance of paludrine . . . [was] very helpful in interpreting the results of certain experiments regarding the action of this drug as a causal prophylactic'.[14]

On 6 November an article under the headline 'New drug, wonder cure for malaria' was published in the Sydney *Daily Telegraph*. This announced the discovery, relayed from London, of a revolutionary new drug discovered by British chemists for the treatment of malaria. The drug, paludrine, was reported as being the 'most powerful antimalarial weapon yet produced'. The article mentioned that clinical trials had been in progress since February at the Liverpool School of Tropical Medicine and that more than 100 cases had been treated successfully. It also stated 'supplies were then flown to Australia, where very extensive clinical trials established that paludrine is not only more effective, but less toxic, than either atebrin or quinine'.

The press report of this announcement came as a complete surprise to the staff of the Medical Directorate at AHQ Melbourne and they did not quite know what to make of it. Members of the Australian Broadcasting Corporation and the press contacted Fairley requesting further information, and this placed him in a quandary. All of the work on the British drugs in England and at Cairns had been carried out under the stipulations of wartime secrecy and, even though the war had ended, it was not clear exactly what information had been released and by whose authority. The press report mentioned that it had been announced by Lord Leverholme, the head of Imperial Chemical Industries, at the annual meeting of the Liverpool School of Tropical Medicine. The British drugs had been synthesised and developed by ICI and their commercialisation rights were not in question, but the wartime work had been co-ordinated under the auspices of the Medical Research Council. The Australian clinical testing program had been formally requested through the MRC, and it would have seemed logical for any press announcements to go through this official channel. Also, the mention of 'paludrine' was quite mystifying. This name had been given to an earlier drug of the series, M.3349, but it had never been made available for testing in Australia where studies had been limited to M.4430 and M.4888. This led Fairley to make an official denial that any work on the newly announced drug had ever been done either at Cairns or on patients with malaria in Australian military hospitals.[15] The press were not pleased with this response, particularly as their British sources mentioned specifically that it had been tested extensively in Australia. It appeared that the local military hierarchy was deliberately withholding information that had already been freely released overseas.[16]

The first official word on the announcement was sent as a signal from Australian Army Staff London to AHQ Melbourne.[17] This made the following points: that M.4888 was now called paludrine; that a statement written by Maegraith had been presented on 5 November at the annual meeting of the Liverpool School of Tropical Medicine; and that the only reference to Australian work was that supplies were flown to Queensland for trial. It concluded with a suggestion that Brigadier Fairley make a statement to the Australian press providing a general description of the Cairns research unit, with special reference to the work done on paludrine, including number of cases involved. A final point was that the Australian representatives of the British press could be requested to forward the statement for publication in England. The signal was dated 6 November, but the press channels carried the news to Australia more quickly than the military ones. It did not arrive until after the *Telegraph* article was published and after press representatives had bombarded the Australian Medical Directorate with questions on paludrine that they could not answer.

Colonel Anderson was caught in the middle of this embarrassing debacle, and he later explained to Fairley how it had come about.[18] During the war, control of information on secret drugs in Britain was handled by the Censorship of Medical Information Sub-committee. It appeared that, following the abolition of wartime censorship, this body simply ceased to function, but Anderson was not informed, even though he was the Australian Army member on the committee. This fact was also not known to another key member of the committee, Dr A. Landsborough Thomson, the Principal Assistant Secretary to the Medical Research Council. The first intimation that Anderson had of a public announcement was mentioned by Dr C. M. Scott of ICI on 26 October. Maegraith wrote to Anderson on 2 November, but this was delayed over a weekend and did not arrive until the day that the announcement was to be made. This letter provided the first advice that M.4888 was to be called paludrine.

Anderson was clearly exasperated with these developments, and wrote that 'as a rule we are able to keep pace with events but in this case I always seem to be a step behind'.[19] He realised that there was no chance of stopping the press announcement so he thought that the best option was to ensure that the medical and lay press knew that work on paludrine was being done in Australia so, at his request, a statement to this effect was inserted in it. He then notified AHQ Melbourne by signal, and thought it best to await full details from Australia before making further comments. This seemed to him to be the best way to ensure that adequate credit was given to the Australian contribution rather than relying on incomplete accounts derived from signals. Anderson had heard that Lord Leverholme initiated the push for publicity and, he added, 'To be quite fair to Maegraith, he naturally thought that I would know of the lifting of the ban'.[20]

The news was announced to the medical community in an article entitled 'Triumph against Malaria' published in the editorial section of the *British Medical Journal* on 10 November 1945.[21] This provided details of the development of paludrine, based on information acquired by the Medical Research Council. The early wartime work on the search for new synthetic antimalarials was summarised, and an outline was given of the British experiments on M.4888. The clinical trials and preliminary pharmacological studies conducted at Liverpool were described, and it was mentioned that supplies were sent by air to Australia for experiments in volunteers at Cairns. This background information was reasonably correct with regard to the British work, but it certainly did not accurately reflect the importance of the Australian contribution. Moreover, comments were made on the action of the drug that were seriously misleading. The article stated that, in the case of sporozoite-induced vivax infections, 'apparently this antimalarial action is a suppressive one, exerted upon the trophozoites as soon as they appear in the erythrocytes'.[22] At that time, the only information known to British scientists on the action of the drug against mosquito-transmitted infections was contained in the first report of the experiments at Cairns received by the Medical Research Council in July 1945. Subinoculations conducted in these experiments had shown that the drug acted in a quite different manner by delaying the initial appearance of trophozoites in volunteers exposed to vivax sporozoites. In a note of unintended irony the concluding paragraph of the article criticised the use of the name paludrine, 'which had already been applied to an earlier less successful product . . . For some time to come this use of the same name for two different substances will cause needless confusion'. The editors did not realise that this situation had already arisen and caused acute embarrassment to the Australian Army Medical Directorate.

The development of paludrine was clearly a triumph of British chemical research, but proof of its value as a malarial drug was overwhelmingly derived from Australian investigations. Clinical trials in England were limited to its use for therapy of naturally acquired infections—predominantly vivax relapses with a smaller number of falciparum cases. The work at Cairns covered the full spectrum of activity against sporozoite-induced vivax and falciparum infections. This included its action as a causal prophylactic, its suppressive activity against the blood stages, its use for treatment of overt attacks, and its ability to protect troops against repeated bites of infected mosquitoes under conditions simulating the stresses and strains of tropical warfare. The latest Australian results were not known in England at the time of the press release. The first report sent to London gave a preliminary account of only the first two months' work at Cairns, but it contained more information on the antimalarial activity of the new drug than all of the British clinical trials conducted in 1945. It was regrettable that this was not accurately reflected in the editorial comments of the *British Medical Journal*. In any case, common courtesy dictated that the Australians should have been informed before any announcement was made.

After receiving the first news on the British announcement the Medical Directorate took steps to placate the Australian press by retracting their earlier comments, and the news media was informed that a statement regarding the work would be issued as soon as it could be arranged. Efforts were also made to prepare an up-to-date report incorporating the latest experimental data for transmission to England. On 9 November Fairley sought information from Cairns requesting the total numbers of volunteers used in all experiments with M.4888, as well as the numbers used in suppressive and therapeutic trials.[23]

A signal was dispatched to Australian Army Staff, London, several days later.[24] Commencing with the statement, 'Fairley reports Cairns investigations definitely confirm superiority paludrine over atebrin', it summarised the major findings derived from the Australian experiments. In the first direct response to the paludrine announcement Fairley wrote to Anderson on 4 December with restrained understatement: 'We took rather a poor view of the way the publicity regarding M.4888 was handled'.[25] He described the difficulties encountered with the local press over this issue, and referred to the summary of the main conclusions cabled to London during mid-November: 'We have been working very hard on the experimental approach at Cairns, and have much additional information which will be incorporated in a progress report and sent [to] you before the end of the year'. Fairley thought that the best way to rectify matters was to suggest that the Medical Research Council write a review of this report for the *British Medical Journal* to bring their first report up to date. He further proposed that statements should be released simultaneously to the Australian and British press.

He was equally restrained but direct in a letter written next day to Maegraith in Liverpool: 'It was unfortunate that this Directorate was not informed beforehand that an announcement was to be made about M.4888, that it had been named paludrine, and that an up-to-date summary of our results could not have been published at the same time and liberated simultaneously in the British and Australian press'.[26] Major General Burston reiterated this view in a formal memo to London at around the same time.[27]

After receiving the memo from the Director General of Medical Services (DGMS), Anderson wrote a letter to Dr Landsborough Thomson pointing out the considerable difficulties the premature news release had unwittingly inflicted: 'There were press accusations that information available elsewhere was being repressed wilfully in Australia; not a pleasant position'.[28] He continued 'Our Medical Directorate feels gratified by its association with the MRC in the prevention of malaria and is pleased at having had the field testing of M.4888 entrusted to it. In consequence, a natural desire exists that the drug should get the full credit its merits warrant'. This was a very diplomatic way of emphasising that credit was also warranted for the Australian research effort without which the full merits of the drug would not have been revealed. The concluding point in Anderson's letter was that the DGMS suggested the simultaneous release of an updated report to the Australian and British press. As it turned out things did not quite happen this way, but ultimately this unfortunate episode was resolved.

One of the key scientists in the ICI research team, Dr D. G. Davey, arrived in Melbourne on 4 December to see the scope of the Australian work on paludrine. After spending several days at the Medical Directorate, he visited Cairns in company with Fairley, and later they both returned to Melbourne. The issue of a suitable news release must have been one of the priority topics discussed with Davey, and it was decided to make an announcement to coincide with his visit. A press conference, called by the DGMS at Victoria Barracks, Melbourne, on 19 December was attended by representatives of the major Australian newspapers. Davey read a prepared statement in which he reviewed the ICI research and screening program that led to the discovery of paludrine:

Our laboratory results were very promising, and then it was quickly confirmed in the Liverpool School of Tropical Medicine that the new drug was a good one. However, special experiments on human beings were required to see if it possessed the particular advantages over atebrin that were being sought. There was only one place in the Empire where these experiments could be done on a sufficiently big scale, and that was in the Research Unit of the Australian Army Staff at Cairns. Thanks to the brilliant work of Brigadier Fairley and his colleagues, and the magnificent help of volunteers from the Australian Army, we have learnt in six months what might easily have taken years in the ordinary way. We in England, and indeed scientists all over the world will always be grateful to Australia for the work which has been done at Cairns.[29]

Fairley summarised the experimental work that had already been undertaken at Cairns, as well as the tests still in progress. In summing up the postwar situation, Major General Burston said that military hospitals would receive the first supplies of the drug when it was available in quantities, and concluded: 'If we can prevent these acute relapses into [*sic*] malaria we will save the cost of maintaining several thousands of beds yearly and prevent the considerable loss of manpower hours in Australian industry'.[30]

Details of the press conference and paludrine were included in Australian newspapers on the following day, but most did not redress the deficiencies of the earlier press reports. For example, a brief article in the Sydney *Daily Telegraph* mentioned that British and Australian scientists had conquered malaria with the discovery of paludrine and that the first large-scale tests had been carried out by the Army Medical Research Unit at Cairns.[31] But very little additional information was provided. A similar cursory account was published in the *Sydney Morning Herald*. The Melbourne *Age* provided one of the few balanced reports that did justice to the Australian research in a double-column article headed 'New Malarial Drug—Amazing results in tests at Cairns'.[32] Fairley's comments were covered extensively, and Davey was quoted as saying: 'but for Cairns we would have been left more or less high and dry in our three years' intensive work'.

The announcement to the Australian lay press was followed up by a special article published in the *Medical Journal of Australia* in February 1946.[33] This presented a succinct overview of the investigations at Cairns, preceded by a fitting background introduction:

> Any army possessing an antimalarial drug which would completely prevent malaria from developing in troops operating in highly malarious areas would have a tremendous advantage over the enemy ... [In the case of paludrine] the difference between the effective therapeutic dose and the toxic dose is very considerable. Taking this into consideration, paludrine is undoubtedly the most potent antimalarial drug known. Its discovery is a triumph for British chemotherapy.

An editorial published in the same issue stressed that 'this article is one of the most important that has been published in this journal' and clarified the events that led to the embarrassing official denials following the first misleading press accounts of the new drug:

> It should be made quite clear that headquarters of the Australian Military Forces was in no way responsible first for its silence, and then for what must have appeared to some persons as an equivocation on its part, when it was denied officially that Paludrine was being extensively investigated in Australia... These happenings do not detract in any way from the value of the work that has been carried out at Cairns by the team of officers from the Australian Army Medical Corps.[34]

Belated recognition in the English medical press for the Australian research was finally provided by an editorial in the *British Medical Journal* on 15 June 1946 that accompanied an article by Maegraith's group at Liverpool on treatment of naturally acquired malaria cases with M.4888: 'The early work on paludrine has recently been confirmed and extended in the field. Fairley and his co-workers in Australia have issued a preliminary report on the results of extensive experiments in volunteers exposed to New Guinea strains of *P. vivax* and *P. falciparum*'.[35] Full scientific credit and priority for the work at Cairns was obtained in October 1946 with the publication of an article in the *Proceedings of the Royal Society of Tropical Medicine and Hygiene*.[36] This publication covered not only the short-term and long-term clinical experiments in human volunteers but extraordinarily detailed and elegant observations that documented, for the first time, the precise stages in the parasite life cycle affected by the drug.

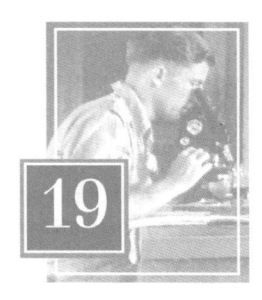

Mode of Action

THE ENTIRE EXPERIMENTAL program at Cairns was dependent upon the continuous availability of infected mosquitoes. Between June 1943 and February 1946 the entomology staff made over 37 000 dissections of salivary glands to determine the presence of sporozoites, and 20 900 infective mosquito bites (8960 *Plasmodium vivax* and 11 940 *P. falciparum*) were given to volunteers.[1] These comprised the largest series of mosquito-transmitted malaria experiments that have ever been undertaken. Jo Mackerras was a meticulous scientist. She painstakingly collated all of this information, which represented the largest set of mosquito-infection data ever accumulated from human malaria experiments. But her contribution was not restricted solely to the mosquitoes themselves, as the infectivity of the gametocytes was a key factor in the whole process. She routinely examined blood slides of the soldier donors, who provided the source of infection for transmission to mosquitoes, and made numerous observations of their asexual blood stages and their gametocytes at the time of feeding. This was then related to the infection rates subsequently observed in the different mosquito batches.

This topic was discussed at a meeting convened by Lieutenant Colonel Blackburn on 1 June 1944 and attended by senior scientific staff of the pathology and entomology sections of the unit.[2] The stages in the blood typically increase to a peak and decline over a period of days or weeks in a parasite 'wave'. Blackburn asked Mackerras to tell the meeting something of the relationship between gametocyte waves and trophozoite waves, and something of the infection of mosquitoes. She said that, as a broad general principle, there was a correlation between the waves. The presence of many gametocytes in the blood usually provided good infective rates in mosquitoes and these rates declined with the fall in the gametocyte wave. However, large numbers of gametocytes did not always guarantee infectivity. She said:

> A man may have gametocytes that readily infect mosquitoes one day, but not so the next, and it is not possible to say which gametocytes would be good and which would be bad . . . sometimes you got 100% infected the first day, 20% the second, and say, none, on the third day.[3]

Mackerras later wrote a vivid description in an unpublished report:

> The developing gams. are very striking being spherical, bright and refractile with madly dancing pigment . . . In vivax the gametocyte wave is usually short and the infectivity can vary in a most harebrained way from day to day.[4]

On the other hand, gametocytes of falciparum persisted much longer, sometimes for several weeks after the trophozoites had been eliminated following drug treatment.

A logical extension of these observations of the parasites in the mosquito was investigation of the direct effects of antimalarial compounds on the parasites in the blood. During the atebrin and quinine experiments in the first half of 1944 it was seen that these drugs exerted an action on the early erythrocytic stages of *P. vivax* within several hours of the patient taking the drug.[5] Parasite growth ceased and the blood stages degenerated but the mature gametocytes were unaffected. Similarly, experiments at Cairns showed that the gametocytes of *P. falciparum* were not harmed by atebrin and quinine, as cases who had been treated with these drugs were still able to infect mosquitoes. But even small doses of plasmoquine rapidly rendered falciparum gametocytes non-infective for mosquitoes.[6]

Thus, the workers at Cairns had acquired considerable experience in the effects of drugs on the blood stages of malaria by the time that the experiments on paludrine commenced. Slides from the first men treated with the new drug were scrutinised with particular interest to see how its mode of antimalarial activity compared with those previously tested. The initial report of the first series stated 'results of treatment of the controls indicate that [in vivax malaria] M.4888 has considerable trophozoiticidal action and a less marked gametocidal action in the dosage used. However, gametocytes show degenerative changes and are rapidly rendered non-infective to mosquitoes'.[7] Later work at Cairns showed that this was not correct, as paludrine acted on later stages of the blood cycle than did atebrin and quinine. The trophozoites were able to grow to their full size in the presence of the drug and the lethal action was exerted against the developing schizonts. The misleading statement in the original report arose because the appearance of these degenerating schizonts was mistaken for drug-affected gametocytes.[8] Further work also showed that paludrine did not affect the formation and appearance of vivax and falciparum gametocytes.

Typical blood slides of falciparum cases only exhibit early ring forms and gametocytes. This is because developing trophozoites and schizonts of *P. falciparum* are restricted to the blood vessels of the internal organs and they are not normally found in the peripheral circulation. The action of drugs on these 'hidden' stages was investigated by a novel technique pioneered at Cairns by a new member of the research team during 1945. The War Establishment of the LHQ Medical Research Unit included a position of captain-physician whose primary role would be to assist the Commanding Officer with clinical examination and management of the volunteers. This position needed to be filled during the second half of 1944, due to the expanded work involving the American drugs, as well as continuing commitments with atebrin and subinoculation experiments. This subject was discussed by Fairley during a visit to Cairns in September and, just before his departure overseas during the following month, he notified Blackburn that 'a suitable Captain is being selected for the unit'. Captain R. H. (Robert) Black marched in on New Year's Day 1945.

Black graduated in medicine at University of Sydney with First Class Honours and the University Medal in 1939. After a year as professorial resident at Royal Prince Alfred Hospital in Sydney, he was appointed senior resident at Innisfail District Hospital in 1941. He joined the militia as a probationary captain in that year, and transferred to the AIF. He was posted to 117 AGH in January 1943, and was transferred to 106 CCS during the following June.

He embarked for New Guinea two months later and worked in Lae, where he first became interested in malaria. It was thought that a number of fever cases in Australian troops may have been due to malaria with parasites present in submicroscopic densities, and Black felt that this might be confirmed if the parasites could be encouraged to grow in test-tube cultures of blood from these patients.[9] He was aware of successful attempts to cultivate malaria parasites under artificial *in vitro* conditions so he attempted to set up a control culture using this method.[10] Some growth of *P. falciparum* ring forms was observed, but the experiment had to be abandoned due to the pressure of other laboratory work.

He was posted out of New Guinea in July 1944 to 2 Aust Blood and Serum Preparation Unit in Sydney, where he had the opportunity to resume the attempts at *in vitro* cultivation. Blood collected from malaria patients admitted to military hospitals was placed into test tubes, and the blood cells were separated by centrifuging. The serum was then placed into a flat culture tube containing glucose solution. Some of the original blood cells were added by pipette and the culture was incubated at body temperature. After 18 unsuccessful attempts Black managed to grow rings of *P. falciparum* through to mature schizonts. The merozoites were liberated and developed to the ring stage in fresh blood cells.[11]

With this background Black would have been a logical choice for the position at Cairns. It is likely that Colonel Keogh heard of his work with parasite cultivation through the medical 'old boy network' and, with Fairley's assent, a posting order was raised. Within four weeks of his arrival Black was detached to 2/2 AGH as medical officer in charge of the volunteers at Rocky Creek. In mid-February he returned to take over the medical supervision of the volunteer patients at Cairns while Blackburn was on leave.

After this introduction to the research work of the unit he continued to support the clinical management of the volunteers, but was also given the opportunity to continue his experiments on artificial cultivation of parasites—initially at Rocky Creek and later at Cairns. For this purpose he was provided with a caravan set up as a mobile bacteriological laboratory. This was equipped with tanks of fresh water, as well as an incubator and refrigerator, and was supplied with electric power from the adjacent main laboratory. It was not needed as a 'mobile' laboratory. All laboratory space was already fully utilised so it provided much needed accommodation for the *in vitro* studies.[12]

Very consistent results with *P. falciparum* cultures were soon obtained using the original method adopted in Sydney. The patients at Cairns were strictly supervised, and they had no exposure to antimalarial drugs before providing blood for the cultures. Black thought that some of his unsuccessful culture attempts in Lae and Sydney may have been due to quinine or atebrin taken by the patients before their blood was collected. This suggested that a fruitful avenue of investigation might be a study of the effects of drugs on the *in vitro* cultivated parasites.[13]

Several previous workers had also believed that quinine in the blood of patients used for cultivation attempts of human malaria had adversely influenced parasite development. In 1922 C. C. Bass, who was the first achieve success with *in vitro* cultivation, reported experiments in which growth of a falciparum culture was prevented by the addition of quinine.[14] There were some other pre-war reports of the inhibition of cultured animal malaria parasites by quinine and atebrin, but such studies yielded little information about the mode of action of antimalarial drugs. These early studies involved the direct addition of the compounds to the culture medium, but drugs are metabolised in the body and they do not necessarily reach the circulation in the original state in which they are ingested. In Black's experiments the action of drugs on the blood stages of falciparum malaria were studied 'in the form in which they circulate in the human body'. This was achieved by a two-step procedure:

(i) cultures were set up from parasites which came from infected donors who had not taken drugs;

(ii) for the test culture, the serum from the donor was replaced with serum from an uninfected healthy volunteer to whom the drug had already been administered. Parasite growth in this medium was compared with a parallel control from the original culture in which the serum contained no drug.[15]

Using this technique Black showed that parasite development was arrested and degeneration occurred at the stage of early ring forms or young trophozoites when cultures were grown in serum from healthy subjects who had taken quinine, atebrin, sontochin or chloroquine. The sulphonamides affected the dividing schizonts but plasmoquine produced inconsistent effects. In cultures containing serum from men who had taken paludrine, the ring stages and trophozoites grew at the same rate as the control cultures, but development then ceased and degeneration was observed at the early stages of schizogony. The complete blood cycle is not normally observed in blood slides from patients with falciparum malaria but all these stages were apparent in Black's test-tube cultures. His results showed that the effects of drugs on the various stages of *in vitro* cultivated *P. falciparum* were very similar to the effects of the same drugs on the corresponding blood stages of *P. vivax* that Mackerras observed in blood films of human volunteers. These results were important as they provided independent confirmation that the drugs affecting the blood cycle of the human malarias did not all act in the same way (see Fig. 12). Thus, *in vivo* observations of *P. vivax* and *in vitro* studies of *P. falciparum* showed that quinine and atebrin acted on the early part of the blood cycle, whereas paludrine acted later when the parasites started to divide and multiply within the blood cells.

In order to maintain a continuous supply of infected mosquitoes at Cairns it was usual for batches to be fed on volunteers who developed gametocyte waves following treatment of their experimental infections. It had already been shown that quinine and atebrin did not prevent *P. falciparum* gametocytes from infecting mosquitoes, so the same practice was instituted during the paludrine experiments. One of the controls in the first test of paludrine against falciparum malaria (Experiment CIII), broke through in the second week of April 1945 and was treated with a fourteen-day course of paludrine. He developed a normal gametocyte wave shortly after his clinical attack was cured. Mosquitoes were fed on this patient on six different days when gametocyte numbers remained high, but subsequent dissections showed that none of them became infected.[16] This was a most unusual finding. The mosquito infection procedures had been refined to a very reliable routine and the large numbers of gametocytes in the patient over the biting period should have ensured that at least some mosquitoes developed oocysts and sporozoites. The gametocytes in this man persisted in the circulation for the usual period of time, and they exhibited no obvious signs of degeneration.[17] So the lack of mosquito infection was intriguing.

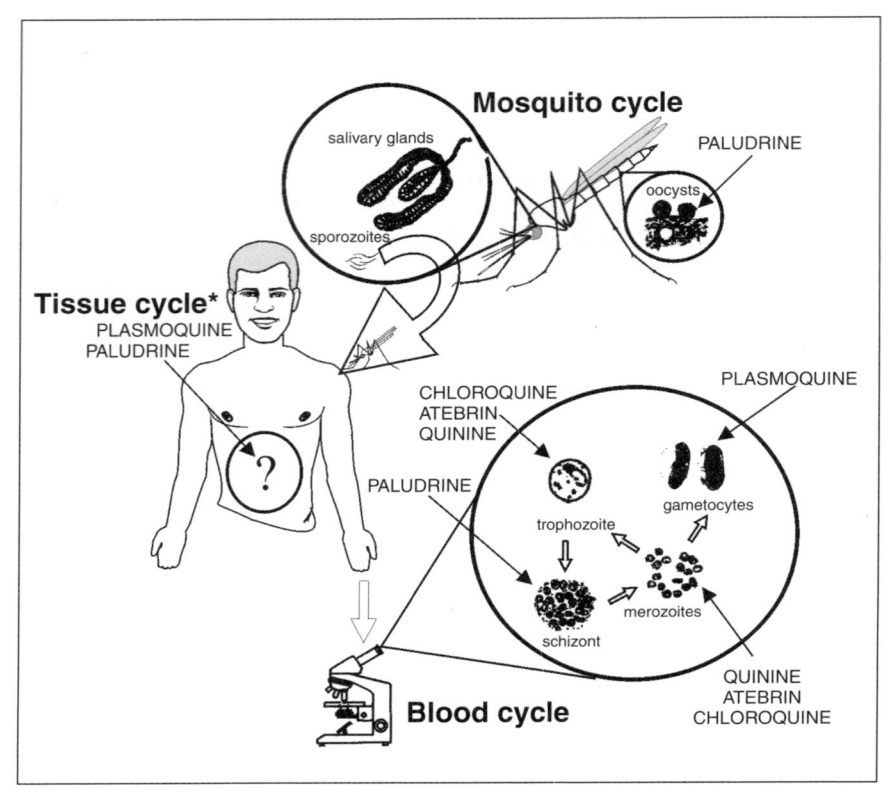

Fig. 12 Sites of action of antimalarial drugs in mosquitoes and humans determined by experiments at Cairns

* The tissue cycle in the liver was discovered three years after the Cairns experiments.

Mackerras made further observations aimed at clarifying this point during the second series of paludrine experiments in July and August. In one such test a batch of mosquitoes was fed on a falciparum case one hour before he received a single 100 mg tablet of paludrine, and another similar batch was fed on the same man one hour after he had taken the drug. The first batch yielded a sporozoite rate of 85 per cent, whereas none of the mosquitoes in the second batch developed salivary-gland infections.[18] Clearly, the drug acted on this part of the parasite cycle and exerted its effects very rapidly—but how did it do this? Did it 'sterilise' the gametocytes in the human host, or was its action manifested at a later stage during development in the mosquito?

In other experiments successive batches of mosquitoes were fed on gametocyte carriers for varying periods after they ceased taking the drug. No infection was recorded when mosquitoes were fed two, four, five or six days after therapy.

Oocysts formed on the mosquito gut, but failed to grow in batches fed between seven and 10 days afterwards. If the gametocytes were sufficiently numerous they sometimes persisted for 12 days or more after ceasing therapy and, in these instances, the oocysts developed normally and sporozoites invaded the salivary glands. This showed that the drug did not produce any irreversible changes in the gametocytes, as these were able to infect mosquitoes when the drug was eliminated from the circulation of the human donor.[19] It was then apparent that paludrine killed the parasite after it had begun to develop in the mosquito.

A final experiment was performed that pinpointed the stage at which this occurred (see Fig. 13). Mosquitoes were allowed to partially feed on a man,

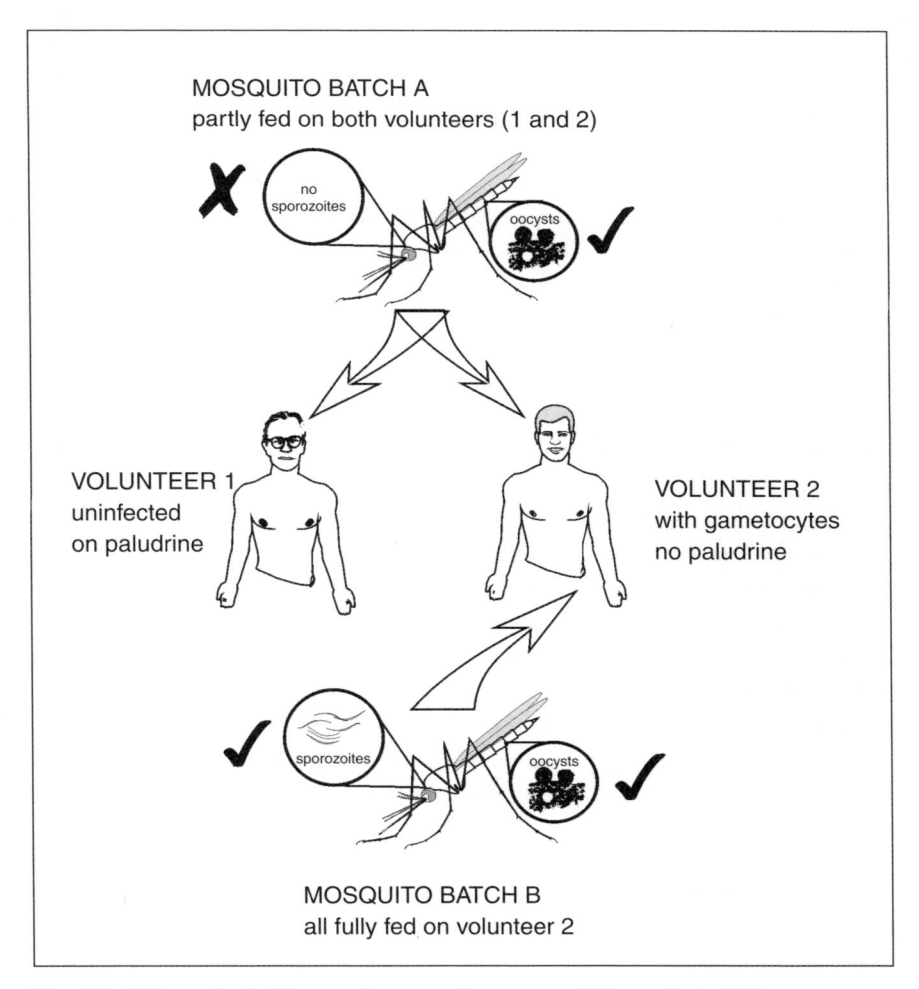

Fig. 13 Effects of paludrine on the mosquito stages of *Plasmodium falciparum*

not infected with malaria, who was taking paludrine. This was achieved by removing the mosquitoes from his arm before they had fully engorged; they were then allowed to complete their blood meal on a patient, who had not taken the drug, with falciparum gametocytes. This procedure ensured that the gametocytes from the infected donor were mixed with drug in the blood from the uninfected man in the mosquito guts. Later dissections of these mosquitoes showed that they had an average of six oocysts per gut, but they did not grow to maturity and none developed sporozoites. A similar batch of mosquitoes was fully fed on the infected patient and acted as a control. The latter batch had an average of 14 oocysts per gut and a salivary gland infection rate of 95 per cent. This experiment showed that paludrine did not prevent the early development of the oocysts, but it arrested their maturation. Other batches of mosquitoes, already infected with developing or almost mature oocysts, were fed on men taking paludrine. In these instances the oocysts continued to develop to form sporozoites in the salivary glands after the usual time interval. This latter result implied that either the drug was not absorbed into the body cavity of the mosquito or, if it was absorbed, it did not penetrate the growing oocyst.

The action of the drug against gametocytes of *P. vivax* was more difficult to ascertain, as these stages do not persist in the circulation for more than a few days after the trophozoites have disappeared. Also, degenerating vivax schizonts could easily be mistaken for drug-affected gametocytes, and this led to some confusion in the first experiments with paludrine. After further observations this matter was soon resolved, and it was shown that the infection in mosquitoes was arrested at the oocyst stage when they were fed on vivax gametocyte carriers several hours after receiving their first dose of paludrine. This indicated that the drug had a similar action on the mosquito phases of vivax and falciparum malaria.[20]

The investigations at Cairns were methodical and systematic but, as often happens in research, luck still played a role. During the last week of June 1945 Staff Sergeant J. W. McNamara and Sergeant J. H. Brockhurst of the Milne Bay detachment of the Medical Research Unit thought they saw the blood stages of quartan malaria in the blood film of a local Papuan man. This is a difficult subject for experimental research as the responsible parasite, *P. malariae*, is uncommon in most malarious regions and is hard to isolate and transmit in the laboratory. Its development in mosquitoes is slower than *P. vivax* and *P. falciparum*, taking four to five weeks for sporozoite formation. This is probably one reason for its scarcity in nature—few mosquitoes live long enough to transmit it. It also reproduces slowly in humans, and the gametocytes are usually few in number. Consequently, it takes a long time for cases to become infectious for mosquitoes but it can persist in the human host for many years, albeit at low levels of parasitaemia, with few clinical symptoms.

The Australian research team tried to establish a mosquito-transmitted strain from the case at Milne Bay, even though they knew that the chances of success were not very great. A batch of *Anopheles punctulatus* reared from locally collected larvae were fed on the Papuan. Normally only larvae were sent by air from Milne Bay to Cairns but, in this instance, the blood-fed adults were sent south to Australia on a RAAF flight. These mosquitoes were held in the insectary at Jungara, and Mackerras found developing oocysts, but not sporozoites, in one dissected 16 days after the original blood meal. Only five mosquitoes of the original batch remained alive after a further eight days, but Mackerras managed to re-feed all of them on an uninfected volunteer. Dissections subsequently showed that three had sporozoites, and blood slides of the volunteer had typical trophozoites of quartan malaria after 24 days. The infection developed slowly, and only small numbers of gametocytes appeared sporadically. Consequently, it was not possible to maintain this strain by sporozoite inoculation, as mosquitoes fed on this volunteer failed to become infected. The parasites were transmitted to two other volunteers by blood inoculation. The three experimentally-induced infections were treated with paludrine. The quartan parasites seemed to be somewhat less susceptible to the drug than *P. vivax*, though it appeared to act in the same way against this species by causing degeneration of the early schizonts.[21]

The primary motivation for the Australian work on paludrine was to investigate its potential for causal prophylaxis by eliminating the parasites during the tissue phase before they invaded the blood. Fairley hoped that it would act in this way to prevent vivax relapses, as this was then the most serious malaria problem facing Allied forces. The first experiments in April 1945 revealed that it did have promise in this regard by delaying the primary attack, but later observations showed that relapses still ultimately occurred. However, during September it was also shown that paludrine completely prevented the development of falciparum malaria if it was taken for the first six days after exposure to sporozoites. This provided the first indication that it was, indeed, a true causal prophlyactic of *P. falciparum*. While this experiment was still in progress another was started in which two volunteers received a single dose of paludrine (one receiving 1000 mg and the other 500 mg) three hours before they were bitten by 10–20 falciparum-infected mosquitoes. Both men remained free of malaria.[22]

This most important finding was the subject of further single-dose experiments to define the relationship between the minimum quantity of drug and the timing of its administration required to destroy the tissue forms before they invaded the circulation. During October the first experiment was repeated, with another two volunteers receiving a single dose three hours before biting, but this time the quantity of drug was reduced so that one received 300 mg and the other 100 mg. On this occasion the man on the higher dose remained free of malaria, but the parasites broke through in the man on the lower dose. On 24 November five men were bitten by mosquitoes with sporozoites of *P. falciparum* and each received 300 mg at various time intervals afterwards. Three of these men who received the drug at either three hours, five days or six days after biting did not come down with malaria, whereas the two men who received their dose on the seventh or eighth day (after the parasites had already been liberated into the circulation) developed overt attacks.

The results described above were summarised by Blackburn in the second week of December.[23] In this report he suggested a logical extension in which single doses of 100 mg would be given to separate volunteers on the first five days after biting to determine 'if there are definite stages of *P. falciparum* (with particular reference to the tissue phase) which are more susceptible to paludrine'. But there was a problem in implementing this last stage of the experimental program at Cairns due to lack of volunteers. The war had ended four months previously, and the Army was rapidly winding down as the Australian armed forces demobilised and returned to civilian life. Christmas was rapidly approaching, and it was anticipated that the work at Cairns would cease early in the New Year. Blackburn was anxious to round off these last experiments, and he realised that the only way to do this was to call for volunteers from among the staff of the unit. Accordingly, the test subjects for the 100 mg single-dose group that commenced in the first week of January 1946 included Blackburn himself, Major J. I. Tonge [who by then had taken over as head of the pathology section from Major T. S. Gregory], Captain R. H. Black, Lieutenants K. G. Pope and S. R. Dunn, CSM W. J. Winterbottom, Staff Sergeant H. E. Davies, and Privates D. I. Bladon, A. R. Birch and K. R. Clarke. The routine work of the unit would be compromised if all these key personnel were hospitalised and subjected to the same clinical follow-up as the other volunteers, so they were admitted as outpatients and it was resolved to treat any breakthroughs as soon as their slides became positive so that they could continue with their normal duties.

Two men in this group took the drug on day Z+6, and both broke through with parasites. The blood slides of the other men who received the drug between days Z+2 to Z+5 remained negative. Subinoculation experiments at Cairns had already demonstrated that falciparum parasites first invade the peripheral circulation on day Z+6, so it was clear that protection was afforded when the dose was taken before this happened.

The experiment was repeated again at the end of January using test volunteers from among the unit staff who did not break through in the previous test. This time they received a dose of 500 mg between Z+2 to Z+5 but, again, there were no breakthroughs. Some of the unit staff were already being demobilised by the time these latter results were established. Nevertheless, it was decided to complete the series with one last experiment using even smaller quantities of the drug.

Blackburn and Black lined up again for a third time with the other negative unit volunteers, and their numbers were augmented by other staff of the LHQ Medical Research Unit and two officers from 116 AGH. The infective bites for the final experiment commenced on 22 February. It involved two single-dose groups, with the drug administered over the same time interval as the previous January tests and with two men on each time/dose regimen: one group receiving 25 mg, and the other 10 mg. Only three out of the 16 test subjects in these groups broke through with parasites: one on the higher dose and two on the lower regimen. This meant that six of the eight men who were given 10 mg only once between the second and fifth day after biting were completely protected. These results were remarkable when it is considered that this dose represented only one-tenth of the usual daily dose administered for prophylaxis.

The work on paludrine at Cairns included the first comprehensive investigations of the mode of action of an antimalarial drug by co-ordinated observations in human patients, test-tube cultures and infected mosquitoes. They revealed that paludrine acted at three discrete places in the life cycle. Mackerras's observations on the action of paludrine against the early schizonts in vivax patients were complemented by Black's studies, which showed that the growth of falciparum malaria *in vitro* was arrested at the same stage of development. The initial records that Mackerras collated on the infectivity of gametocytes were expanded to provide important baseline information on transmission of malaria from human to mosquito. This provided a foundation for understanding drug action against this part of the parasite life cycle. It culminated in a highly sophisticated experiment that showed that, under conditions involving brief exposure of gametocytes in the mosquito gut to tiny quantities of the drug, paludrine exerted its action with remarkable precision against a specific stage of parasite growth in the mosquito. Finally, the elegant series of single-dose experiments directed by Blackburn confirmed the action of the drug against the tissue stages.

The last experiment of the Cairns group furnished an impressive demonstration that a single minute dose of paludrine administered during the incubation period was able to completely prevent the development of falciparum malaria. This phase of the work was well advanced when the British press announcement on paludrine was made. It is not surprising, therefore, that Fairley was displeased, as this premature disclosure was based on inadequate information. It did not do justice to the drug nor to the Australian research that had revealed its true value.

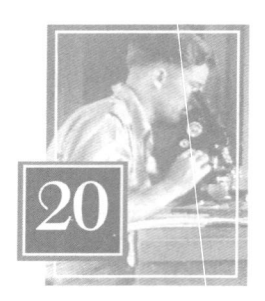

Tolerance and Immunity

MALARIA EXACTS A savage toll of mortality among infants and children in areas where the disease is endemic, but the survivors acquire an immunity that moderates the debilitating effects of later attacks. This immune response was appreciated by malariologists in the early part of the twentieth century. It may be manifested by an increased tolerance to a given level of infection (so that the individual does not feel as ill in later attacks as during the first attack); or by the appearance of immunity that enables the immune system to directly deal with the infection by limiting the extent to which the parasites multiply within the red blood cells. There were numerous reports of tolerance and immunity amongst populations living in endemic areas. Observations made by workers involved in malaria therapy of syphilis patients implied that a level of tolerance developed before immunity, but long-term studies on the relationship between clinical and parasitological phenomena in malaria patients had not been systematically undertaken before World War II.

Lieutenant Colonel Blackburn became interested in this subject before he was appointed Commanding Officer of the Medical Research Unit at Cairns. In June 1943, while he was at 113 Australian General Hospital (AGH) in Sydney, a patient with an unusually persistent infection of *Plasmodium vivax* came to his attention. This man, P. K., had served in the Middle East and was later attached to the Headquarters of 7th Division in New Guinea during the advance across the Kokoda trail to Buna. Quinine was used for prophylaxis during this campaign and, as the research in Cairns subsequently demonstrated, it was not able to prevent attacks of South West Pacific strains of vivax malaria. Those who were too ill to remain in the fighting line were evacuated to Port Moresby. The soldier treated by Blackburn at 113 AGH was one of these cases. He was evacuated to 2/9 AGH in Moresby and, early in 1943, was transferred to a non-malarious area in Australia. On four occasions between March and May 1943 he received quinine, atebrin, plasmoquine (QAP) treatment for vivax relapses at 115 AGH in Melbourne. In June 1943 he was admitted to 113 AGH in Sydney with a severe attack of vivax malaria and was given another full course of QAP treatment. Blackburn observed that the man's symptoms were relieved during this treatment but parasite densities in his blood remained unchanged.[1] His blood films became negative after the administration of intravenous quinine and the arsenical compound neosalvarsan. Two weeks later, however, parasites reappeared in his peripheral blood, even though he had no appreciable symptoms of malaria. Blackburn was most interested in this case, as parasites had persisted in the blood for a long time, despite repeated treatment courses with a variety of antimalarial drugs. He would have liked to study the patient further but lacked the facilities to do so.[2]

Blackburn's interest in the relationship between clinical symptoms and parasite density in the blood was stimulated again during May 1944 when he summarised the experimental data of the first group of volunteers taking quinine. He wrote:

> An attempt is being made at the present time to relate the degree of reaction to the combined effect of parasite density and time (i.e. degree of reaction to total, involvement) in *P. vivax* controls. It appears that the man who takes a longer time than the average to reach the degree of reaction regarded as requiring therapy has a lower parasite density than the man who reaches that degree rapidly.[3]

The clinical reactions of the test and control volunteers were followed closely as this experiment continued. One of the *P. vivax* infected test volunteers taking 650 mg of quinine each day was of particular interest. He received 10 infected bites on 27 May 1944; parasites broke through in his blood on day Z+13; and he had a prolonged attack of malaria, despite the fact that he continued to take quinine each day. Parasites persisted in his blood, and he had periods of fever and shivering almost every day for the next seven weeks. For the last fortnight of this period he felt quite well in the mornings and regularly went fishing in a stream about 3 km from the unit. He returned each afternoon to have his paroxysm around 3 p.m., and spent the evenings playing cards or billiards. He commenced QAP treatment on 31 July, and his blood slides were negative until 26 August, after which parasites built up again to reach the same levels as in his primary attack. However, his symptoms during this relapse were relatively mild—so much so that treatment was delayed for five weeks after its onset.[4]

Soon after the quinine groups commenced, Blackburn remembered P. K. whom he had treated at 113 AGH 12 months previously and recognised the advantages of making further observations of his parasites.[5] He discussed this with Fairley who requested P. K.'s transfer from his present posting in Western Australia to Cairns. This soldier, an older man known as 'Old Paddy', willingly came to Cairns and was very contented to remain there for more than 18 months. He was the longest-serving experimental subject, and became somewhat of a 'mascot' at the unit. P. K. arrived at the Medical Research Unit on 26 June, and slides showed that he had a low level of *P. vivax* trophozoites in his blood but no symptoms of malaria. He remained well for the next six weeks, during which time parasites persisted continuously in his circulation, and, on 7 August, 10 ml of his blood was inoculated into another volunteer. P. K. was then given quinine for 11 days, after which his blood films remained negative for the next three weeks. Meanwhile, the recipient of his blood developed a full-blown symptomatic attack of vivax malaria with typical trophozoite and gametocyte waves. On 7 September 10 ml of the recipient's blood (containing 130 million parasites) was inoculated back into the original donor (P. K.). The latter developed a small trophozoite wave without symptoms of malaria, but his blood films became negative after 18 September. On 25 September P. K. was bitten by seven mosquitoes infected with sporozoites derived from feeding on the recipient of his blood while the recipient had gametocytes in his circulation. A small trophozoite wave occurred from 14 to 18 days after he was bitten but no clinical symptoms were observed (see Fig. 14).

This experiment demonstrated that P. K. had a high level of tolerance and immunity to his own strain of parasites. He did not feel sick or develop a normal trophozoite wave after he was inoculated with large numbers of parasites and after he was bitten by infected mosquitoes. This was radically different to the severe clinical symptoms and parasitological response that invariably followed blood inoculation and sporozoite inoculation of 'virgin' volunteers at Cairns who had not previously been exposed to malaria. This man had been treated for nine separate attacks of malaria in the 18 months between the acquisition of his natural infection in New Guinea and his arrival at Cairns. However, in the intervals between these attacks his clinical and parasitological condition had not been closely monitored, so it was not possible to accurately chart the course of his immune response. It clearly was of considerable interest if further observations were to be made on the development of tolerance and immunity in cases that were continuously subjected to the meticulous daily scrutiny given to the volunteers at the Medical Research Unit.

Blackburn discussed these results with Fairley, who responded on 14 October 1944, shortly before his departure for the United States and England. He said 'it would be very interesting when the opportunity arises to see if a proven latent [vivax case] is resistant to his own strain when inoculated with the dose of parasites of the magnitude we employ'.[6] The outline of an experiment to

20 Tolerance and Immunity 217

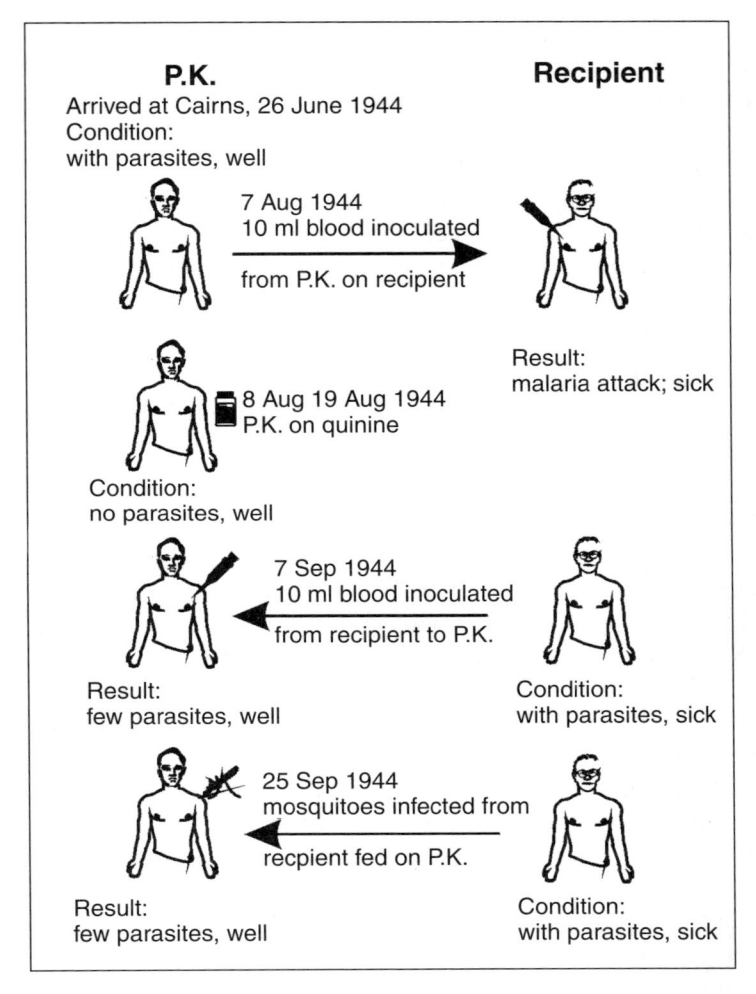

Fig. 14 Clinical experiments on naturally acquired immunity to vivax malaria

examine this question was proposed. The plan involved infecting a group of four volunteers via the bites of vivax-infected mosquitoes and permitting their attack to remain untreated for 10 to 14 days so that they could develop some immunity. They would then be given a 10-day course of quinine to eliminate the blood stages, and after a further five days subinoculated to recipients to determine whether they were still harbouring submicroscopic levels of parasites within their bloodstream. Soon afterwards on the same day three of the men would receive an injection of blood from a patient having a high density of parasites of the same strain to see whether they would develop another attack.

Fairley realised that there was a small chance that such attacks might represent a relapse of the original mosquito-induced infection, but he thought that this was unlikely to occur in less than three weeks after treatment ceased. But in order to lesson the likelihood of this possibility the fourth man was not to be inoculated with infected blood to see whether or not he developed a relapse.

In a report dated 18 November, which was addressed to Fairley in London, Blackburn said that this experiment had commenced after preliminary observations were made to confirm that there were no significant amounts of quinine remaining in the circulation five days after the proposed course of treatment was completed:

> They have all had considerable reaction . . . high fever for over a week with marked sweating etc. and considerable loss of weight. Response to therapy has been rapid. The chief difficulty is one of timing—to have a suitable donor with high density of *P. vivax* ready on the 5th day after ceasing therapy.[7]

On the designated date, 30 November, 200 ml of blood from each of the four men was subinoculated into a separate recipient. All four recipients of the subinoculations developed overt attacks of vivax malaria, thereby indicating that the donors had submicroscopic levels of parasites in their blood, even though they had completed a 10-day course of treatment with quinine just five days previously, and their blood slides at the time of the subinoculations were negative. Much to Blackburn's relief a suitable donor with a sufficiently high parasite density was available so, immediately after the subinoculations, 18 ml of his blood (containing approximately 50 million trophozoites) was inoculated intravenously into three of the four volunteers. Each of the three test volunteers who received the 50 million trophozoites developed an overt attack of malaria, but the symptoms were milder than the primary attack. Their attacks all developed more than a week earlier than the relapse of the fourth man who was not inoculated, so it was considered that these attacks had possibly developed as a direct result of the inoculation. One aim of this experiment, stated in the title of Blackburn's report, was to 'test subinoculation and subsequent inoculation of trophozoites as a criterion of cure in volunteers who have had experimental mosquito-transmitted benign tertian malaria'.[8] There was the possibility that men who had submicroscopic densities of parasites in their blood might not develop a frank attack of the disease if additional blood stages were directly inoculated into their circulation. The results indicated that this hypothesis was not correct, and Blackburn concluded that 'It is questionable, therefore, if the development of an attack of [vivax] malaria following inoculation of trophozoites is an adequate criterion of cure of a previous sporozoite induced infection with the same strain of *P. vivax*'.[9]

Two of the men inoculated with 50 million trophozoites were subsequently treated with quinine, but the third man, whose symptoms were even milder than the others, was not treated for this attack.[10] His parasites persisted continuously at relatively high levels for the next two months. Throughout this period he was well, with only intermittent minor symptoms on a few occasions, and on 2 February 1945 he received another inoculation of 470 million trophozoites of the same strain. He subsequently developed another large parasite wave, but his clinical symptoms were very mild. In the published report of this work Blackburn wrote:

> This experiment illustrated a further stage in development of tolerance to infection. After some 90 days a stage had been reached at which the volunteer had not only developed considerable tolerance to his trophozoites but, while he was able to keep the parasite densities down to levels at which they caused no reaction, he could not reduce them to insignificant levels ... Superinfection, however, broke down his resistance, and a clinical attack developed when trophozoites reached high densities. His tolerance had developed to a greater extent then his antiparasitic mechanisms (or immunity).[11]

One question arising from these observations was whether the immune response was stimulated by parasites within the tissues or by the continued presence of circulating blood stages. Blackburn designed an elegant experiment to investigate these possibilities (see Fig. 15).[12] Three volunteers were each subjected to 50 infective bites from mosquitoes infected with the same strain of *P. vivax* on 2 May 1945. One man received a four-day build up on atebrin before biting, and was then placed on continuous prophylaxis using the standard daily atebrin dose of 100 mg per day. Another was not placed on suppressive therapy, and each attack was allowed to develop for several days before he was given a 10-day course of quinine treatment. The third volunteer did not receive any antimalarial drugs and his attacks were allowed to develop normally without any clinical intervention though he was monitored very closely, as were the other men. The man on prophylactic atebrin continued to take the drug until Day Z+147 without any evidence of parasites in his daily blood slides. Trophozoites were first observed in his blood on 27 October (Z+178), and he developed a major parasite wave with severe symptoms.

The second man received quinine treatment for three attacks during the first three months after biting. The first two attacks were quite severe in terms of parasite densities, as well as clinical symptoms. The third attack was also accompanied by a large parasite wave but, on this occasion, the symptoms were moderate. Parasites appeared again from Z+106 and increased to a mild fourth attack, which was not treated. The blood stages persisted at low levels until Z+175, and intermittently thereafter. The untreated volunteer developed a primary attack with fever for 16 consecutive days commencing on Z+12, accompanied by typically severe shivering and sweating. His symptoms moderated from Z+30 but increased again to a second attack from Z+38, with his last

220 *Malaria Frontline*

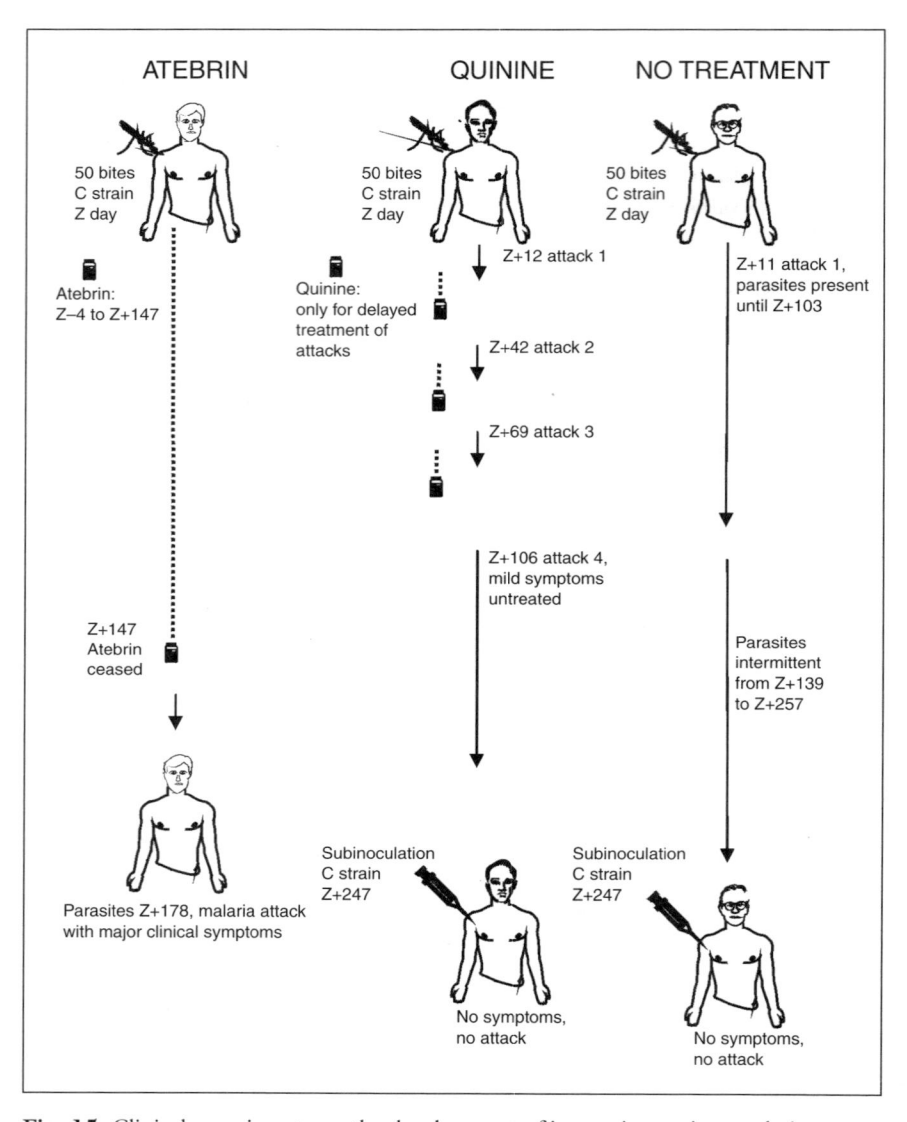

Fig. 15 Clinical experiments on the development of immunity to vivax malaria

episode of malaise recorded on Z+54, after which he remained well. Parasites persisted in his blood until 13 August (Z+103), when he went on compassionate leave because of his father's death. He had no antimalarial treatment while away from the unit, and returned to Cairns after a month with low densities of parasites still present. These persisted for a week after his return, and the odd trophozoite was seen thereafter.

On 4 January 1946 (Z+247) the volunteer who received quinine treatment and the untreated volunteer both received an intravenous inoculation containing 200 million parasites of the same strain of *P. vivax* to which they were originally exposed. The two men did not develop a parasite wave, though a few trophozoites were in their blood, and both remained well and entirely free of malaria symptoms. When reviewing the results of this experiment, Blackburn noted that the man on atebrin prophylaxis developed a typical and severe attack of malaria soon after he ceased taking the drug, whereas the other two men, who had already had considerable exposure to the blood stages in previous attacks, 'were experiencing no clinical phenomena of malaria infection by this time'.[13] He considered that all three volunteers should have had similar exposure to the tissue forms of *P. vivax*. This implied that the immune response to malaria was stimulated by the presence of parasites within the blood and not by the stages within the tissues.

Another relevant consideration was the degree of specificity of immunity. Did its development to a particular strain of malaria confer a degree of protection to other strains of malaria from other geographical areas that might have different biological and immunological characteristics? Up until this time the Cairns experiments on tolerance and immunity had been made with the 'C' strain of *Plasmodium vivax*. This was isolated in May 1944 from a soldier attached to Headquarters of 3rd Division who acquired the infection while in New Guinea between February and November 1943. During this period the division was engaged in operations in the Wau–Salamaua campaigns on the north coast of New Guinea. It is very likely that this man acquired his infection somewhere in this area and that it was suppressed by atebrin until January 1944 when he ceased taking the drug after returning to Australia. He was admitted to the Medical Research Unit at Cairns in May 1944, and his strain of parasites was transferred to recipient volunteers by the bites of infected mosquitoes. It was maintained via sporozoite transmission as well as by blood inoculation, and was used during the next two years for a number of experiments. In early 1946, in the closing days of the research program, the finding that several volunteers had acquired both tolerance and immunity to the 'C' strain prompted an experiment to see how they would react to infection by a strain of vivax malaria from another area.

The response of different malaria strains to drugs was an important matter in mid-1945 during the investigations of atebrin-resistant falciparum parasites from Aitape–Wewak. In the course of this work a strain of vivax malaria, designated the 'A' strain, was isolated at Cairns from a soldier who was infected during this campaign. On 14 January 1946 the untreated man from the previous experiment and the man who received delayed treatment with quinine were inoculated with 140 million parasites of the 'A' strain.[14] These two volunteers had already shown no clinical and little parasitological response to blood inoculation with the 'C' strain, but they both developed large trophozoite waves with the 'A' strain though their clinical symptoms were relatively mild. The soldier P. K., who had been shown in previous experiments to have acquired immunity to a naturally acquired infection, was also inoculated with the 'A' strain at the same time as the other men. He developed a moderate trophozoite wave, but his only clinical manifestation was a feeling of slight malaise on the ninth day after inoculation. These most interesting results showed that tolerance was not strain-specific, as previous prolonged exposure to infection originating from the south-eastern part of New Guinea afforded considerable protection from clinical symptoms following inoculation with a strain from a different geographical area. On the other hand, this experiment implied that immunity was highly specific as the three volunteers developed their highest trophozoite densities after exposure to the second strain, even though it did not make them very sick.

Finally, Blackburn carried out a retrospective analysis of the records of 91 vivax-infected volunteers at Cairns. This confirmed the observations made on individual cases and clearly demonstrated that the degree of tolerance and immunity was directly related to the duration and density of their parasite waves in the blood. In summarising the results of this work he wrote:

> No subjects ever developed any syndrome that could be called 'low fever' . . . The excellent health of the volunteers who were tolerant and immune to their continued slight parasitaemia clearly placed them in the category of malaria infection without malaria disease. The failure to disturb their equilibrium by severe chilling and alcoholic excess, together with the complete absence of fever or splenomegaly, made a diagnosis of 'chronic malaria' untenable. One should be sceptical about a diagnosis of 'chronic malaria' given to minor illnesses characterised by malaise, headache, and perhaps slight chilliness and fever, simply because the patient had vivax malaria sometime in the past.[15]

21

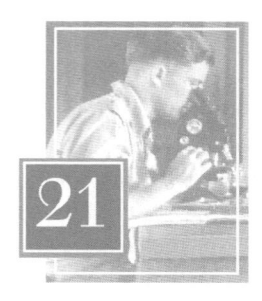

Guinea Pigs

THE WHOLE RESEARCH program at Cairns depended on the continuing availability of adequate numbers of suitable and co-operative volunteers. The first groups were recruited from convalescent depots in southern Queensland. All of the men from this source had recently been ill (though not from malaria, hepatitis, or other relevant diseases) but had recovered and were awaiting reposting to another unit. They arrived at regular intervals in drafts of eight to 12 men and were promptly assigned to the sulphonamide experiments at either Cairns or Rocky Creek. It was thought at the outset that some recompense should be offered and it was proposed that 21 days' leave should be granted at the end of their detachment. Soon after the first men arrived Major R. R. Andrew sent a signal to Fairley requesting that he arrange the necessary authority.[1] A minute from the DGMS to the Adjutant General was raised in support of this recommendation. Although the extra leave had not been promised there was 'a natural expectation of some recompense', and it was pointed out that the volunteers would undergo a voluntary period of close confinement, many would contract malaria, and some would have an unpleasant illness, after which some period of leave would be reasonable.[2] A period of 21 days' extra leave was subsequently granted to the volunteers after completion of their experiments.

The original scope of the research was directed solely towards clinical evaluation of the sulphonamides, and it was envisaged that the total requirement for the project would probably be for about 200 experimental subjects. The initial call for volunteers had yielded about 100 men within a month, but the source of supply from southern Queensland was rapidly becoming depleted, so a memorandum was sent to Army headquarters in Victoria and New South Wales calling for volunteers from convalescent depots in these States.[3] The full implications were to be explained to prospective candidates, as well as the risks of malaria to which they would be exposed. Secrecy was to be observed, including the use of the code word 'NEILL' in signals referring to the experiment. It was stressed that 'no inducement will be offered. Although it is probable that leave will be granted at conclusion of the test, this is not to be used as an inducement to volunteer'.[4] This communication resulted in a steady stream of volunteers during the latter half of 1943 and the first few months of 1944, which permitted the implementation of the A-S experiments, the combined series involving sulphonamides and atebrin, and the short-term and long-term atebrin experiments.

Most had overt attacks of malaria at some stage of their experiments, for periods ranging from several days to two weeks or more, during which time they were quite ill. It was common for those in the fever phase to perspire so copiously that the mattress became saturated and pools of sweat formed under the bed.[5]

In a report to Fairley in February 1944 Blackburn remarked that 'it is very rarely that disciplinary action has to be taken against the volunteers—when necessary great care and tact must be used to avoid loss of co-operation with experiments in progress'.[6] One of the very few exceptions was a man in the atebrin experiments whose plasma levels of the drug were very low and who, it was strongly suspected, was not taking his designated dose. He was discharged from the experiment after he absented himself without leave for the whole of one day. This experience led to a tightening of the conditions for drug administration associated with the experiments. The men were lined up on a formal parade each morning in one of the wards or in the recreation hut under the supervision of CSM Winterbottom or Blackburn himself. The tablets were broken in half by a nursing sister and the drug was seen to be placed on the tongue. Half a mug of water was then drunk, and the men remained standing at attention or at ease until five minutes elapsed after the last volunteer had his drug. Blackburn said: 'I do not think that a man can now miss his atebrin'.[7]

By mid-1944 volunteers from the convalescent depots were becoming scarce, and some of those arriving in Cairns were not of the required standard. Blackburn wrote:

> The draft-conducting N.C.O. who recently came up told a member of the unit that they did not so much call for 'volunteers', as select those people, who were, to use his own words, 'no hopers'. This seems most undesirable, and [is] obviously the explanation why our men are now not up to standard. It also implies that the supply from Sydney has reached 'bedrock'. [8]

This shortage came at a crucial time, as it coincided with the need to expand the experimental work to commence the experiments on sontochin. Fairley made a visit to Adelaide to seek volunteers from South Australia, and on 9 August a memo from the Adjutant General was sent to Army headquarters in

Victoria, South Australia, Tasmania, and Western Australia. It stated that volunteers were urgently required to participate in tests to evaluate 'a new antimalarial drug which is regarded by American scientists as definitely superior to atebrin'.[9] Unlike the previous recruitment drive this call was not restricted to convalescent depots nor to troops who had never lived north of 17°S latitude. Men who had been stationed in New Guinea or other malarious countries would not be eligible, but 'residence in potentially malarious areas on the mainland of Australia will in future NOT preclude acceptance provided such volunteers have never suffered from an attack of malaria'. It was specified that 'B' Class men with physical disabilities such as defective hearing, vision, and joint problems would be acceptable, but a proportion of 'A' Class volunteers capable of prolonged physical exertion would also be required for field types of experiments. In order to ensure an orderly and steady flow of volunteers, headquarters in the different States were requested to meet specific monthly allocations from units under command to make up totals of 60 men in September and 20 per month for the following five months. The memo concluded: 'As in the past, this work will be given the highest priority. The discovery of a new antimalarial drug which would cure benign tertian relapsing malaria would be of inestimable value from the military viewpoint in the rapid rehabilitation of troops'. The contents of this memo were circulated in unit routine orders throughout Australia and resulted in a favourable response.

Assistance in recruitment of volunteers was also obtained from another unexpected source. On 1 July 1944 an article headed 'Volunteers help experts to fight dreaded malaria' was published in the *Australian Women's Weekly*. After a brief introduction to the problem of malaria in the present war and the experiments at Cairns, the article focused on the role of the volunteers and their important contribution to the research. The Commanding Officer was quoted extensively and there were several photographs that showed volunteers feeding mosquitoes, taking atebrin and providing blood for slides under the supervision of staff members.[10] This article was published after the Atherton Conference when the results of the Cairns work on atebrin were widely disseminated throughout the army. Presumably the censors judged that the need for secrecy that shrouded the formation of the unit had diminished to the extent that the research could then be revealed to the public at large. Blackburn, however, was most unhappy with certain aspects of the story. He wrote to Fairley that he was quoted inaccurately as calling the volunteers 'guinea pigs'. In fact, the volunteers commonly referred to themselves as 'guinea pigs', but Blackburn scrupulously avoided the use of this term as he considered that it would be disparaging for him to do so.[11] The article also said that the volunteers 'very rarely actually get malaria . . . because scientific tests and treatments have been so perfected that the parasites are rendered ineffective by the time they have provided the data in each experiment'. This, of course, was entirely wrong and completely misleading. It appears that Blackburn's complaint about this press coverage was heeded, as Army censors later decreed that due to exaggerated publicity no further references to the work of the unit were to be published unless released by Land Headquarters.[12]

During the next month Blackburn received a number of letters from soldiers in various parts of Australia who wished to volunteer for the malaria experiments. He replied to all these men and to their Commanding Officers, providing details of the experiment and the requirements that they would need to meet before being accepted. Blackburn mentioned this in a letter to Fairley and requested that he expedite the transfer of these men through official channels, as a rapid response should encourage their mates to follow their example. He concluded: 'In passing, most of these men mention that they have read about the unit in the Women's Weekly [*sic*]—its an ill wind—'.[13]

The recruitment of volunteers kept pace with the experimental requirements through the remainder of 1944, although some minor problems were experienced due to misunderstandings in the administrative arrangements. For example, the Adjutant General's memo directed that the volunteers should proceed to 116 AGH at Cairns rather than to the Atherton Tablelands, as was the practice since the inception of the malaria experiments. The mosquito-proofed quarters at Jungara were only sufficient to accommodate volunteers during their experiments, so arrangements had to be made to move the new arrivals to Rocky Creek to avoid the risk of locally contracted malaria.[14] Also, some men recruited in New South Wales were allocated first-class rail travel, which was normally only provided for hospital patients.[15] Army movement authorities in Queensland objected that special travel arrangements were not needed as the volunteers were fit for normal travel on troop trains. In at least one instance the extra leave provisions were denied a volunteer after he returned to his unit. This man, from 1 Infantry Training Battalion, wrote a personal letter to Fairley respectfully requesting clarification because the 21 days' leave, which he had already received at the completion of his detachment, had been reduced by 14 days.[16] His unit advised him that, in accordance with General Routine Orders, only seven days' sick leave should have been granted. An amendment to the Adjutant General's memorandum was raised in December 1944, which addressed the foregoing concerns. It specified that volunteers were to move by normal troop train to 2/1 Convalescent Depot in the Atherton Tablelands and not to 116 AGH. The 21 days' sick leave was not to be debited against members' annual recreation leave as it was in addition to the normal leave entitlements.[17]

Private A. R. (Ray) Chittleborough was assigned to the group taking Diamadino Stilbene, and was bitten by mosquitoes infected with *P. vivax* in October 1944. He broke through with blood stages during the first week of

November, and parasites remained continuously in his blood during the following month. Over this period he had episodes of typical malaria symptoms, including sweating, fever, headache and malaise, but the course of his attack was relatively moderate and he was only confined to bed for a few hours on several days. On 13 December he felt well, and went fishing after lunch in a creek about 2 km from the unit. He had an attack of colic around 3.30 p.m. and returned to the unit. His cramps increased in severity that night and he was given mild sedation and fluids. Next day he felt better but developed a mild attack of malaria that was treated with intravenous quinine. However, Chittleborough had appendicitis. He was admitted in the afternoon to 116 AGH where his appendix was removed by the senior surgeon in an operation involving considerable technical difficulty. After the operation he was given penicillin at three-hourly intervals and sulphamerazine, but his condition deteriorated and he died on the morning of 16 December. Private Chittleborough was the only volunteer to die during the entire experimental program at Cairns and Rocky Creek. An autopsy revealed that the cause of death was due to complications arising from the appendectomy, and a detailed report on this case was sent to Colonel Keogh at the Medical Directorate in Melbourne and to Fairley in England.[18] The patient had been given two intravenous injections of quinine before the operation and, even though he still had a low density of parasites in his blood, 'his malaria was unquestionably controlled'. Private Chittleborough was given a full military funeral with 50 of the volunteers on parade at their own request, as well as his brother-in-law who was also in the area. This tragic incident did not seriously affect the morale of the other volunteers nor impede the progress of the experimental work. Blackburn pointed out to Fairley: 'The other volunteers do not appear to be much upset as they all realise that he had an acute appendix and was treated by 116 AGH where he died'.[19]

The importance of maintaining a steady flow of volunteers was stressed in another memorandum from the Adjutant General that was circulated through the chain of command in February 1945.[20] Formations were allocated quotas ranging from one per month in Tasmania to seven per month in New South Wales to provide an Australia-wide monthly total of 25 men. Two weeks later a signal from Land Headquarters doubled this quota for March and April after advice was received from Fairley in London that newly discovered British drugs were available for clinical evaluation.[21] The response to this request was not encouraging. Military Headquarters in Hobart replied on 27 February that the list of men who had volunteered in Tasmania was exhausted.[22] Returns from units in Western Australia indicated that the full quota for March would not be met. Advice was received that New South Wales would be able to fulfil the April quota but no further volunteers were available for the May quota.[23] Queensland also had difficulties, and provided a table showing the breakdown of men who had volunteered and the loss due to various reasons: of 61 original volunteers, 12 were claimed by units as key personnel, four were disqualified because of Middle East service, and three were unavailable for other reasons.[24] After meeting the March quota, only 26 men were available for future commitments. The above position was presented to Lieutenant Colonel Blackburn by the Director General of Medical Services in early April with the suggestion that 'nothing further be done in this matter until Brig. N. Hamilton Fairley returns to Australia'.[25]

The need for volunteers was then greater than ever. The entire program of research at Cairns was aimed at finding a drug that would solve the malaria problem not only by protecting troops while they were operating in malarious areas but also by preventing relapses of *P. vivax* after their departure. Preliminary experiments at Cairns in April and May 1945 had already suggested that paludrine was the most promising antimalarial drug to be discovered since the synthesis of atebrin. There was a good chance that it might be the first practical causal prophylactic against falciparum malaria and that it might also prevent vivax relapses. The LHQ Medical Research Unit was the only clinical facility available to the Allied forces with the capacity to quickly evaluate this drug. The shortage of volunteers was an urgent problem that had the potential to completely disrupt this research.

Fairley quickly responded to this state of affairs on his return from Britain and South East Asia at the end of May 1945. He went to Cairns in June to review progress of the current work and, while there, prepared a report for the Adjutant General that summarised the present situation and highlighted the reasons for which the volunteers were needed. Some of the volunteers told the staff at Cairns that there were many other men in their units who were willing to volunteer but they were not being encouraged to do so. Fairley said:

> A volunteer coming to Cairns in February from one of the Workshops in Victoria stated that a captain in his unit told him that six volunteers had died as a result of experimental malaria infection at LHQ Medical Research Unit, Cairns. Such a statement is absolutely untrue and its effect is to prevent men volunteering.[26]

He confirmed that there were no deaths from malaria at Cairns, and only one volunteer had died as a result of complications following an appendicitis operation. The possibility was raised that Fairley himself could make a tour of the different States to recruit volunteers if this became necessary but this would need to be deferred until his investigation of the Aitape–Wewak malaria epidemic. In the meantime he requested that the Adjutant General exert 'relevant pressure' through the chain of command in the various States.

The conditions of acceptance were subsequently amended to allow members who had served in the Middle East to be accepted as volunteers, provided they had no malarial history. Formations were instructed to bring these revised conditions to the notice of all troops under command and to stress the urgent need for volunteers.[27] This resulted in an increase in the numbers of men coming forward, but more were still needed. In an attempt to make up the shortfall from Army sources Fairley then decided to seek permission to recruit volunteers from the Royal Australian Air Force (RAAF). In mid-July the Medical Research Unit was informed of this proposal and was instructed to indicate by signal the numbers urgently needed in the next four weeks, as well as the monthly requirements to the end of 1945.[28] The unit replied that no extra men were required for the next month and that subsequent needs were 25 per month.[29] The Director General of Medical Services, RAAF, had previously told Fairley that it might be possible to raise 20 volunteers per month, with most coming from partly-trained aircrews who had not seen service in New Guinea. A formal submission outlining the background to this request was then instituted by the Adjutant General to RAAF Headquarters.[30] This pointed out that the supply of men from the Army was practically exhausted and that, if these additional numbers were forthcoming from RAAF, then the vital malaria research could be completed. The Air Member for Personnel subsequently agreed to supply 20 volunteers per month for six months, but this decision was revoked when the war ended. Senior RAAF officers raised this matter again in early September following discussions with Fairley, but it was still turned down.[31]

It was then no longer possible to argue that the malaria research was required to defeat the enemy, but the prospect of vivax relapses in returned men remained a major problem. Strenuous efforts to recruit volunteers continued, even though most men were now looking forward to getting out of the Army and returning to civilian life. In calling for volunteers from Army units within Victoria during this period it was stressed that it was important to complete the malaria experiments for the benefit of the large numbers of prisoners of war who were returning to Australia, many of whom were debilitated by malaria.

On 6 September a signal was circulated to Army headquarters in the different States calling for all available volunteers to proceed to Cairns.[32] Those accepted were required to formally agree to continue service during the period of demobilisation, and the last drafts moved during October. The men from these final drafts, together with volunteers recruited at Cairns from among the staff of the Medical Research Unit and 116 AGH, were sufficient to complete the final experiments on paludrine and the Aitape–Wewak resistant strains of falciparum malaria.

What of the volunteers themselves? One may presume that they viewed the whole enterprise from a somewhat different perspective than those who participated in the technical or administrative aspects of the work. A total of 889 men were involved between June 1943 and April 1946.[33] Apart from the fact that they had not previously suffered from malaria, they were a heterogeneous group as they were recruited from Australian Imperial Force (AIF) and militia units with diverse backgrounds in terms of such criteria as age, education, military experience and civilian qualifications. They were advised about the conditions that were required for acceptance as volunteers, and they appreciated the need for the Army to win the fight against malaria, but they were not informed of the background of the project and their precise role in the experiments. The local authorities responsible for recruitment would not have known any more than the brief details provided in the memoranda calling for experimental volunteers. In addition to the 'virgins' who had not had malaria, there were 301 soldiers with malaria infections acquired during service in New Guinea who were either employed as gametocyte carriers or admitted for special investigations (such as those involving the Aitape–Wewak strains).[34]

Donald Friend, one of Australia's most talented artists, was among the volunteers during 1943. He was stationed at Greta, NSW, as a gunner in 2 Australian Anti Tank Regiment, a role he loathed. In volunteering he did not reveal that he had previously been infected with malaria while living in West Africa during the late 1930s, as this would have disqualified his participation in the experiment, which he saw as an opportunity to escape from the mindless boredom and intellectual isolation he felt in the regiment. He kept a diary in soft-cover exercise books, lavishly illustrated with pen sketches and watercolours, which are now in the manuscript collection of the National Library of Australia. Three volumes entitled 'Decline and Fall of a Guinea Pig' are devoted to the period of his involvement with the malaria experiments.[35] Gunner D. S. L. Friend was certainly not a typical soldier nor, for that matter, a typical volunteer, but his spontaneous comments provide an interesting contemporary chronicle of some of the early volunteers at Rocky Creek.

Friend was in a group of volunteers who travelled by train to Brisbane on 2 September 1943, where they were told by a sergeant major that the experimental course would last for approximately six weeks, with 14 or 21 days' sick leave at its completion. There was considerable uncertainty about the details of the experiment, and this encouraged speculation and rumours. One of the group 'who specialises in the more scare-brain tales' said that he had heard that 'whilst none of [the earlier volunteers] expired from malaria, a lot had gone down with blackwater fever. The Sgt Major here holds that over four hundred had been treated so far without a single casualty.'[36] They left Brisbane on 6 September for a train journey to Townsville that lasted three days. After another night they detrained at a staging camp at Redlynch, near Cairns, and were then taken by truck to the Atherton Tablelands where they were accommodated at 2/1 Convalescent Depot, a sprawling conglomeration of tents and sheds in arid surroundings. They soon learned that some of the volunteers were allocated to Cairns where they 'not only have a permanent leave-pass but are experimented on with mosquitoes instead of hypodermic needles'.[37] This appeared to be a much more attractive option, and Friend confided to his diary:

> We are resolved to try to wangle the Cairns show. Everyone is eager to get out of this place as soon as possible. Some of them are already bellyaching at the prospect of getting needles, which seems pretty ludicrous, as we knew when we volunteered that there was a fair chance of pegging out as a result of this jaunt, so a few hypodermic jabs en route won't make much difference.[38]

However, they did not go to Cairns but were allocated instead to the blood-inoculated sulphonamide series at 2/2 AGH.

A primary motivation of Friend's participation was the prospect that he might have ample spare time when he could sketch and paint. He was not disappointed, as there was little to do while they waited for their experiment to commence. During the first week he persuaded one of the nursing sisters to show him a cage of guinea pigs (laboratory animals used by the pathology laboratory), which he wished to use as subjects for a drawing. The result was 'Los Medicos'—a highly imaginative ink sketch with a blue watercolour-wash background depicting a sword-bearing Roman soldier sitting astride an enormous elephant-sized guinea pig.[39] Two other soldiers hold needles, as big as pneumatic drills, which are poised near the back of the rodent while Japanese soldiers cower in the background. He became friends with some of the hospital staff, one of whom was familiar with his artistic work before the war, and was invited to join their gramophone club and to attend a staff picnic. His social contacts among the officers and nursing sisters were not shared by the other members of his group, but some of the notes in his diary reflect the experiences of those involved in the subinoculation experiments.

> The sister announced with rather grisly humour—'well, this is the beginning, boys'—and packed us off to a hall of horrors called the Blood Bank. Here we waited nervously (It was worse than the dentist: we died a thousand deaths over and over again) in a grim ward where all the patients lay in weird beds, their limbs supported in intricate pulleys. Each of us had a blood giver—a man of the same blood group who had already been through the treatment, who had been pumped full of drugs and malaria, but on whom the malaria had not taken.[40]

After the transfusion, which Friend found particularly nerve-racking, there was the usual four-week period during which they were examined daily for signs and symptoms. His donor was one of the 'A-S series' test volunteers infected with *P. falciparum* by blood inoculation and who had received sulphamezathine. The subinoculation of 200 ml subsequently proved to be negative, and Friend was one of the very few volunteers who did not experience an attack of malaria. Before being discharged from the experiment he received the usual QAP treatment, during which he found that the high doses of quinine and plasmoquine affected his nerves and made his hands shake so much that he found it difficult to draw. His last assignment was to paint the sets for a theatre production staged by the hospital.

Donald Friend enjoyed his sojourn in the Tablelands, and later wrote that it was one of his few 'sunny interludes' before he was commissioned as an official war artist in 1945.[41] Unlike almost all of the other volunteers, he did not have episodes of fever and he certainly had an easier time than the men who were subjected to the exhausting physical conditions of the long-term field experiments that commenced in 1944.

Donald Friend was not the only artist associated with the unit. Nora Heysen, a distinguished Australian artist and winner of the Archibald Prize in 1938, was an official war artist who was attached to LHQ Medical Research Unit in August 1945. She spent the next two months sketching and painting the staff and volunteers in the wards and laboratories.[42] Some of her works during this period are reproduced as illustrations in this book from the art collection of the Australian War Memorial, Canberra.

Corporal E. E. (Ted) Viant was in one of the groups from South Australia who responded to the call for volunteers in the second half of 1944. He was a member of the militia who decided to volunteer for the malaria experiment as his 'bit to humanity'.[43] His group of volunteers joined this enterprise in a very sober manner as they did not expect it to be a bed of roses. They travelled by interminably slow troop train from Adelaide via Melbourne (bypassing Sydney) to Brisbane and then on to Townsville, and ultimately to 2/1 Convalescent Depot, Rocky Creek. Several weeks passed pleasantly while they awaited allocation to the experiments and they were taken to many tourist spots around the Atherton Tablelands. After the compulsory parade each morning, they were free to roam around the area at will, provided they returned by curfew in the evening.

In due course Viant and other members of his group were transported by truck to Cairns, where he was assigned to the short-term experiment to evaluate SN-7618 against mosquito-induced vivax malaria. After a four-day build-up on the drug, his group were assembled in the evening and ordered to roll down their sleeves and fasten all buttons. They were taken out of the mosquito-net-enclosed area of the unit to a laboratory where they were bitten by 20 vivax-infected mosquitoes, after which they were escorted back to be locked into their mosquito-proof accommodation. Their dusk-to-dawn curfew within this area was enforced throughout the experiment as a precaution to prevent the chance of inadvertent transmission from local mosquitoes.

The volunteers were allocated to various routine duties. Viant and another man were assigned to clean one of the laboratories each morning before attending the closely supervised parade during which their designated drug was administered. They were then free to do as they pleased for the rest of the day. Sometimes they spent the day swimming in one of the nearby creeks or exploring the local area on foot. Various excursions for the volunteers were organised from time to time. These included launch trips to Green Island and picnics to Ellis Beach. Transport for the latter excursions were by truck, with a food hamper provided by the cooks, and the billy was boiled at the beach. Amenities provided at the unit included a library, a workshop for those interested in woodworking, and facilities for handicraft activities. Viant came down with vivax malaria 39 days after ceasing medication.

> I . . . remember shivering to extreme and what felt like a ton of blankets on me but I still shivered uncontrollably. I lost consciousness and knew later that I had perspired to such an extent that it went through the mattress and formed a pool under my bed on the concrete floor of the sick bay.[44]

Private K. G. (Ken) Glover and Corporal R. W. (Ray) Whiteley were mates at 129 AGH in Darwin from June 1942.[45] Their unit was disbanded in early 1945, and they were sent to a staging camp at Narellan, NSW, to await reposting to another unit. After remaining there for some weeks with little to do, Glover saw a letter on the notice board requesting volunteers for medical research. Shortly afterwards there was an announcement on parade, during which it was mentioned that those volunteering would receive three weeks' extra leave at the end of the assignment. As they were both bored with their present situation, Glover and Whiteley decided to volunteer. They arrived at 2/1 Convalescent Depot at Rocky Creek on Anzac Day, and during the last week of May moved down to Cairns where they were assigned to the last long-term field-type experiment (Number CXX) with paludrine. They were not explicitly briefed about the research and the purpose of the work for which they had volunteered, but they soon learned what it was about from other volunteers and various staff of the unit when they settled into Cairns.

After they were put on their drugs and bitten by mosquitoes, they started a strenuous exercise program. This consisted initially of marches lasting for one day, but these were built up to become forced marches rather than normal hikes, and they increased in duration and degree of difficulty in subsequent weeks. CSM Winterbottom was a hard taskmaster and their daily marches were often up the railway line (over the sleepers and ballast) to Kuranda and back, a round trip of 30 km. Longer marches included a 145 kilometre return trek to Atherton, and marches along the coast road to Port Douglas, Mossman and back to Cairns (160 km). Their longest march, taking three days, was a trek from Cairns through the mountainous terrain of the Atherton Tablelands, then to Gordonvale, and finally back to Cairns. They marched at a heavy pace for 50 minutes in the hour with a 10-minute break. For their overnight marches they were issued with rations and would carry a water bottle and a haversack with blanket, groundsheet, change of socks, towel, and shaving gear. On these trips they would march well into the night and would sleep on the ground wherever they stopped. They knew that the purpose of all this was to see whether or not the parasites would break through the drug under these conditions, which were designed to simulate battle fatigue as closely as possible.

Glover and Whiteley said that the men were not discouraged from drinking beer, but they had to walk 15 km to the hotel in Cairns; the military police were instructed to drive them home as they were not permitted to stay out after dusk. Lieutenant Colonel Blackburn took a dim view of drunk and disorderly behaviour but, on the other hand, he was known to occasionally 'lend a quid' to a man going for a beer in town. They formed the opinion that he was willing to turn a blind eye on their alcoholic indiscretion in order to see whether or not they would break through the drug after imbibing to excess. 'But the drug was too good and none of us had an attack—until the use of the drug was discontinued and then we all had very severe attacks'.[46] They were subsequently given a course of treatment, and were discharged from the experiment after their weight had built up to its original level.

In addition to an extra 21 days' leave at the end of their assignment all of the volunteers received a card signed by the Commander-in-Chief, which stated: 'Your Commanding Officer has brought to my notice your name for recognition of your valuable contribution to the war effort by voluntarily submitting yourself to experiments in Army medical research' (see Fig. 16).

Towards the end of the war there was a belief in the minds of some volunteers that they were also entitled to other additional benefits. Approaches were made to Army Records Offices in several states to claim service chevrons and badges that were issued to men returned from service in operational areas. The members said that they had been told that their action in volunteering for the malaria experiments would entitle them to receive these awards. The Records Office staff refused these requests on the grounds that they were unaware of any such entitlement.[47] But the notion persisted in certain quarters that participation in the experiments qualified for repatriation benefits that were granted to men returned from active service. During 1983 a memorandum was circulated to the various state offices of the Department of Veterans' Affairs drawing attention to enquiries 'by, and on behalf of, veterans regarding their eligibility for service pension solely on the basis of their participation in malarial experiments during the 1939–1945 War'.[48] Some of the veterans presented their Commander-in-Chief's Card as evidence that they were volunteers. They said that they had been told that their involvement in the experiments would entitle them to the same benefits as servicemen who had returned from a theatre of war.

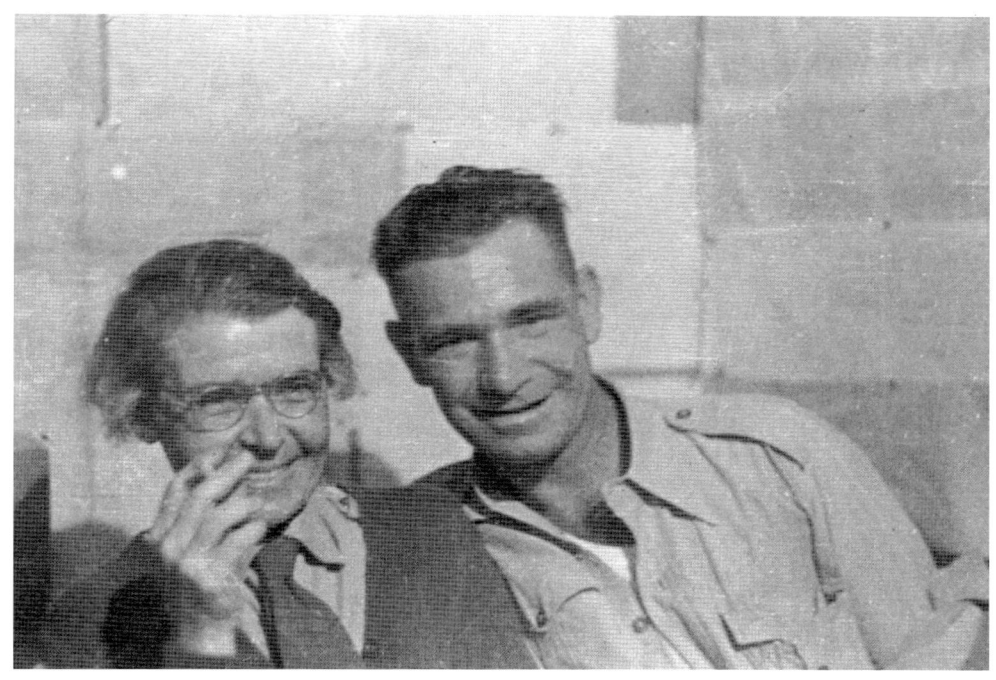

Major Jo Mackerras and Warrant Officer Bill Winterbottom in a social setting

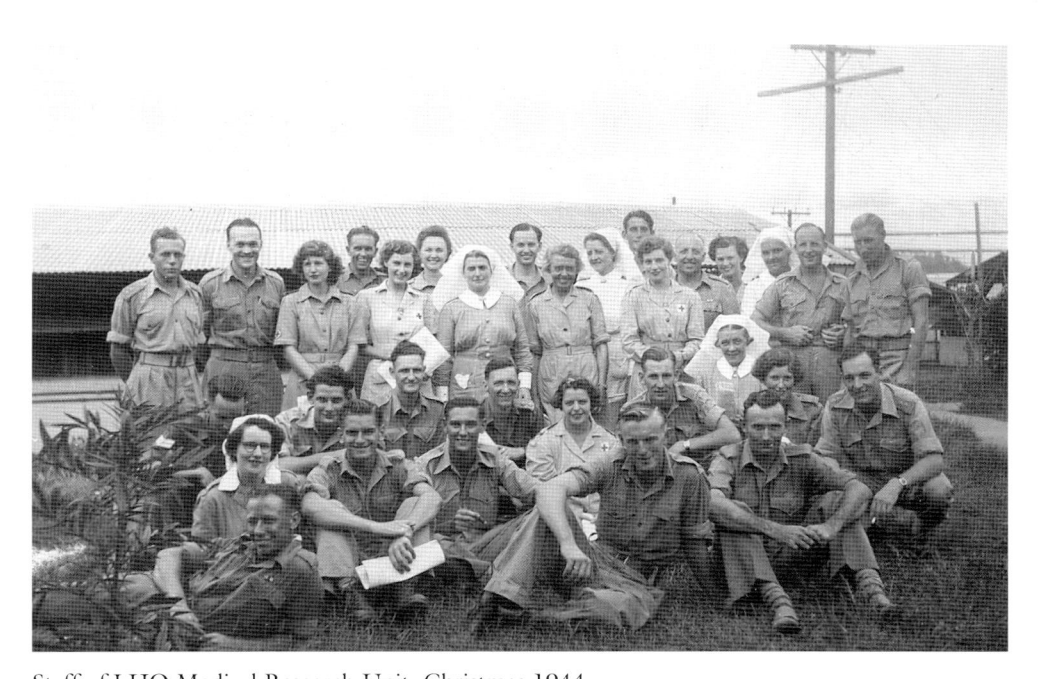

Staff of LHQ Medical Research Unit, Christmas 1944

'The little yellow atebrin tablet issued by an officer was taken with a great deal of ceremony', from 6th Div. Sketches by James Wienecke

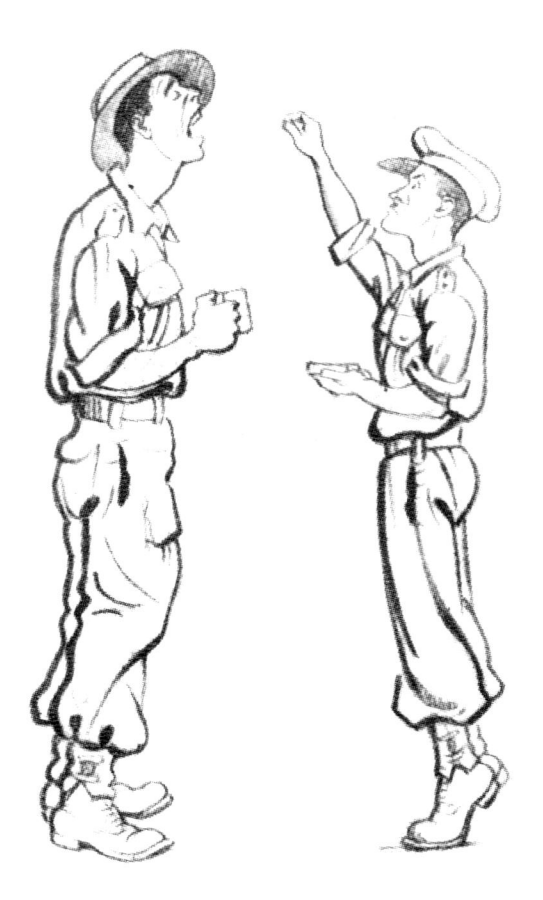

Lieutenant J. J. Garrick, 2/6 Cavalry (Commando) Regiment, placing atebrin tablets in the mouths of his men during the daily 'atebrin parade' while on operations in the Aitape–Wewak campaign in 1945

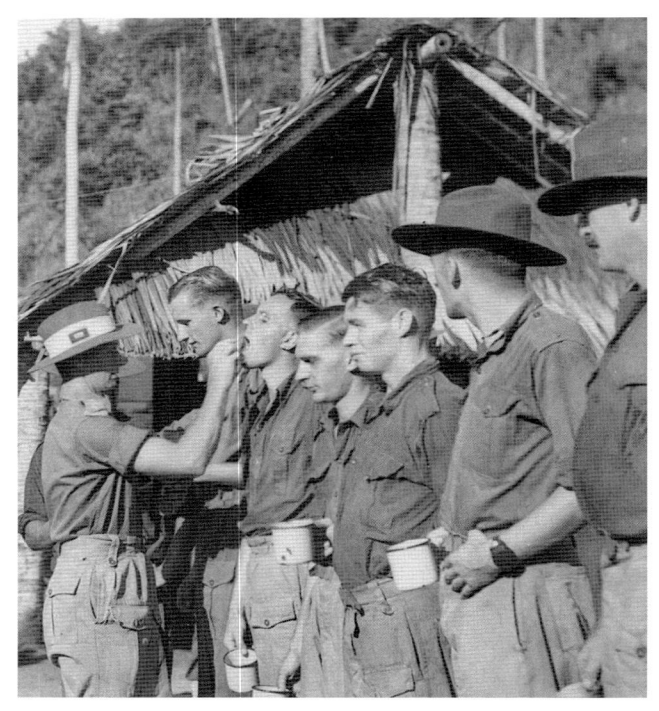

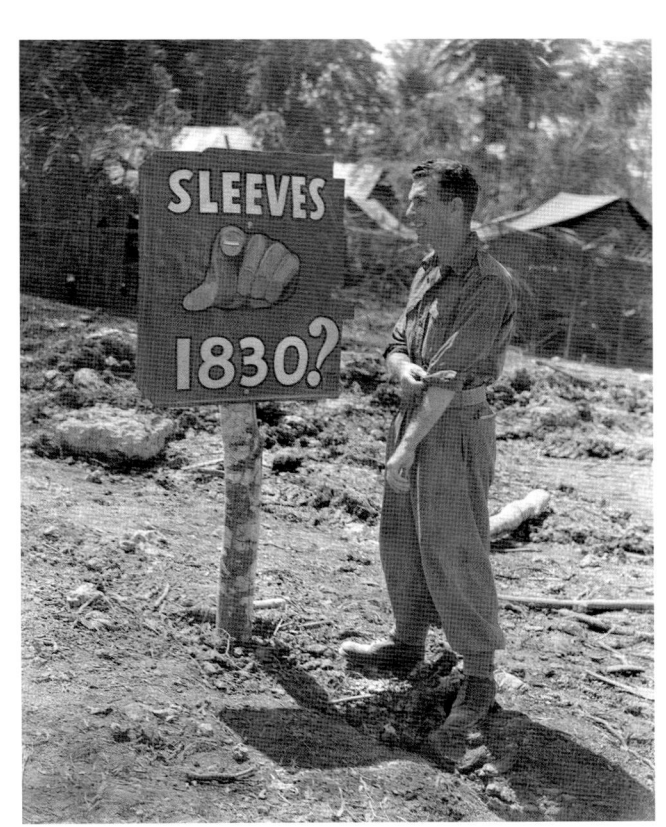

Private J. P. Merity of Headquarters 9 Division in Morotai during 1945 heeding the anti-malaria sign to roll down sleeves after 1830 hours

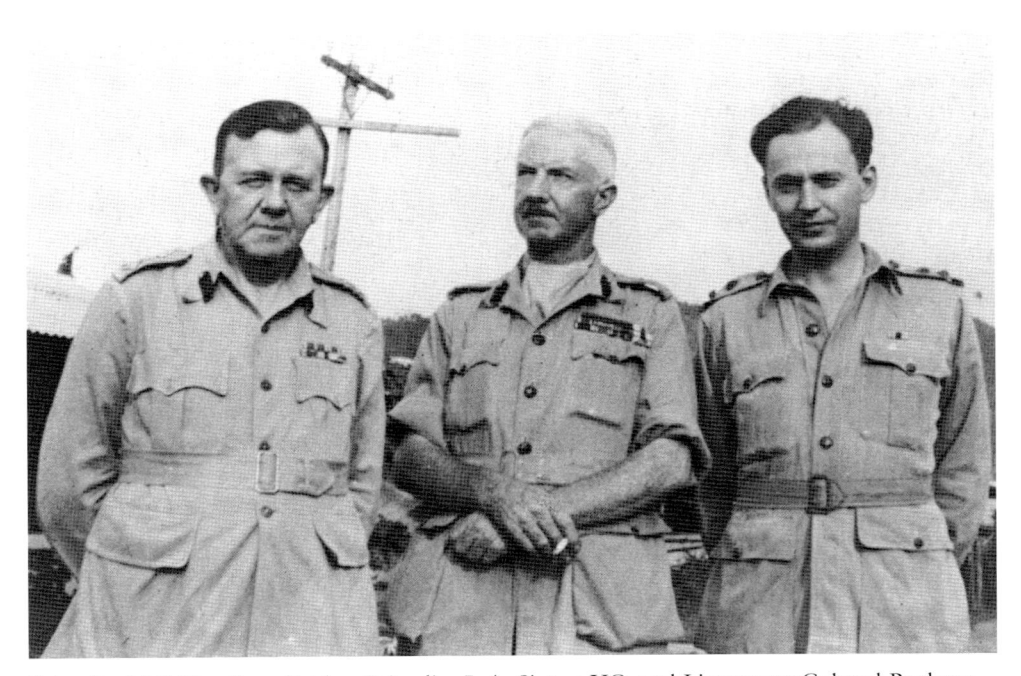

Brigadier Neil Hamilton Fairley, Brigadier J. A. Sinton VC, and Lieutenant Colonel Ruthven Blackburn at Cairns in June 1945

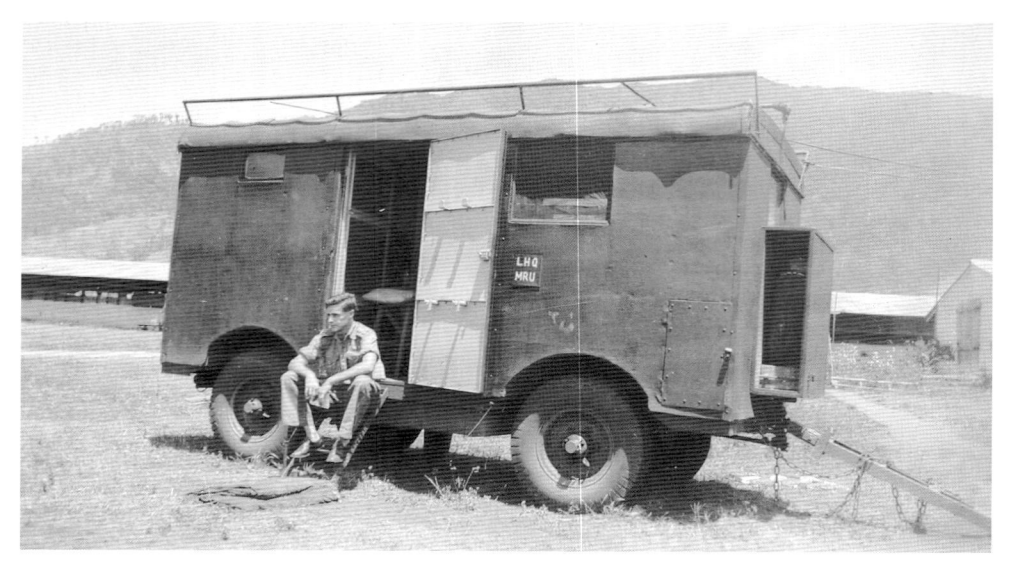

Captain Robert Black and the mobile laboratory in which he grew malaria parasites in test tubes

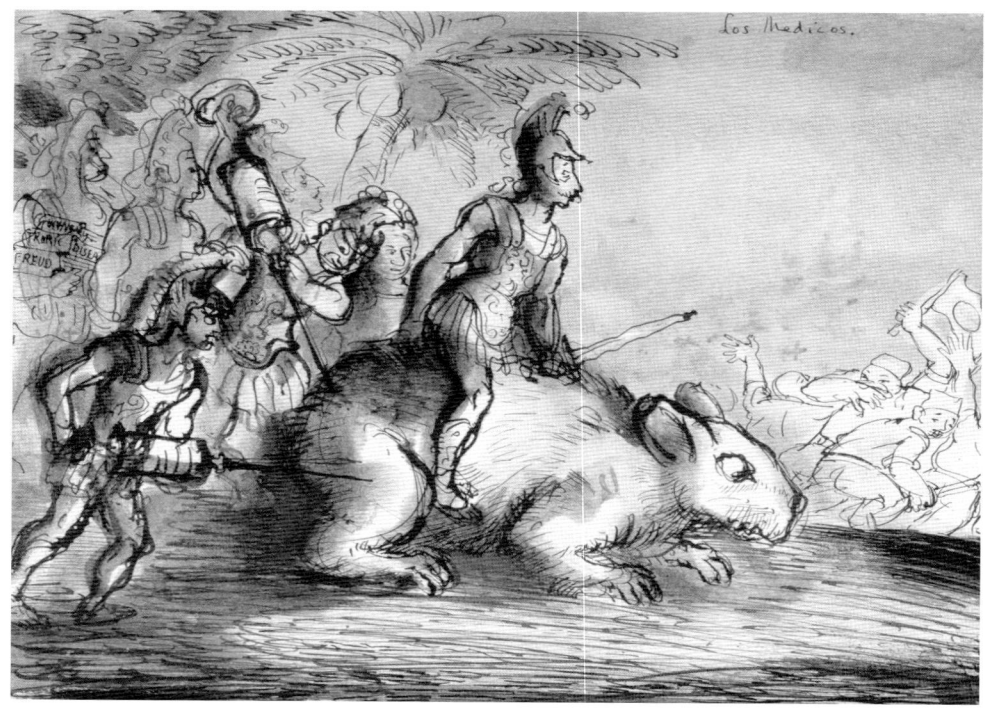

Ink sketch, 'Los Medicos', from the diary of Gunner Donald Friend, 15 September 1943

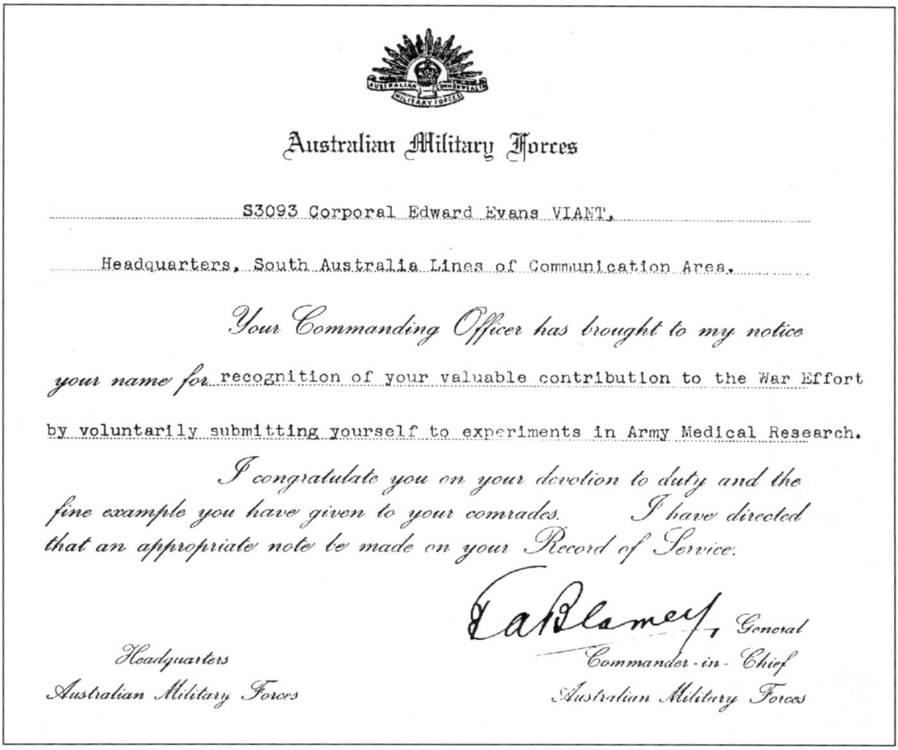

Australian Military Forces

S3093 Corporal Edward Evans VIANT,

Headquarters, South Australia Lines of Communication Area.

Your Commanding Officer has brought to my notice your name for recognition of your valuable contribution to the War Effort by voluntarily submitting yourself to experiments in Army Medical Research.

I congratulate you on your devotion to duty and the fine example you have given to your comrades. I have directed that an appropriate note be made on your Record of Service.

T. A. Blamey, *General*
Commander-in-Chief
Australian Military Forces

Headquarters
Australian Military Forces

Fig. 16 The Commander-in-Chief's card signed by General Blamey, awarded to Ted Viant after his participation in the experiments

Examination of the documentary record suggests how this situation may have arisen. The memoranda calling for volunteers, which were circulated through Army channels in July and August 1944, stated:

> They will be exposed to malaria infections of malignant tertian and/or benign tertian types while taking antimalarial drugs, and a proportion of them will develop malaria. The malignant tertian malaria, which is the dangerous type, will be cured before they leave the Cairns area, but relapses of benign tertian malaria will probably occur in some volunteers after returning to their units. *In this respect, such volunteers will be in the same position as many thousands of Australian troops who have seen service in New Guinea* [my emphasis].[49]

Some might have interpreted the last sentence to mean that the conditions of service of the volunteers would be considered to be the same as troops who had been to New Guinea, and that they would therefore be entitled to the same benefits as New Guinea veterans. But it is clear that the entire thrust of this paragraph is to inform potential volunteers of the experimental conditions to which they would be exposed. The last sentence explains that 'such volunteers [who subsequently get benign tertian relapses] will be in the same position as many thousands of Australian troops [who are also subject to benign tertian relapses]'. This misunderstanding may have arisen among the volunteers themselves, but it might also have been misread by staff in some units who were responsible for processing recruitment of volunteers. In any case the Department of Veterans' Affairs did not consider that participation in the experiments was service in a theatre of war as defined in the repatriation legislation.

During World War II there were no internationally accepted guidelines for the use of volunteers in medical research. The infamous medical experimentation involving brutal mishandling, torture, and often death of non-consenting inmates of Nazi concentration camps was considered at the Nuremburg Trials after the war. This led to the enunciation of the Nuremburg Code, which addressed the ethical considerations of permissible medical experiments on volunteers: 'The voluntary consent of the human subject is absolutely essential'.[50] It was stressed that this consent should be based on 'sufficient knowledge and comprehension of the elements of the subject matter involved as to enable [the volunteer] to make an understanding and enlightened decision'.[51] The memos calling for Australian Army volunteers explained the essential facts in broad terms: they would probably be sick with malaria and would receive treatment with drugs. On arrival at Cairns they learned that they would be exposed to malaria either by the bites of infected mosquitoes or by receiving blood from an infected donor. So by the time of allocation to a particular experiment the men knew what to expect.

The Nuremburg Code formed the foundations for the Declaration of Helsinki (adopted by the World Medical Assembly in 1964), which laid down recommendations for doctors involved in experimental research using human subjects. The basic principles were that the research should be based on laboratory and animal experiments or other scientifically established facts; that it should only be conducted by medically qualified persons; and that it should only be carried out if the importance of the objective was in proportion to the risk to the experimental subject. The Helsinki Declaration was revised in 1975 to include recommendations that proposals for research should be documented in a written experimental protocol that should be considered by a specially appointed independent ethics committee. There should also be a provision for the volunteer to withdraw his consent.

The clinical experiments at Cairns were undertaken at a time of global conflict when men were called on to volunteer for perilous military missions. These contemporary conditions underline the importance of the research objective that was succinctly argued in the following terms: 'The Pacific campaign has been fought and probably in the future will continue to be fought against two enemies; on the one hand the armed forces of Japan, and on the other, malaria. To defeat the armed forces of Japan, we must first defeat malaria'.[52] Another relevant consideration was the risk associated with the drugs that they received. The doses of quinine and atebrin administered in the experiments were the same as therapeutic and prophylactic doses already in widespread use throughout the world. Plasmoquine is a potentially toxic drug that can cause massive breakdown of red blood cells in certain individuals. This idiosyncrasy was known at the time, though the cause (deficiency of the enzyme glucose-6-phosphate dehydrogenase) was not discovered until after the war.[53] Preliminary drug sensitivity tests were made in volunteers selected for the plasmoquine experiments so that anyone with a sensitivity to the drug could be excluded. The routine drug-screening procedures in both the American and British programs included a range of animal toxicity tests to evaluate mammalian safety. Those compounds with sufficiently high antimalarial activity and low toxicity were then tested for safety in humans before being considered for clinical trial. Fairley insisted that the newly developed drugs produced by the Americans and British would only be tested in Cairns in doses that had already been shown to be safe for humans. This applied to sontochin, chloroquine, M.4430 and paludrine.

There was no question that the research was crucially important to the war effort, but what about the disease risks to which the volunteers were exposed? Infection with *P. vivax* is not potentially lethal, even if it remains untreated, but falciparum malaria is a life-threatening disease without proper treatment. However, under the clinical conditions of the experiments at Cairns and Rocky Creek, the volunteers were constantly monitored by blood examination each day. If the test drug failed to prevent or cure *P. falciparum* infections, it was eliminated by timely treatment with quinine before potentially dangerous densities of parasites developed. The men infected with sporozoite-induced vivax malaria were subject to relapses for up to three years after their primary attack was cured, but, in this regard, they were no different to the thousands of combatant troops who served in the Pacific and Asian theatres of operations.

Were the men given sufficient information to make an informed decision to volunteer in accordance with principles of the Nuremburg Code and the Helsinki Declaration? The memos calling for volunteers explained the essential facts in broad terms: they would probably be sick with malaria and would receive treatment with drugs. The volunteers did not find out the precise details until after they arrived at Rocky Creek or Cairns when they soon learned that they would be exposed to malaria either by the bites of infected mosquitoes or by receiving blood from an infected donor. So by the time of allocation to a particular experiment the men knew what to expect. Although they were not given the opportunity to consent in writing they were not pressured to participate against their will. For example, one of the volunteers who arrived in September 1944 refused to have anything to do with blood transfusions, and he was discharged from participating in the experiments.[54] The researchers at Cairns could not have been expected to anticipate guidelines drawn up 20 or 30 years afterwards. Nevertheless, the experiments were conducted with due consideration for the ethical criteria of the day and were in sympathy with the spirit of both the Nuremburg Code and the Helsinki Declaration.

None of the foregoing comments should be allowed to trivialise or understate the severity of the actual experimental conditions and the clinical effects of malaria suffered by the volunteers. A full-blown attack of malaria is an exceedingly unpleasant experience. Most men had episodes of high fever, severe chills, splitting headaches, and vomiting. Volunteers in the long-term experiments were regularly subjected to the most arduous conditions of physical exercise until they reached the point of exhaustion. The extent of their contribution was well recognised by contemporary researchers. In the discussion following the first scientific presentation of the Cairns research during Fairley's visit to London in January 1945 the eminent British malariologist Colonel S. P. James said that 'a tribute is also due to the volunteers for their self-sacrificing cooperation'.[55] In his speech of acceptance for an award from the American Foundation of Tropical Medicine in New York during 1946 Brigadier Fairley said:

> Human volunteers made a major contribution to the solution of tropical disease problems in the South West Pacific. Without their voluntary assistance and full co-operation rapid answers to essential questions concerning the control and transmission of disease could not have been given to the high command.[56]

In 1997 Ted Viant had discussions with the committee of the Rocky Creek Memorial Park as he wished to see a monument erected in commemoration of those who volunteered for the malaria experiments.[57] This park had been established in 1995, adjacent to the Kennedy Highway at the original site of 2/2 AGH, to commemorate the troops who were stationed in the Atherton Tablelands during World War II. He subsequently donated a plaque but was unable to attend the commemoration ceremony due to ill health. The plaque was unveiled by another volunteer and local resident, L. T. E. (Mick) Hendersen, on 15 August 1998.[58] The caption reads:

> This memorial honours the contribution of the army personnel who volunteered for the malaria experiments conducted by LHQ Medical Research Unit at Cairns and in this Rocky Creek area at 2/2 AGH, 2/1 ACD and 47 ACH from 1943 to 1946.

The Military Value of the Cairns Research

CAPTURED JAPANESE DOCUMENTS and statements by Japanese prisoners of war showed that malaria was their greatest wartime disease. The rate of malaria in the Japanese Army in the area was close to 100 per cent, with a death rate of around 10 per cent. The Japanese Medical Department was unprepared to cope with this disastrously high disease toll.[1] There was no set scheme for suppression of malaria—originally this was left to the individual whims of medical officers, and almost every possible combination of quinine, atebrin and plasmoquine was used. It is certain that a large number of deaths were due to insufficient early treatment.[2] The debilitation of Japanese troops by malaria must have severely impaired their fighting efficiency. This was in contrast to the condition of the Australian forces in the final year of the New Guinea campaigns.

By mid-1944 the research conducted by LHQ Medical Research Unit provided conclusive proof that atebrin was able to provide complete protection against the disease. This proof was presented to the Army during the Atherton Conference. During the next few months the incidence of malaria among the Australians in New Guinea fell to the lowest levels yet experienced, anywhere in the world, by non-immune troops operating for extended periods in highly malarious areas (see Fig. 17). This was a remarkable achievement, which must have been an important contributing factor to the Australian military successes during the last year of the war when the soldiers remained fit and healthy while many of the enemy died of malaria and the survivors were weakened by recurrent bouts of fever and sickness.

It is also remarkable that the experimental results were applied so quickly and effectively in the field. While he was in the Middle East, Fairley wrote a

240 *Malaria Frontline*

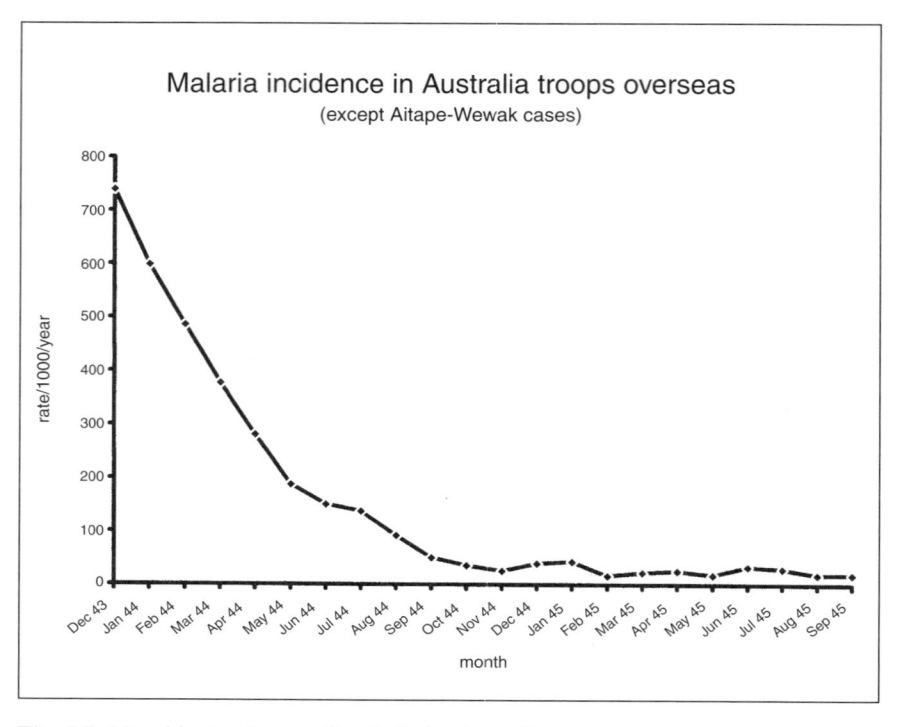

Fig. 17 Monthly incidence of malaria in Australian troops on overseas operations December 1943 to September 1945

pamphlet on malaria that was printed in 1941 and issued to all officers with the instruction that the information it contained should be conveyed to the men under their command.[3] The pamphlet included an introductory section on the importance of malaria in war, with particular emphasis on the havoc that it could cause in a military force. The ways and means of its prevention by protective measures (nets, protective clothing, repellents, and insecticidal sprays) were described, as well as the prophylactic use of quinine that was 'not a preventive of infection but a method of suppressing the symptoms of malaria and keeping men on their feet'.[4] It was the duty of every officer, NCO, and soldier to do all in his power to see that all these measures were thoroughly carried out with strict attention to detail: 'Failure to observe such precautionary measures is tantamount to self-inflicted injury'.[5] Even though malaria was not a major problem at that time, the dissemination of this information prepared the AIF for the crisis that it was to face in New Guinea. Routine Orders issued during 1943, after atebrin was adopted for prophylaxis, reinforced the message that malaria was a military, rather than a medical problem, and that the responsibility for its control rested on the Commanding Officer of every unit and on every individual soldier. During this period it was not known that atebrin could entirely protect an army in the field, so the orders were prudent in not saying that the prophylactic measures were invariably effective, while emphasising that the control methods had to be applied as rigorously as possible in order to avert a military catastrophe.

After the results of the atebrin experiments were presented at the Atherton Conference there was an immediate change in the attitude to malaria throughout the Army, and this was followed by a rapid and massive reduction in malaria casualties. The decline in malaria rates was brought about not by the adoption of new methods of protection against malaria but rather by the meticulous application of existing measures. If it were accepted that atebrin was able to completely prevent malaria in jungle warfare, it followed that the only explanation for the continuing cases among the Army, after atebrin was adopted in early 1943, was the failure to take it scrupulously each day. For commanders, the admission of the validity of the evidence presented at the Atherton Conference was to acknowledge that the Army was not correctly following the current atebrin regulations. One may imagine that this was not an easy admission to make, for it implied that the commanders themselves were remiss in not ensuring that the regulations were rigorously followed. It is not surprising therefore, that General V. A. H. Sturdee said, in his summing up of the conference, that 'there was no doubt that many officers came with little enthusiasm, if not hostility'. During the course of the conference, however, the Army commanders responded so positively that they 'appeared to be desirous of pressing the medical services further even than the latter were prepared to go'.[6]

It is tribute to the leadership throughout the command structure of the Australian Army that there was a full and frank admission of previous deficiencies in antimalarial measures and an overwhelming resolve to ensure that the situation was immediately rectified. Thereafter, Army orders in New Guinea asserted that 'success in fighting malaria will be treated as just as important as fighting in the field. Failure to fight malaria will be regarded in the same way as failure in the field due to neglect or incompetence'.[7] Malaria control became a ritual in every unit, and was treated as an essential duty like weapon cleaning and kit maintenance. It was considered to be an integral part of all operations and was never overshadowed by the military component of any task. All patrols were briefed on malaria control before departure, and were interrogated on return. In their written reports patrol commanders included a paragraph on the malaria precautions taken. There is little doubt that Fairley himself, with the support of Major General Burston and other key officers of the Medical Corps, was responsible for stimulating this dramatic change in the Army's attitude.

Fairley has been described as having rugged, determined features and a 'bulldog' expression but, in contrast, his speech and manner were gentle and considerate.[8] Several of Fairley's close friends and colleagues who knew him well have commented that there was an element of shyness in his personality, and that he was not a gifted speaker. Nevertheless, he was impressive in the way that he expressed himself: clearly and directly with transparent sincerity, using simple words. At the Atherton Conference Lieutenant Colonel Ted Ford said that Fairley 'presented his case, in his usual, quiet orderly way'.[9] He knew that 'the purpose of his address was to get action based on understanding', so he said what was needed without cajoling or 'talking down' to his audience.[10] It obviously produced the desired effect:

> He saw that the facts were translated into action in the Allied forces and the dramatic results were his accolade. Few are able to set up experiments, to get useful results, to confirm these results, to apply them to large numbers of people and to see their increased health. Neil Fairley was one such [person].[11]

As CO of the unit from 1944 to 1946, Lieutenant Colonel Blackburn had a unique opportunity to appreciate how this was accomplished. In reviewing the historical setting he later said that the important elements were 'at the right time, the right man was in the right place with sufficient facilities'.[12] The time was right because of the critical war situation and also because, at that time, there was sufficient pre-existing knowledge about the malaria parasite and the drugs available to make such a study feasible. Cairns was a suitable place where adequate resources were provided for the experiments, but there is no doubt that 'the right man' was the most important factor in this great enterprise. Blackburn wrote that Fairley believed 'that the best way to get things done was a combination of believing that they could be done, his credo, . . . selecting people to work with him who had a similar credo and delegating to them and their staff with complete confidence'.[13]

In two world wars and many other smaller conflicts Australian soldiers have been noted for their lack of reverence for military hierarchy and intolerance of 'top brass' while, at the same time, they have demonstrated an outstanding capacity to respond to good leadership. This has been well documented as part of the ANZAC legacy. The present account provides another aspect of this response to leadership in war. Fairley's leadership 'inspired deep loyalty in those who worked with him and under him . . . because he took pains to further their interests and never failed to give credit where it was due':[14]

> To work with him was a continuing pleasure. He never spared himself physically or mentally and expected his staff to do the same—very hard work, completion of everything on time, excellence of scientific performance, and honesty. Everyone always gave of their best to Neil, who was their leader, not their director or boss.[15]

Fairley's great talent for scientific leadership was also complemented by military leadership in the Australian tradition. This is exemplified by his personal efforts to recruit volunteers for the experiments. One such visit for this purpose was made to Adelaide in July 1944 when there was a shortage of test subjects for the forthcoming experiments on sontochin and chloroquine.[16] Colonel Keogh later observed:

> A rather shy man ... it seemed unlikely that he would impress the Australian private soldier ... but his judgement was right, the fact that he himself troubled to explain personally the objects of his experiments evidently appealed to them, and he quickly recruited the necessary numbers.[17]

The benefits of the research at Cairns were not restricted solely to the Australian forces. Many malariologists from England, India and the United States saw for themselves the background to the experiments at Cairns and the impressive results of their practical application in the field in New Guinea. Subsequently the Australian methods were applied in other areas, and malaria rates declined among Allied forces. Brigadier G. Covell was a senior medical officer of the British Army who wrote the standard manual on mosquito control that was used throughout India during the war.[18] As Consulting Malariologist in South East Asia Command he visited Cairns and New Guinea to investigate developments in malaria research and control in the South West Pacific in August 1944. He reported:

> The overall rate [of malaria] ... *per week* for all the forces operating in New Guinea and the adjacent islands is slightly less than the overall rate *per day* recorded in the Assam–Burma theatre ... A point which struck me most forcibly in my conversations with senior commanders ... was the acceptance *in toto* of the principle that the prevention of malaria in the field is a function not of the medical services but of the command ... I was present at one of the daily anti-malaria parades of [an] Australian infantry battalion at which each man takes his mepacrin [*sic*] and applies repellent in the presence of an officer, who at the same time inspects the men's clothing and mosquito nets, and can testify to its thorough nature. The whole procedure was accomplished in a surprisingly short time, obviously the result of long practice ... At the risk of repetition the following extracts from the notes made by a commander of one of the brigades which operated in the Ramu Valley during the early months of 1944 are given below. Their significance lies in the fact that they express the opinions of a combatant officer with long experience of battle conditions, and not those of a medical officer: 'The brigade moved in to the Ramu Valley conscious of the dangers of malaria, and with a determination to keep their sickness casualties down to a minimum ... The men must carry on their backs the necessities for fighting and living. Each night they must construct new rain shelters, erect nets, take mepacrin [*sic*] and apply repellent. All this is not easy when all ranks are wet through, hungry and exhausted. Weapon pits must be dug, patrols go out and sentries posted; but still the malaria precautions must be carried out.'[19]

In January 1945 a memo was circulated throughout the South East Asia Command:

> The incidence of malaria in SWPA is now less than 1 per 1000 per week, the lowest figure in military history. This reduction has been effected by (a) discipline in the observance of anti-malaria precautions, including a marked awareness of the dangers to health and wastage to man-power resulting from malaria, [and] (b) the acceptance by commanders at all levels of the results of the human experiments conducted at the LHQ Medical Research Unit, Cairns, Queensland, under the direction of Brig. N. Hamilton Fairley, Director of Medicine, LHQ . . . There is no reason why troops within this theatre of operations should not be able to reduce the incidence of malaria to the figures achieved in the South West Pacific.[20]

It was stressed that 'the implications of the Australian experiments must be understood and accepted by all commanders'.[21] Two months later Lieutenant General Christison, British Army Commander in South East Asia, wrote to all formations under his command: 'As the result of our drive our figures have now fallen to just twice those of the Australians in New Guinea. That is good but not good enough . . . I want all ranks to know that we are out to beat this record'.[22]

Brigadier J. A. Sinton was a distinguished malariologist who first discovered that plasmoquine had activity against relapsing vivax malaria.[23] He was also an 'iron man' in the military sense. The citation for his Victoria Cross in the World War I, when he was a captain in the Indian Medical Service in Mesopotamia, states: 'Although shot through both arms and through the side he refused to go to hospital and remained as long as daylight lasted attending to his duties under very heavy fire'.[24] His views on the implications of the work at Cairns are therefore worthy of consideration from both medical research and military points of view. After visiting the Australian Army in New Guinea and the Cairns Unit in June 1945, he wrote to Fairley:

> Before leaving, I must express my extreme admiration of all the antimalarial work I have seen. It has been most excellent and I only wish that our troops will reach such a high standard without having to learn by experience. The malaria consciousness and discipline among the Australians in most of the areas I visited had to be seen to be believed. I never met such a keen and energetic crowd as your malariologists and anti-malaria personnel—good practical men. They tackle their problems not by rule of thumb but with common sense based on an extensive knowledge properly applied. Your propaganda and that of your helpers have raised the level of the combatant outlook on conservation of man-power by health measures to a most remarkable state of efficiency. They and you are to be congratulated. As for the Cairns Unit, I cannot tell you how much I was impressed. This unit is absolutely unique in its facilities and I cannot imagine a better, more competent and enthusiastic team of workers than those you have gathered together. I

only wish I could have spent a longer time there. I was in my element getting back again to a laboratory, and such a laboratory, and such material. This research must be continued at full pressure without any curtailment of its facilities. It is of inestimable value to the war effort all over the world ... to old soldiers in future and to peace-time conditions. Any question of abolishing or curtailing its activities would be, in my opinion, most disastrous at this stage. We are all dependent on Cairns for the answer to many vital questions not only immediate problems but also those which are bound to arise in the future. Nowhere else in the world are there the same facilities combined with such a remarkable team ... It is a great achievement and a most notable one for Australia.[25]

The focus of the Australian Army's fight against malaria changed direction after the cessation of hostilities. The need to protect soldiers who continued to serve in malarious areas still remained, but there was an urgent requirement to consider the ramifications of relapses in thousands of men after they came back to Australia and ceased taking atebrin.

A dramatic illustration of the scope of the malaria problem in returned troops was provided by the experience of the 6th Australian Infantry Brigade. The battalions of this brigade spent 21 continuous months in operations against the Japanese in malarious areas from October 1943 until June 1945. After a year on the north coast of New Guinea in the Buna and Lae campaigns they were redeployed to New Britain. The average weekly incidence of malaria in the brigade during the last year of the war was well below one case per thousand men per week. These low rates led some observers to assert that New Britain was 'not very malarious', even though this was the island in which the 2/22 Battalion was decimated by the disease in 1942. Two battalions of the 6th Brigade returned to Australia in June 1945, and the third battalion left New Britain for the mainland during July. Only a few cases occurred in the month after their departure while they were still on atebrin, but a major epidemic commenced six weeks after they disembarked in Australia. Over the following eight weeks there were 976 reported cases of malaria; all but four of which were confirmed *P. vivax*. This represented a 45 per cent overall malaria rate, but it did not reflect the full extent of the epidemic as no allowance was made for men who were on leave and transfer, and there was insufficient time for all suppressed cases to develop.[26]

The treatment of demobilised soldiers was covered under the provisions of the Repatriation Commission, the terms of which were explicitly covered in a General Routine Order issued to army units soon after hostilities ceased in August 1945. This provided instructions for any ex-members who became ill with malaria after discharge. Those living in a capital city were to report to a Repatriation General Hospital for examination and treatment. Those living in country areas were advised to contact the nearest Repatriation medical officer.

If this were not practical, then consultation and treatment could be undertaken by a local civilian doctor whose fees would be paid by the Repatriation Commission.[27] The number of cases in ex-servicemen treated under these arrangements soon exceeded those within the Army.

Based on the findings at Cairns, paludrine offered clear advantages over atebrin, but it was not then commercially available and had not been released onto the open market. In January 1946 Imperial Chemical Industries (ICI) supplied 225 kg free of charge to the Australian Army[28] so that work on paludrine for treatment could be continued, but this was not enough to meet all the Australian requirements. It was estimated that over the next 18 months there would be a need for at least 750 kg (7.5 million tablets each of 100 mg), of which 400 kg would be for the armed services and 350 kg for repatriation cases.[29] It was then arranged that a further 225 kg should be supplied free of charge, and that the balance would be supplied at the current price for atebrin.[30] In a personal note that accompanied the official letter Dr D. G. Davey explained that ICI would gladly provide all of Australia's requirements free of charge, but there were political concerns that other countries, particularly India, would complain if this were done. A nominal charge was made to circumvent this possibility.[31]

It was important to adopt the most efficient treatment regimen to provide rapid cure of the present attack and to minimise the chance of future relapses that were not prevented by the standard therapy of quinine, atebrin and plasmoquine (QAP). The key to preventing further relapses in returned men was a treatment regimen that would not only cure the present attack by destroying the blood stages, but which would also eliminate the tissue stages responsible for subsequent relapses. Of all the drugs tested at Cairns only plasmoquine and paludrine were shown to have some effect on the tissue forms of the parasite. The subinoculation experiments had demonstrated that the blood stages of vivax malaria first appeared eight to nine days after inoculation of sporozoites by infected mosquitoes. Invasion of the blood was delayed by at least several days if plasmoquine or paludrine were administered during the first week after biting, and the primary attack of malaria developed about one to two weeks later than in untreated cases. None of the four test subjects in the plasmoquine series had relapses during the nine-month observation period after their initial attacks were cured.[32] Even though relapses subsequently occurred in the paludrine test cases, Fairley thought that if they were both given together for treatment they 'may produce a higher proportion of radical cures than any other combination of antimalarial drugs'.[33] An experiment designed to investigate the combined effect of using the two drugs was undertaken in Army hospitals in Brisbane (112 AGH), Sydney (113 AGH) and Melbourne (115 AGH). Soldiers who were admitted with vivax relapses received 10-day treatments with either a combination of paludrine (300 mg daily) and plasmoquine base (30 mg daily), or a combination of quinine (2000 mg daily) and plasmoquine base (30 mg daily).[34] Records were kept of all men who received both treatment courses in the three hospitals so that any subsequent relapses could be documented.

The final experiments at Cairns were completed in March 1946, and the unit was disbanded during the following month. Lieutenant Colonel Blackburn returned to Sydney and took up an appointment as a physician at Royal Prince Alfred Hospital. At Fairley's suggestion, he continued in the Army on a part-time basis and maintained an involvement in the ongoing malaria treatment experiment, for which he prepared a progress report during the first week of June 1946.[35] At this stage of the study some soldiers had completed their treatment course up to six months previously, whereas others had only been discharged from hospital for a week or so. But this time factor was the same for both treatment groups at 112 AGH and 113 AGH, and an analysis of the reported relapses in both groups showed that the relapse rates were around 13 per cent for both the paludrine/plasmoquine and quinine/plasmoquine treatment groups. Blackburn noted that the interval between treatment and relapse appeared to be longer in those treated with the former regimen.

Fairley left Australia in May 1946 and was appointed to the Chair of Tropical Medicine at the School of Hygiene and Tropical Medicine in London. Before his departure, he suggested treatment regimens for repatriation cases that were based on those to be adopted by the armed services. It was decided that the standard treatment for both vivax and falciparum malaria was to be a 14-day course of paludrine and plasmoquine.[36] A single tablet of each drug (100 mg for paludrine and 10 mg for plasmoquine) was to be taken three times a day after meals. The instruction specified that acute haemolytic anaemia was known to occur in a small proportion (1 in 10 000) of cases treated with plasmoquine. For this reason the patient was to be in hospital as a bed-case under strict medical supervision throughout the treatment period, and plasmoquine administration was to cease immediately if his urine became blackish or red coloured. The results of such treatment were followed up, and the data were compiled for the statistical survey of Army malaria cases. Those treated as inpatients in repatriation hospitals in the various states received the specified 14-day course of paludrine and plasmoquine. None of these patients was permitted to leave hospital until the course was completed. Cases treated in country areas received the QAP regimen adopted by the Army during the war. All repatriation patients were supplied with 50 tablets of paludrine on the completion of treatment, and were instructed to take two tablets each week on Wednesdays and Sundays for six months.

In February 1947 a progress report was prepared by the Repatriation Commission on the cases treated under these arrangements throughout Australia between August and December 1946.[37] This information was presented to the Army, and Lieutenant Colonel Blackburn flew to Melbourne to review the data and evaluate the results.[38] Over this period almost 12 500 men had received treatment for malaria and been issued with a six-month course of paludrine. There had been 58 reported recurrences since the initial treatment course but deficiencies in procedures adopted in the various states were already apparent. Of the 40 recurrences reported from New South Wales the blood films were negative in 14 films, and in another 14 cases it was not stated whether a positive film was obtained. Thus, it was not known for certain whether all of these reported cases were due to malaria. Also, two of the men who relapsed in South Australia admitted to not taking their prophylactic paludrine twice a week on a regular basis. The Repatriation Commission ceased the systematic compilation and analysis of their malaria treatment and relapse cases at the end of June 1947. The final figures included 21 588 cases, of whom 1670 relapsed after treatment.[39] In South Australia and Tasmania there were 2250 cases, but the drugs used during treatment of the acute attack were not recorded. Total figures in the other states indicated a relapse rate of 2.5 per cent of 3500 cases treated with paludrine and plasmoquine, and a relapse rate of 8 per cent in 15 000 cases following atebrin or QAP treatment. However, there was no information concerning the length of time between cessation of the six-month period on prophylactic paludrine and the time of relapses. There were suggestions that men relapsed while they were still taking paludrine for prophylaxis, but this was not explicitly recorded (drug levels in the blood were not measured) and it was not possible to know whether the men actually took the drug punctually twice a week. It is possible that some men only took the drug when they felt the onset of an attack. Under these circumstances the results of the survey could not be considered to represent the true comparative value of the various drug combinations in preventing relapses.

In addition to his position as Professor of Tropical Medicine in London, Fairley was chairman of the Malaria Subcommittee of the Colonial Medical Research Council and British representative on the Malaria Committee of the World Health Organization at Geneva. In these latter appointments he played a key role in advising on drug schedules for prophylaxis and treatment. He was most interested in the results of the post-war Australian experience in the use of paludrine for treatment and suppression of relapses, as there were no equivalent observations in Britain and the USA on follow-up of large groups of vivax cases treated with this drug. He wrote to the Director General of Medical Services in Melbourne in April 1947 requesting the results of cases treated by the Repatriation Commission. He also asked for the follow-up information on the comparative study involving paludrine/plasmoquine and quinine/plasmoquine for treatment of soldiers in Australian Military Hospitals that he understood to be in the process of analysis by Lieutenant Colonel Blackburn.[40]

A month later Blackburn replied with a summary of the relapse data compiled from Army records.[41] All cases had proven vivax malaria before treatment commenced and, unlike the repatriation cases, a six-month prophylactic course of paludrine was not administered. The summarised data for the three hospitals showed an overall relapse rate of 21 per cent in 642 men who received paludrine and plasmoquine and 23 per cent in 491 men who received quinine and plasmoquine. Blackburn said that

> these relapse rates, of course, do not necessarily represent true rates—the only relapses known are those who reported to either an Army or Repatriation Medical Officer and they may not have all done this. This factor should have affected patients receiving both courses in a similar manner and the comparison of rates seems quite justified.[42]

The only appreciable difference was in the time elapsing between treatment and first relapse—the mean interval following the paludrine course was 2.8 months, whereas that following the quinine course was 1.6 months.

The relatively high relapse rate following both treatment schedules was a considerable disappointment, as there were initially good grounds to suggest that the concurrent administration of paludrine and plasmoquine might have had a synergistic effect against the tissue stages of *P. vivax*. Even though this drug combination was not able to prevent vivax relapses, paludrine alone proved to be very effective for prophylaxis and treatment. The remarkably rapid and thorough clinical evaluation of the new British drug was a tribute to the team at Cairns, and it is fitting that Australia was the first country in which it was used on a large scale for treatment of malaria in men returned from the war. This was a direct benefit of the Australian research effort that contributed to minimising malaria casualties in the immediate post-war period while the country was making the transition to peace.

23

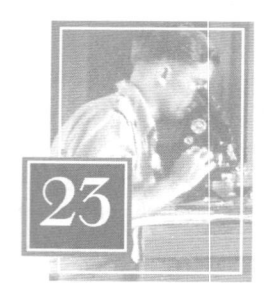

A Glorious Gamble in Science

During the first half of 1945 clinical trials in the United States showed SN-7618, chloroquine, was the most active of the 4-amino-quinoline compounds screened against human malaria. Tests indicated that a single weekly dose of 300 mg of the drug should be adequate for prophylaxis.[1] Subsequent field trials in malarious areas confirmed the validity of these observations. This was considerably less than the doses that had produced toxic symptoms in humans and around half the minimum effective dose of atebrin required to provide adequate suppression of vivax and falciparum malaria. Additional advantages of SN-7618 were that it did not discolour the skin after prolonged administration and did not cause the occasional gastrointestinal side-effects of atebrin. However, it was not developed in time to become available for operational use by US and other Allied forces during the war.

In the last stages of the war in Europe an American military intelligence team visited Elberfeld to obtain information on German pharmaceutical research and development. Dr Kenneth Blanchard participated in this mission, and reported to the Board for the Co-ordination of Malarial Studies at a Panel of Review meeting in June 1945 that SN-7618 was identified as resochin, a compound first synthesised by Andersag in 1934, but that the Germans believed it to be inferior to SN-6911. Blanchard said: 'In point of fact, SN-7618 prepared by the Germans appears never to have been given an adequate clinical trial. It seems that this drug was found by Sioli to be too toxic for practical use'.[2]

During 1946 the US Council on Pharmacy and Chemistry (acting in response to a request from the Board for the Co-ordination of Malarial Studies) published a brief note in the *Journal of the American Medical Association*.[3] This recognised that the compound chloroquine, 'a non proprietary name for the antimalarial substance sometimes described as SN-7618', was covered by a German patent, but noted that the work in developing its antimalarial properties and usage was done under the auspices of the wartime co-operative program.

A brief outline of the American co-operative wartime research program was announced to the scientific community in the journal *Science* in January 1946.[4] This article described the huge scope of the program, involving co-operative efforts of large numbers of university investigators supported by the Office of Scientific Research and Development contracts and the participation of industrial firms. Over 14 000 compounds were screened for antimalarial activity in avian parasites, of which about 80 were subjected to clinical evaluation against human malaria. Described by the senior US Army member of the Board, Brigadier General J. S. Simmons, as 'one of the most glorious gambles in science',[5] it involved an enormous effort and expenditure, and was only surpassed as a scientific enterprise by the Manhattan project that developed the atomic bomb.

Nevertheless, the senior scientists associated with the board were somewhat ambivalent about the advances that had been achieved. On the one hand, they had developed chloroquine to the stage of practical use in the field. This was shown to be a highly effective prophylactic when administered only once a week; it rapidly cured clinical attacks of vivax and falciparum malaria and did not have the side-effects of atebrin. But, on the other hand, the Americans could not take the credit for the discovery of this drug as it was a compound originally synthesised by German chemists before the war. Moreover, chloroquine only acted against the blood stages of the parasite, and was unable to prevent vivax cases from relapsing. This was identified by the Board during 1944 as the most important problem facing the US malaria program, and in the immediate post-war period it assumed even greater prominence. The Americans were then in exactly same situation as the Australians with the return from the Pacific campaigns of thousands of servicemen who were subject to recurrent attacks of vivax malaria.

The major emphasis of drug screening during the final months of the American program was to seek analogues of plasmoquine that would eliminate *Plasmodium vivax* relapses.[6] There were about 500 8-amino-quinolines in the survey records, of which 60 were in the process of being evaluated in animals for antimalarial activity and toxicity, but there was still the problem of deciding which ones should be selected for clinical trial.[7] It was decided that only those with less toxicity to animals than plasmoquine would be considered for tests in humans and, in order to provide sufficient margin of safety, they would initially be administered in amounts estimated to be only one-sixth of the maximum-tolerated dose based on toxicity tests in monkeys.

Dr A. S. Alving's group at University of Chicago was then the principal institution in the United States involved in clinical evaluation of drugs against sporozoite-induced malaria. This work was undertaken with the Chesson strain of vivax malaria using prisoner volunteers at Stateville Penitentiary. Six compounds within the 8-amino-quinoline series that met the selection criteria were allocated to the Chicago testing unit at the end of July 1945. One of this group, code numbered SN-13,276, was included because it had high antimalarial activity against *P. lophurae* in ducks and low toxicity in animals, being only one-quarter as toxic as plasmoquine in monkeys.[8] At a subsequent meeting of the Panel on Clinical Testing on 16 October 1945 it was reported that this compound was the most promising among those tested to that date.[9] It had been administered for 14 days at a dosage of 60 mg in combination with quinine and there had been no relapses for 41 days after drug administration ceased. A longer period of observations was required before it would be known whether or not breakthroughs might still occur, but Alving was most encouraged by his experiences with SN-13,276 and other related compounds. He said that even when breakthroughs occurred with some of these 8-amino-quinolines the attacks were more easily cured than breakthroughs following causal prophylactic trial of any other drugs that he had tested. He thought that, even if the 8-aminos did not result in causal prophylaxis, 'they exerted an effect on the underlying tissue forms and thereby modified the subsequent course of the disease'.[10]

The activities of the Board for the Co-ordination of Malarial Studies were terminated in June 1946. At the last meeting of the Board a motion was passed that Dr E. K. Marshall should communicate with the Council on Pharmacy and Chemistry of the American Medical Association suggesting that the chemical known as SN-13,276 be registered as 'pentaquine'.[11] This proposal was adopted in anticipation that the drug would soon be available for trial in service installations. In summarising the work of the Chicago unit in his final report to the Board Alving wrote:

> Eleven 8-amino-quinolines of the 22 tested apparently cured at least 1 patient who presented severe challenge to the drug. Five compounds other than plasmoquine have cured more than one patient. The most effective compound studied to date is pentaquine (SN-13276) which is approximately $1\frac{1}{2}$ times as effective as pamaquin but is $\frac{1}{2}$ as toxic.[12]

This finding vindicated the American efforts to seek a better drug against the tissue stages of malaria from among compounds related to plasmoquine. It was realised that there may be more effective drugs in this series, but there was insufficient time to bring this exploratory work to a logical conclusion before the termination of the program. However, this promising lead was followed up in the immediate post-war years by Dr Leon Schmidt and his colleagues at the Christ Hospital Institute for Medical Research, Cincinnati, Ohio, and at the

University of Alabama in Birmingham. During 1947 Schmidt's group evaluated some 8-amino-quinoline derivatives that had been synthesised during the wartime program but not tested in humans. They used a screening system based on the primate malaria parasite, *P. cynomolgi*, in rhesus monkeys, which has a relapse pattern similar to *P. vivax* in humans. This led to the identification of primaquine (SN-13,272) as being the most promising of the series.[13] Primaquine was later shown by Alving's group to be effective in preventing relapses of the Chesson strain, and it is still the standard drug for radical cure of vivax malaria.[14]

The Australians played an indirect, though important, role in improving the efficiency of the malaria research effort in the USA during 1945–46. The research at Cairns convinced the Americans that South West Pacific strains of vivax malaria had an early relapse pattern quite unlike their standardised experimental strains. This stimulated the isolation of the Chesson strain, which provided a crucial research tool to permit rapid evaluation of drugs against the tissue stages of the disease. This strain was used by Shannon in New York to confirm the pre-war British work on plasmoquine, and it was then adopted by Alving in Chicago for clinical evaluation of other related compounds. The rapid results achieved by the Americans during the closing stages of the war set the stage for the post-war commercial development of primaquine, the most active of these compounds. It is unlikely that this line of research would have been carried on to fruition if the clinical evaluation of malaria drugs in the United States had continued to rely on strains of *P. vivax* with delayed relapses. Under these circumstances the pace of the work would have been so slow that promising leads could not have been followed up before the American program was terminated.

The universally accepted benchmark for priority in scientific discovery is the date of first publication of the findings in a peer-reviewed scientific journal. Many American publications on chloroquine were published in the 1940s, including the causal prophylactic studies of G. R. Coatney's group in Atlanta that were published in the *American Journal of Hygiene* in 1949.[15] These publications, and the fact that chloroquine was subsequently marketed by American pharmaceutical companies, have subsequently tended to overshadow the Cairns work on chloroquine, which was not published until 1957.[16] This delay occurred because Fairley suffered a cerebral thrombosis in December 1947. He subsequently made a good, but not absolute, recovery as he did not fully regain his tireless intellectual energy and prodigious capacity for demanding scientific work. Nevertheless, a summary of the Australian work on sontochin and chloroquine was published in 1946.[17] This explicitly stated that the experiments at Cairns demonstrated that these drugs act on the blood stages and are not causal prophylactics. These findings were reiterated in the following year in the paper describing the subinoculation experiments.[18]

Coatney's 1949 article cited all relevant American studies with chloroquine but, curiously, did not mention the ground-breaking Australian work. However, American historical accounts have accorded full credit to the significant part played by the Australians in the clinical evaluation of the 4-aminoquinolines. The history of the American co-operative wartime program stated that 'the Board was particularly indebted to Brigadier Fairley for the extensive and brilliantly thorough trials of SN-6911 and SN-7618 in Australia'.[19] The official history of the US Army Medical Department in World War II acknowledged the prominent role of Fairley's group in confirming the suppressive activity of sontochin and chloroquine, and credited the subinoculation experiments at Cairns with demonstrating that these drugs did not act as causal prophylactics.[20]

The mutually beneficial co-operation between the American and Australian malaria research teams was not always evident in the wartime relations between the Americans and the British. During 1944 there was an unfortunate breakdown in liaison between the US Board for the Co-ordination of Malarial Studies and the British Medical Research Council. Fairley was told of this during his visit to Washington in October 1944. The British had suggested that some of the American malaria research workers should come to Britain, or alternatively that certain British malaria research workers should visit the USA. The Americans declined the offer to visit Britain. Dr A. N. Richards, Chairman of the US National Research Council, asked Fairley to act as an intermediary by informing two influential members of the British Medical Research Council, Sir Edward Mellanby and Sir Henry Dale, of the American difficulties in this regard. Richards explained that, due to factors outside his control, there would be certain things that the British workers would not be shown if they visited the USA.[21]

The reason for this breakdown in co-operation is not precisely clear from the documentary record but it is likely that it stemmed from commercial rivalry between competing American and British interests. In April 1944 Shannon reported tests in his laboratory in New York using the ICI compound M.3349.[22] The US Board for the Co-ordination of Malarial Studies later approved a contract for the American firm, Dupont, to produce analogues of this drug. ICI and Dupont had a pre-war commercial arrangement, and the Americans hoped this might assist integration of the development programs between the two companies. The Board sent a cable to Dr Hamilton Southworth, the scientific liaison officer of the US Committee on Medical Research in London, asking him to contact ICI and request that copies of the ICI reports on synthesis of this group of compounds be given to Dupont.[23] Southworth replied that 'ICI was all in favour of closer integration with Dupont' but the release of reports had to be cleared by the British Medical Research Council (MRC) and the Patents section of the Ministry of Supply:

Personally, I feel that we can make no complaint about this when we haven't furnished all of our material of commercial origin to the British group. It is quite possible that a good deal of the work now being planned for Dupont has already been done over here [in Britain]. Isn't it full time we arranged things in the States so that a situation like this would not occur?[24]

Dale was the chairman of the MRC's 'inner group', and he told Southworth that direct exchange between ICI and Dupont could not be made without MRC clearance.[25]

A probable contributing factor to this impasse was the sequence of events leading up to the commercial development of penicillin. The antibiotic value of this drug was discovered in England by the Australian scientist Howard Florey, and was subjected to preliminary clinical evaluation and development by his research group at Oxford during the early years of the war. Due to the grave wartime situation there was then little chance that British firms could or would undertake commercial development, so, with a grant from the Rockefeller Foundation and with encouragement from Mellanby, Florey visited America in 1941 to solicit the support needed to mass-produce penicillin for clinical use. Subsequently, the US firm Merck & Co. devised methods for industrial production, and patented the stages in the process. By 1945 British firms had to pay royalties on their penicillin production. This must have been a source of considerable resentment by British authorities, including Mellanby and Dale, who had both told Florey before he went to America that penicillin should not be patented in Britain. They felt strongly that it would be unethical to do so because discoveries by medical researchers should be made freely available to the world.[26]

The American interest in exploiting the British discovery of M.3349 and its analogues contrasted with their reluctance to reciprocate by sharing their fortuitous capture of the German drug sontochin with their British allies. They were eager for the Australians to have the drug, knowing that the superior set-up for clinical testing at Cairns would permit its evaluation more promptly and more thoroughly than could be done in the USA, but they did not make it available to the British until several months later.[27] After delivering a sample of sontochin to Dr Harold King of the National Institute of Medical Research at Hampstead in August 1944, Southworth wrote a letter to Dr George Carden, Secretary of the Board for the Co-ordination of Malarial Studies. It throws a revealing light on the commercial considerations that were an undercurrent between the malaria programs of the two countries.[28] Southworth was surprised to learn that King already had the drug in his laboratory, and had even suggested to ICI that they produce some for clinical testing. King was a senior British scientist who was responsible for directing much of the experimental work on malaria undertaken in British universities and the MRC during the war. He was also an informal adviser to the synthetic chemists working at ICI.[29] After hearing that the Americans had captured a drug from the Germans in North Africa, he managed to obtain some of the captured material through the Foreign Office and worked out its formula without any help from the United States.[30] Southworth's letter emphasised 'that there was no leak of information supplied by us to King. In fact, if King had known that we were working with the material he would probably not have taken ICI into his confidence'.[31]

The minutes of the Board for the Co-ordination of Malarial Studies indicate that one of the American firms, Winthrop, refused to provide information to the Australians and the British. This refusal could have had unfortunate military consequences for the Australian forces in New Guinea. Dr Carden reported that in early November 1944 he had received requests from Australia and Britain for data concerning the tabletting of atebrin.[32] Considerable difficulty was being experienced with atebrin tablets in humid tropical environments, as they became soft and were prone to disintegrate before use. The request was for technical details on the tabletting and shellac coating so that the problem could be dealt with. On receipt of this request Carden wrote to Dr C. M. Suter of Winthrop requesting these details for transmission to the Director General of Medical Services in Australia and MRC in England. Suter replied:

> At the present time we do not feel free to send this information for the research councils in Australia and London. The request is an interesting one in view of the long experience which the British have had in the manufacture of atebrine tablets, which so far as we know, are as satisfactory as the ones manufactured in this country.[33]

On receipt of this refusal Dr Carden consulted Dr Elderfield, who approached Dr Volwiler of the Abbott Laboratories. He received a prompt favourable response with details of the Abbott process by mail two days later. The members of the Board were most unhappy with Winthrop. Elderfield said that, 'even though government contractors are devoting a great deal of time and effort to the exploitation of the Winthrop Chemical Company's patented compounds, [the company] continues to display an uncooperative attitude'.[34] Carden wrote to the Directors of Winthrop:

> The problem faced by the Australians is of considerable military importance. As indicated by the attached letter from Colonel Downie of the Australian Military Mission, a second request was submitted to your company. In a letter to Dr Suter, 8 December, I enclosed a copy of Colonel Downie's letter and asked, in view of the possible operational significance in the difficulties with atebrin tablets experienced by the Australians, if the Directors of Winthrop Chemical Company might not care to reconsider their decision . . . Because the problem is an urgent one and has both military and diplomatic significance, a prompt reply to the second request submitted over two weeks ago would be greatly appreciated.[35]

Winthrop's reply to this letter is not recorded in the Board minutes. Also, it is not clear whether the Australians and the British were told of the company's attitude or whether they were simply given the information provided by Abbott Laboratories.

In a letter to Major General S. R. Burston, sent from London in February 1945, Fairley said that the Americans 'have come to the conclusion it would pay them to get together again' following the discovery of paludrine by ICI. The British had received a formal request for R. E. Loeb, S. R. Shannon and E. K. Marshall to visit England during the following month:

> Sir Edward Mellanby and Dr Scott (I.C.I.) have asked my opinion on this question, and I had no hesitation in strongly advising them to agree to their coming. In the long run it will lead to a better understanding and more cordiality between research workers in the two countries, and that really is more important than any other consideration at the present time.[36]

Loeb and Shannon subsequently visited England for two weeks in April 1945. On their return they reported favourably to the Board on the British malaria research program. During an executive session Loeb said:

> Tentative arrangements for the exchange of information on developments in the fields of synthesis, pharmacology, and clinical testing of antimalarials, including information held 'in confidence' was arranged with the MRC in London. It was generally agreed that the inner group of the MRC and Board for the Co-ordination of Malarial Studies and CMR should become repositories of all information. It was also agreed that information classified 'in confidence' in the States would be withheld from British commercial firms and likewise material of a confidential nature submitted by British firms to the MRC would be withheld from American commercial firms.[37]

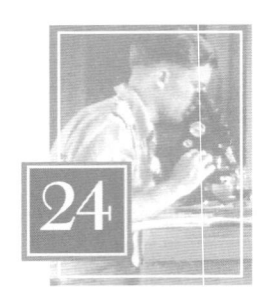

Press Reports

BRIEF REPORTS IN several Australian newspapers broke the first news of malaria experiments in Australian soldiers 'at a research hospital in northern Australia' following comments by the Minister for the Army, Frank Forde, in Canberra on 5 February 1944. The Sydney *Telegraph* ran the story under the lurid heading '1000-bite-an-hour men in malaria test':

> Thousands of larvae of the New Guinea malarial mosquito are regularly brought to the hospital ... reared ... and allowed to bite malaria patients so they will become carriers of the disease. Then they are turned loose on the volunteers ... Before exposing themselves to the mosquitoes, the soldiers take a new preventive drug. Details and results of the experiments are secret, but the excellent results already achieved will be increased when the present investigations are completed.[1]

These details, including the grossly inflated mosquito biting rate of 1000 bites/hour, were also reported in the Brisbane *Mail* and the Melbourne *Age*.[2] The latter newspaper quoted Forde as saying that the men were fully informed of the risks they incurred, but this had not prevented them from volunteering.

Four months later Senator J. M. Fraser, then Acting Minister for the Army, released further details of 'how effectively the service medical experts had tackled the problem of malaria'.[3] He revealed that the Australian Army Medical Research Unit was established in Cairns in June the previous year to investigate the efficacy of antimalarial drugs in the control and treatment of the disease: 'At this research centre large numbers of volunteers have been experimentally infected with malaria under controlled conditions'. The names of the drugs tested were not revealed, but the results of the experiments with atebrin were summarised:

Some of the volunteers have been repeatedly infected by mosquitoes with both malignant tertian and benign tertian malaria for a period of three months—just as they would in jungle fighting. Throughout this period various antimalarial drugs have been taken regularly under supervision ... The researches at Cairns have shown it is possible with adequate medication to prevent volunteers continuously exposed to malaria developing either malaria fever or parasites in their blood while taking the antimalarial drug. In addition, with malignant tertian malaria, fever is not only prevented but the disease is actually cured.[4]

This information, which was reported widely in the Australian press,[5] was disclosed to the public just before the Atherton Conference at which the far-reaching implications of the atebrin experiments were explained to senior Army officers.

In October 1945, two months after the end of hostilities with Japan, there was another batch of press articles revealing how malaria was beaten in the war.[6] Several Australian newspapers quoted a 'previously secret report' by Brigadier Fairley that showed 'the reduction of malaria service casualties from 90 per cent to 2.4 per cent'. The articles indicated that this was 'one of the greatest stories of the war' and was primarily due to Australian scientists, as well as to 'Australian servicemen voluntarily subjecting themselves to the disease in its most virulent form at the Cairns laboratories'. The article in the Perth *News* said that 'so successful have been the researches at this unit that the Medical Research Council in Britain and a similar U.S. organisation have selected it as the medical centre for the testing of their most recent drugs'. The Adelaide *News* reported that 'two new drugs, still on the secret list, have been proved as effective as atebrin ... One of [them] under test on volunteers in Cairns has proved superior to atebrin in some respects.' The 'secret' drugs referred to in this article were clearly chloroquine and paludrine. As explained in Chapter 18, the ICI press release naming paludrine during November 1945 caused considerable embarrassment to the Australian Army Medical Directorate, as Australian journalists thought that information freely released in England was being withheld in Australia. This could have been avoided if the British authorities had forewarned the Australians of the impending announcement. All of the essential facts about the experiments at Cairns had already been reported in Australian newspapers by that time so that this new information would have been readily accepted by all concerned.

The Cairns research continued to attract regular press attention for some time after the war. This often coincided with significant events such as Fairley's departure from Australia in 1946: 'Regret at the departure of another distinguished Australian scientist, Brigadier N. H. Fairley, who will take up two important appointments overseas, must give place to gratitude for the services he has rendered his country during the war'.[7] Similarly, a lengthy article in the *Bulletin*[8] paraphrased, for the lay reader, the significant scientific paper 'Malaria in the South West Pacific' published in the *Medical Journal of Australia* in August 1946.[9] There were occasional newspaper reports in Australia and overseas in later years. A graphic description of the atebrin experiments at Cairns was given in 'How we won the war with malaria', a feature article of the London *Guardian Weekly* in 1992:

> Some [volunteers] chopped wood all day long, five days a week, others had to swim upstream until they were tired out—or sank—while others were marched over hills as fast as possible by a specially trained sergeant major ... Not one of them developed malaria and it was considered that the case for atebrin had been proved.[10]

In the lead-up to Anzac Day 1999 there were several feature articles in the Melbourne *Age* and *Sydney Morning Herald* on the World War II malaria experiments. The *Age* coverage commenced on 19 April with a front page 'exclusive': 'The Hidden Experiments' under the heading 'Army used soldiers, Jews in experiments':

> Disabled soldiers and Jewish refugees fleeing Nazi Germany were used as human guinea pigs for medical experiments by the Australian Army during World War II. Giant British and United States drug companies profited from the experiments that involved deliberately infecting volunteers with malaria. Former human guinea pigs say the experiments damaged their health, but many have been unsuccessful in claiming war service benefits ... Documents indicate that the work was carried out in Australia because America and Britain were reluctant to risk using their own soldiers ... When new British and US drugs needed testing, the Australian Army trawled convalescent depots and military hospitals for volunteers ... German and Austrian Jewish refugees interned and forcibly sent to Australia by Britain on board the ship Dunera ... were recruited for the experiments after joining the army's 8th Employment Company.

The story, which was expanded over more than two pages in this edition, was pieced together 'by interviews with former guinea pigs and staff and documents held at the Australian Academy of Science, the Australian War Memorial, army personnel records, the Archive of Australian Judaica at the University of Sydney, international medical journals and the Australian Government Archive'.[11] On the same day an almost identical page one introduction, 'Troops and refugees given malaria', and feature stories on the 'Frontline Guinea Pigs' were published in the *Sydney Morning Herald*.[12]

Both newspapers published further articles on this subject during the following two days.

> A report published in the *Age* yesterday indicates how subservient Australia remained to its great and powerful friends. British and American pharmaceutical companies such as ICI and Winthrop wanted subjects for malarial experiments, and because Britain and US were reluctant to risk the lives of their own soldiers Australia provided the human guinea pigs.[13]

The *Age* also reported:

> A leading international Jewish human rights organisation yesterday described the Australian Army's use of Jewish refugees as guinea pigs in World War 2 medical experiments as a 'scandal' . . . 'The use of Jews—forced to flee their homes due to the Nazis' racial policies—as the subjects of medical experiments which seriously affected their health, reflects the cynical attitude of the Australian authorities towards Hitler's victims' the director of the Simon Wiesenthal Centre, Dr Efraim Zuroff, said in a statement issued in Jerusalem.[14]

An editorial in the *Sydney Morning Herald* said that their investigation 'has revealed a shameful story of the exploitation of the volunteers, to the point where there seemed to be little concern that the experiments virtually ensured long-term damage to their health'.[15]

The articles were written by two journalists, Gary Hughes of the *Age* and Gerald Ryle of the *Sydney Morning Herald*. In March 1999, the month before the stories were published, I received an email letter from Hughes. He had heard of my interest in the activities of the Medical Research Unit at Cairns and wished to discuss certain aspects of the experiments. There followed an exchange of email correspondence and several telephone calls. Hughes asked why the research continued into new drugs after the remarkable success of the atebrin experiments and the subsequent decline in malaria casualties among Australian troops. He was also interested to know why the Americans and British had left it up to the Australians to do the research on healthy volunteers, and why they were reluctant to use their own men as guinea pigs. Also, why the work on paludrine continued for more than six months after the war when the immediate beneficiaries appeared to be ICI.

I provided lengthy replies to these queries based on my archival investigations in Australia and overseas. All of the research at Cairns was aimed at protecting the Australian Army from malaria. The threat did not end with the cessation of hostilities. The efforts to find better drugs were driven by the need to combat the problem of relapsing vivax malaria after the troops stopped taking atebrin on their return from malarious areas (see Chapter 14). I described how the Americans and British lagged behind the Australians in their human trials of new drugs, as they initially put the major emphasis on large-scale screening of drugs against bird malaria parasites (see Chapters 10 and 16). The programs in both countries did not have the resources to rapidly increase human clinical tests. They lacked the elegant experimental set-up at Cairns, and they did not have the rapid relapsing strains of vivax malaria used by the Australians. After they found out about the research approach at Cairns the Americans were happy to provide their newest drug, chloroquine, for testing by the Australians because they appreciated that the team at Cairns had the means to find out how good it was before the Americans themselves could do so. Similarly, the Australians were able to evaluate paludrine quickly, whereas the British could not.

I explained that a more reasonable explanation for the failure of the Americans and British to promptly evaluate their new drugs was that they did not have the foresight or perhaps the sense of urgency to establish the kind of experimental program that was put in place at Cairns. After Japan entered the war all of the Australian land forces were engaged in tropical areas where malaria was an overwhelming problem. The urgent need to defeat this disease was appreciated by Army leaders and the Australian government to be of paramount importance in winning the war. Accordingly, the highest priority was accorded to the fight against malaria. This was in contrast to the situation facing the bulk of the British and American forces who were occupied with the war in Europe where malaria was not a major problem. Difficulties due to this tropical disease were probably considered to be remote (except, of course, among the Americans in the Pacific and the British forces in Burma).

An editorial in the *Age* said that the use of Jewish refugees was 'an especially cruel twist ... People who fled Nazi Europe, where they might have been forcibly subjected to medical experiments, found themselves caught up in experiments here'.[16] A different view was provided in a letter to the editor of the *Sydney Morning Herald* by Henry Lippmann:

> The sensational reporting of the Australian malaria tests during World War II has caused some misunderstanding locally as well as overseas. As a 'Dunera Boy' and an ex-serviceman who served with the 8th Australian Employment Company I wish to make a comment. It cannot be said that Jewish refugees were particularly targeted for these malaria tests. The number of Jewish refugees who volunteered for these experiments was in proportion to the larger total number of participants in this undertaking. The 8th Australian Employment Company was a regular unit of the Australian Military Forces Southern Command. It had a strength of approximately 500 other ranks. These men were all refugees from Nazi Europe, mostly Jewish, who had been mistakenly interned in England in 1940 and then deported to Australia on S. S. Dunera. As aliens, the soldiers of the 8th Australian Employment Company were not allowed to join combat units, although they had enlisted with the idea to fight the common enemy. When these fellows learned about the malaria tests, many of them saw this as an opportunity to join other units and, further, they wished to do their valiant best for the common cause. Therefore they volunteered. They were not coerced. A certain limited quota had been allocated to this company which was quickly filled. Whatever, the fellows of the 8th did the job that was allocated to them with an extraordinary zeal. In the words of their commanding officers 'They have done their duties second to none'. We remember this with pride. Especially on Anzac Day'.[17]

The nominal roll of volunteers in the malaria experiments (see Appendix 3) lists seven men from 8 Employment Company. Thus, the proportion of former Jewish refugees from this unit in the experiments was less than 1 per cent of the total number of volunteers.

Following the adverse media reports in the *Age* and the *Sydney Morning Herald*, the Minister for Veterans' Affairs, Bruce Scott, announced that 'the health effects of these experiments' was to be referred to the Repatriation Medical Authority (RMA). On 12–13 July 1999 the RMA convened a workshop in Brisbane to 'assist the RMA members in clarifying and considering the short and long term side effects of the antimalarial agents and the Australian Army malarial experiments testing those agents'. The history of the trials was also considered. The drugs used had been subjected to pharmacological and human toxicological evaluation in America and/or Britain before being tested in Australian volunteers. The workshop considered that the 'medical supervision was vigilant and of a high standard, and high quality medical records were maintained and kept for each individual volunteer and are still available'. Moreover, 'there was no sound medical-scientific evidence concerning possible adverse health effects'. It was concluded that the experiments were 'a remarkable piece of Australian history with overwhelming positive outcomes for the nation and the Allied forces in general'. It was also noted that 'the antimalarial trials were widely and accurately reported in the media of the day'. The workshop participants 'were saddened that media reports earlier this year were inaccurate and incomplete in their reporting and served to denigrate the role of the volunteers in this important contribution to Australia's military effort in World War II and to world public health knowledge' (see Appendix 4).[18]

Epilogue
The Rise of Drug Resistance

THE NEW GENERATION of antimalarials, developed by the wartime British and American programs and clinically tested at Cairns, came into widespread use after the war to completely replace atebrin by the end of the 1940s. Paludrine was used widely for prophylaxis and treatment of malaria in the former dominions and other countries that had trade links and historical ties with Britain, whereas chloroquine was initially employed in those areas under American influence. Both drugs were relatively cheap, very safe in therapeutic doses, and effective for prophylaxis and for treatment of human malaria. It appeared that malaria would cease to be a military problem, and Fairley had high hopes that the new drugs might also play an important role in controlling the disease among civilian populations in malarious regions.[1] But within a few years doubts were raised about paludrine.

In 1947 two separate groups of workers in England showed that *Plasmodium gallinaceum* in chickens was able to develop resistance to paludrine.[2] Wartime chemotherapeutic work had shown that the action of drugs against human malaria could not always be predicted by their activity against avian parasites. Consequently these findings did not give rise to serious concern that such resistance might also develop in human parasites. However, in 1949, researchers at the Liverpool School of Tropical Medicine detected paludrine resistance in a Hong Kong strain of *P. vivax* and in a West African strain of *P. falciparum* following repeated blood inoculation in successive subjects and challenge by small doses of the drug.[3] Nevertheless, as this resistance was developed under highly artificial conditions it was considered 'unlikely to give rise to a serious degree of resistance to strains . . . in the field'.[4] Hopes that the development of such resistance may be limited to artificially-induced laboratory conditions were dashed following the gradual accumulation of data that documented the appearance of paludrine-resistant parasites in Malaya.[5] Initially, the confirmed case reports of resistance emanated from only a few areas, and paludrine continued to be used for prophylaxis. But its use for treatment, particularly for falciparum malaria, declined in favour of chloroquine. During this period there was no evidence of the development of chloroquine resistance of human malaria, and by 1960 it came to be accepted as the drug of choice for both prophylaxis and treatment.[6] Shortly afterwards, the first substantiated cases of chloroquine-resistant falciparum malaria were reported from two widely separated parts of the world, Colombia[7] and Thailand.[8]

During the Malayan Emergency Australian troops took paludrine as a suppressive, originally at a dose of one tablet (100 mg) per day. From their initial deployment in 1955 until 1960 the numbers of malaria cases in the Australian infantry units were low, around 20–30 per 1000 men per year, a similar result to that achieved in 1945 in New Guinea. The incidence of the disease increased during the malaria season from 1958, and it was thought that paludrine resistance might have been a factor in some of these cases.[9] This was not conclusively demonstrated, even though such resistance had been reported previously among British troops in other parts of Malaya.[10] As a precautionary measure the daily dose of paludrine was increased to 200 mg. The 2nd Battalion, Royal Australian Regiment, suffered a major outbreak of falciparum malaria while on operations in North Perlis, Malaya, in 1962. It was not known whether these cases were due to paludrine resistance but some of them were not cured by the standard treatment course of chloroquine.[11] This was a major concern, as there were then doubts about the invariable efficacy of paludrine, the first-line drug used by the Australians for prophylaxis, and chloroquine was the drug of choice for treatment.

The incidence of chloroquine-resistant falciparum malaria spread through most of South East Asia during the 1960s. This had serious implications for US and Australian forces during the Vietnam War. The Americans were taking a suppressive regimen of chloroquine and primaquine, with incidence rates in different units ranging from 350 cases to 1000 cases per 1000 men per year, and a case fatality rate of about 1 per cent.[12] The Australians, on paludrine, experienced sporadic cases of falciparum malaria within a few weeks of their arrival at Bien Hoa, Vietnam, in 1965. The incidence of the disease increased with the onset of the malaria season in the latter half of each of the following four years.[13] There were 25 cases in December 1965, with one death. Robert Black, who had served in the Cairns Unit as a captain-physician during 1945, was the only member of the LHQ Medical Research Unit, apart from Fairley, to spend the rest of his working life in the field of malaria. He became Professor of Tropical Medicine at the University of Sydney, and was appointed Army

Consultant in Tropical Medicine with the rank of Colonel. The rise in malaria cases among the Australian force was viewed with concern by the Director General of Medical Services, and Black was sent to Vietnam to report on the situation in January 1966. In discussions with senior US Army medical officers Black was told that the US Commander in Vietnam, General William Westmoreland, considered malaria to be an enemy equal to the Viet Cong. In order to combat chloroquine-resistant falciparum malaria the Americans were using a combination of quinine, pyrimethamine (a new antimalarial developed after the World War II) and dapsone (a sulphone compound) for hospital treatment of falciparum malaria. They were also evaluating the addition of dapsone to chloroquine and primaquine for routine prophylaxis. Black suggested that, if the results of the American trials were favourable, the use of daily dapsone, in addition to paludrine, should be considered by the Australians.[14]

In 1968 there was a dramatic rise in malaria, with 440 cases between July and November.[15] This was the most serious medical threat faced by Australian troops since the dark days of World War II. At one stage the numbers of malaria patients exceeded the capacity of 1 Australian Field Hospital in Vietnam and some had to be treated in US Army facilities. In spite of this help from the Americans, some patients had to be transferred to the RAAF hospital in Malaysia, while others were evacuated to Australia.[16] This alarming sickness wastage placed a heavy toll on the fighting strength of the force, and there were grave concerns that, if the epidemic continued unchecked, there could be serious manning problems among operational units. This was reminiscent of the manpower difficulties that arose from the malaria wastage in New Guinea during 1942. In response to the 1968 epidemic the Army Medical Directorate decided to conduct a field trial in which part of the force took a combination of dapsone and paludrine and the remainder continued with paludrine alone. After a month there were no malaria cases in the dapsone–paludrine group, but new cases continued to emerge amongst the rest of the force. The data were not scientifically conclusive at this stage but it was decided, due to the urgency of the situation, to terminate the trial and put the whole force on the combination.[17] Apparently, this ad hoc measure had the desired effect of curtailing the epidemic.

Black presented a paper on 'Malaria as a military problem' at the Royal Military College, Duntroon, in August 1963.[18] This provided the background to emerging drug resistance and in particular to the situation facing Australian troops in North Perlis during that year. He said that the position then was 'somewhat similar to that in the Second World War before the researches on atebrin were carried out at Cairns'.[19] Black pointed out that the wartime success after the atebrin findings was due to the application of laboratory research, and he later suggested the formation of an Army malaria research laboratory to

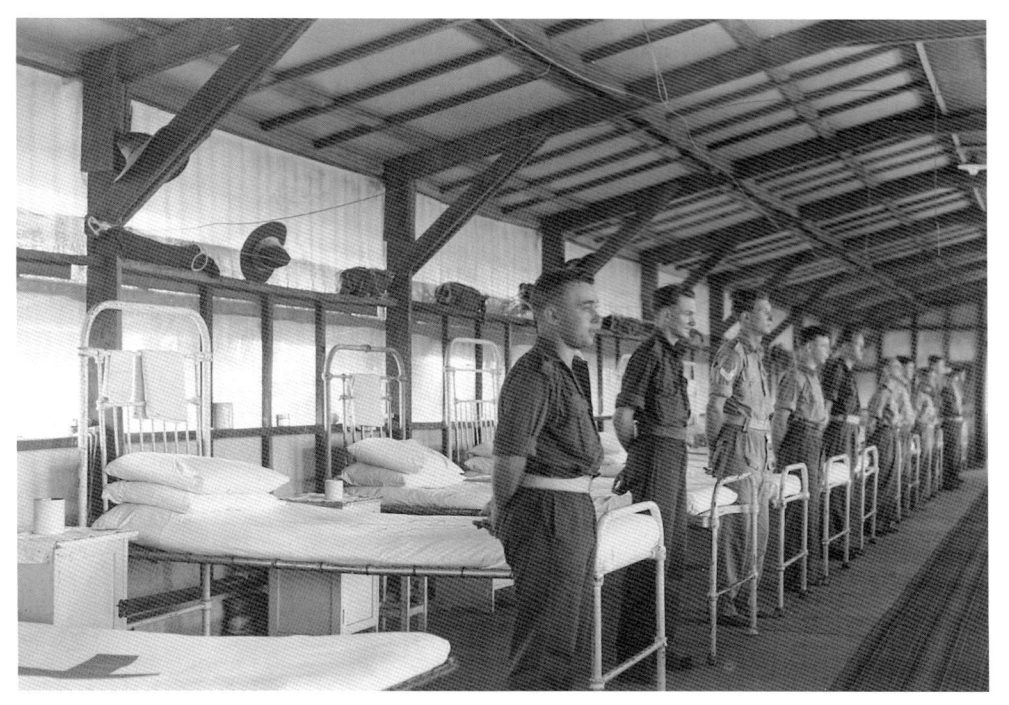

Soldiers who have volunteered for malaria research lining up for inspection in a mosquito-proof ward at LHQ Medical Research Unit.

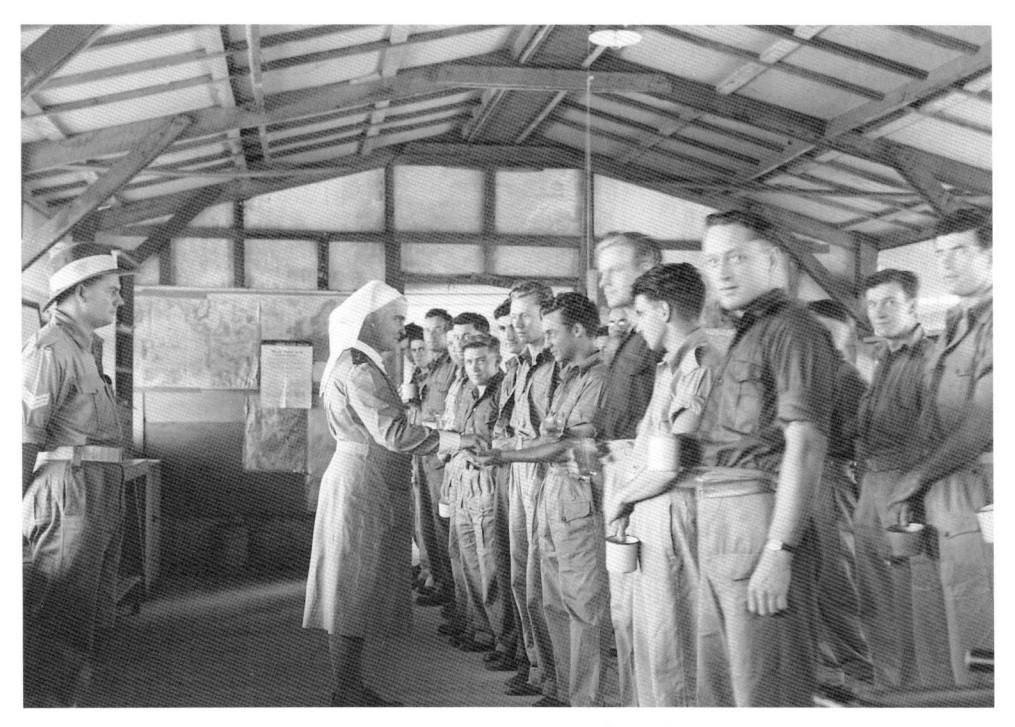

Drug parade: volunteers lining up to receive their drugs from the matron, Captain Beryl Burbidge, under the watchful eye of the duty sergeant

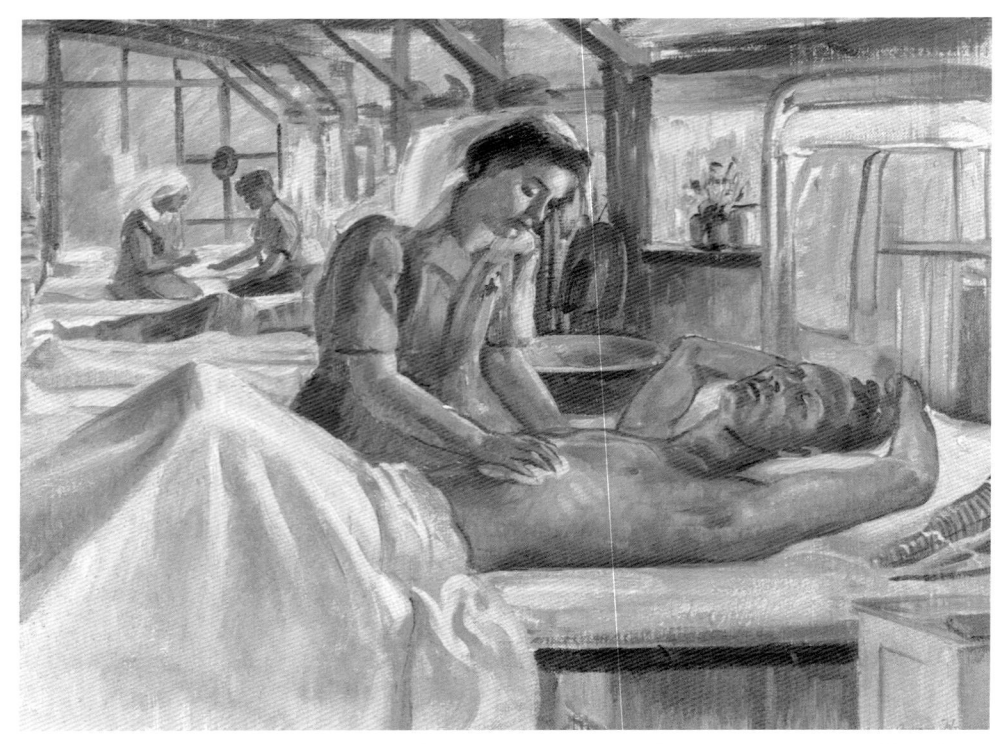

AAMWS nursing orderly (Private Hazel Lugge) sponging a volunteer (Private Ken Glover) suffering an attack of malaria (oil painting by Nora Heysen)

Volunteers pausing by a waterfall during a march up the railroad track from Cairns to the Atherton Tablelands as part of a 'long-term field experiment' in which they were subjected to prolonged and strenuous exercise after being infected with malaria suppressed by daily atebrin. From left: Corporal R. B. Graham, Craftsman W. F. West, Private W. D. Mitchell, Warrant Officer Bill Winterbottom, Private B. I. Hagan

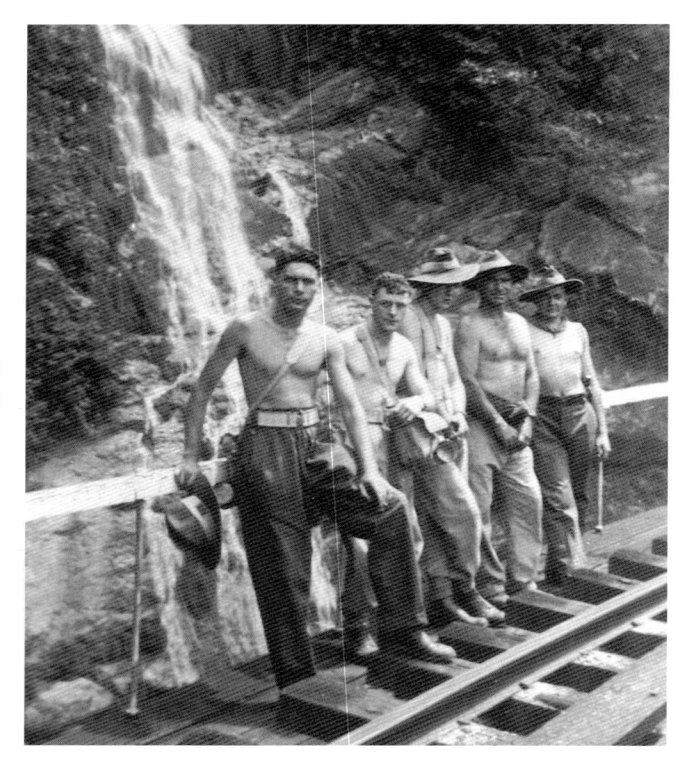

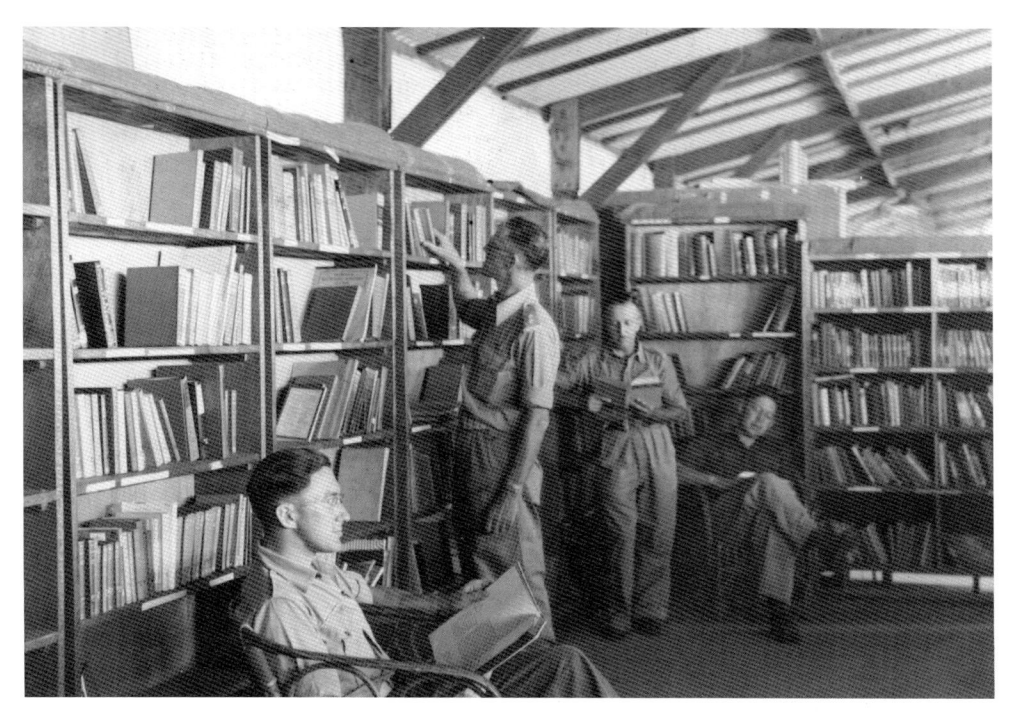

Volunteers in the library at LHQ Medical Research Unit

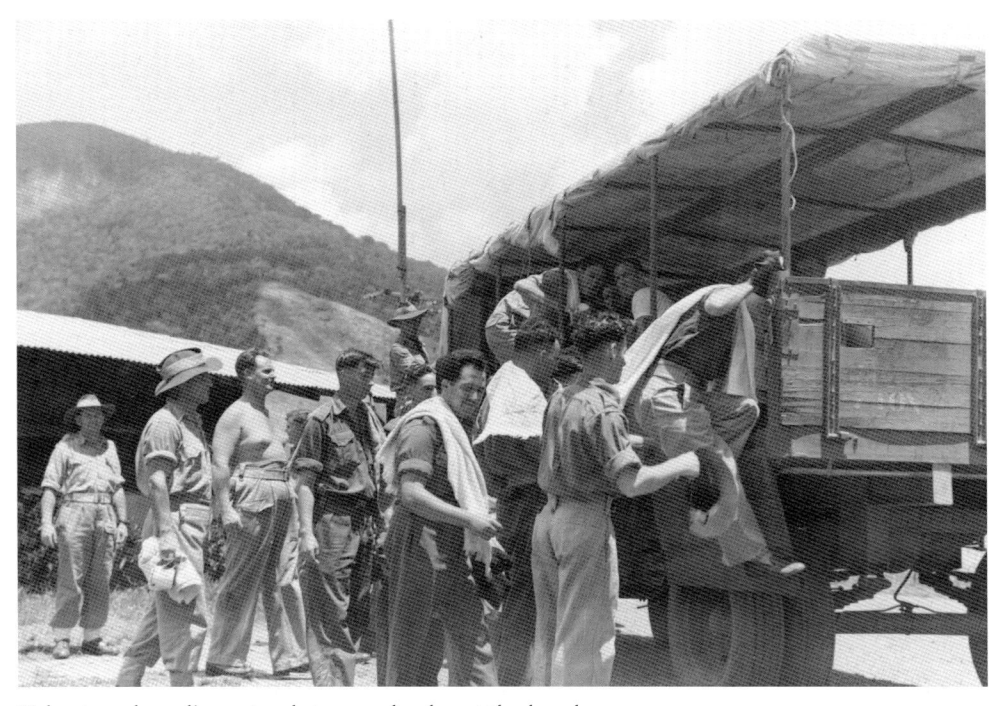

Volunteers boarding a truck to spend a day at the beach

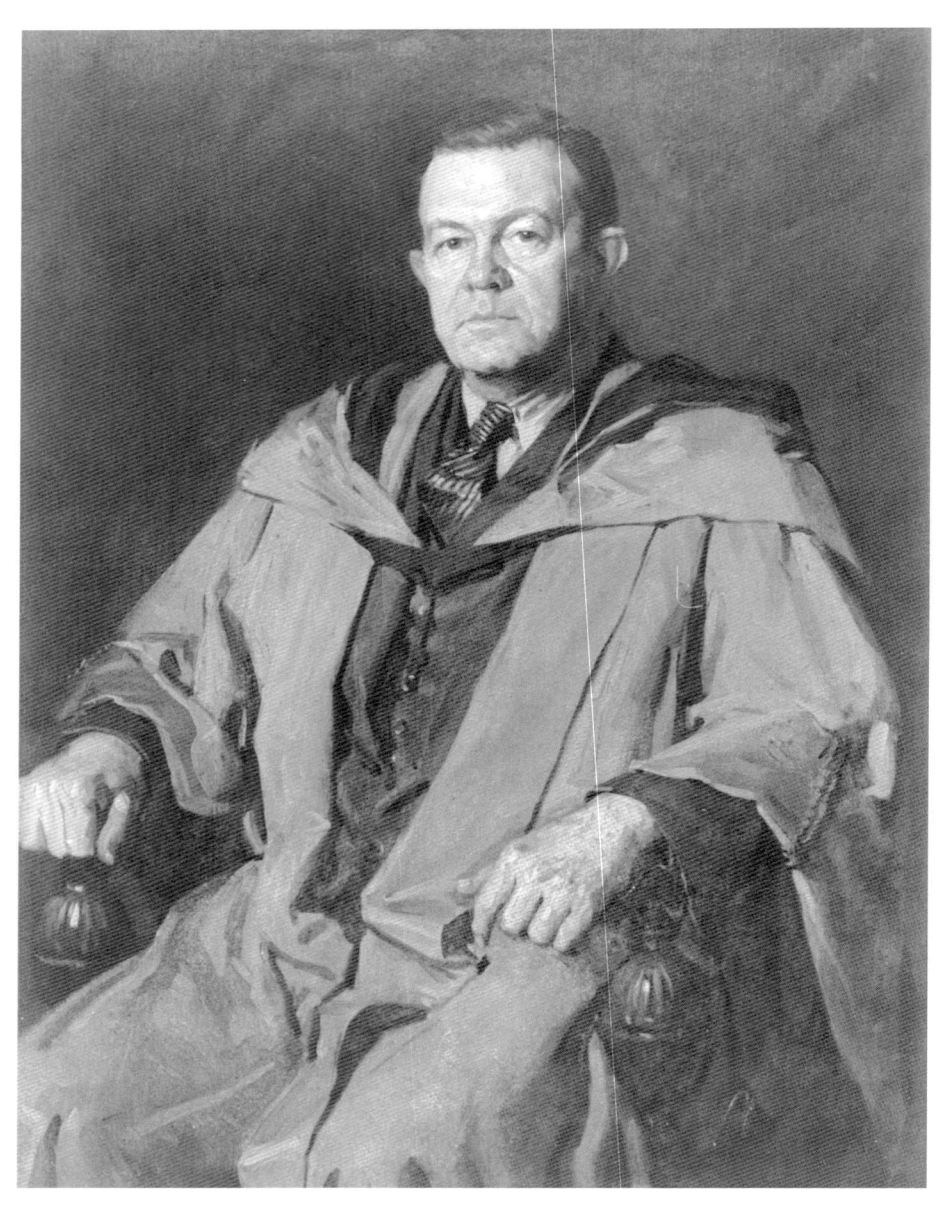

Professor Sir Neil Hamilton Fairley (oil painting by William Dargie)

combat the resurgence of the disease among troops on operations in South East Asia. After some delays this proposal received a favourable response, which coincided with the increasing malaria threat in Vietnam, and 1 Malaria Research Laboratory was established in 1967. It was initially accommodated within Black's department at the School of Public Health and Tropical Medicine, and moved to purpose-built laboratories at Ingleburn, western Sydney, in December 1973. The name was later changed to Army Malaria Research Unit. (In December 1996 the unit moved again to a modern laboratory complex at Enoggera, Brisbane, and was renamed the Army Malaria Institute.)

For more than two decades after the Vietnam War there were no large-scale operational deployments of Australian troops in malarious areas overseas. Australian soldiers were, however, regularly involved in training exercises in tropical countries, particularly in Papua New Guinea. In 1989 the Army Malaria Research Unit confirmed the presence of chloroquine-resistant *P. vivax* in two soldiers who acquired their infections in New Britain.[20] This was the first documented evidence of chloroquine-resistant vivax malaria in the world. The Army Malaria Institute later monitored the ongoing malaria threat to Australian troops during deployments in Bougainville and East Timor.

Hopes that the new drugs that came out of the wartime research programs would eliminate malaria as a military problem have been forestalled by the increasing spread of drug-resistant parasites. By the end of the 1980s cases of chloroquine-resistant falciparum malaria had been reported from most malarious countries of the world.[21] The antimalarial drug mefloquine (also known as lariam) was introduced in 1984 following clinical trials that demonstrated high activity against blood stages of vivax and falciparum malaria.[22] A significant number of failures of this drug to cure *P. falciparum* infections in Thailand were reported within five years.[23] It has been suggested that *P. falciparum* may have the ability to develop resistance to any compound with which it is challenged.[24] Nevertheless, continued efforts are being made to develop new antimalarial drugs and drug combinations. The use of a tetracycline antibiotic, doxycycline, was first recommended for malaria prophylaxis by the Army Malaria Research Unit in 1993.[25] This antibiotic drug is now widely used as an alternative to mefloquine for malaria prophylaxis and, at the time of writing, parasite resistance to this drug has not yet developed.

A number of other newer drugs are being assessed by the Army Malaria Institute and other institutions, and it is possible that one or more of them may play a role in the prevention of drug-resistant malaria in the future. Research studies on malaria vaccines are being undertaken in a number of academic institutions in several countries but none have been developed to the stage at which they can reliably prevent the disease in the field. It appears that it will be many years before an effective vaccine can be contemplated.[26]

During World War II there was another scientific advance of relevance to malaria control. This was the discovery of the insecticide DDT. In 1955 the World Health Assembly advocated global malaria eradication by country-wide 'residual spraying' campaigns involving the systematic application of this insecticide to the interior walls of houses to reduce the longevity of the anopheline vectors and interrupt transmission of the disease. Malaria eradication programs based on DDT spraying were undertaken in many malarious countries in the 1950s and 1960s. There were some initial successes. Transmission of malaria was interrupted in some countries, and the incidence of the disease was substantially reduced in others. However, the goal of global eradication was not realised.

Operational difficulties were reinforced by an increasing backlash against the widespread use of broad spectrum organic insecticides, particularly DDT, by environmentalists. Moreover, the ongoing financial burdens of continued spraying as a malaria control measure could not be continued indefinitely. Insecticide resistance of mosquitoes also developed in some areas. It was not a universal phenomenon, though it was enough to blunt the progress that might have been achieved.

During the 1970s many of the early gains were lost, and the worldwide malaria situation deteriorated to pre-spraying levels.[27] Insecticide-impregnated mosquito nets have been shown to give protection in field tests in some malarious countries, and their use by communities has been advocated by the World Health Organization as part of the global strategy against malaria.[28] However, their operational effectiveness in providing a sustained reduction in the incidence of malaria in any country has yet to be demonstrated. The world will continue to rely on drugs for prophylaxis and treatment of malaria for the foreseeable future.

The experiments at Cairns were said to have 'brought a greater advance in the knowledge of chemoprophylaxis than had occurred in the previous 50 years, or was to [occur] in the subsequent 20'.[29] As Brigadier Sinton predicted,[30] the scientific work of the LHQ Medical Research Unit formed the solid foundations on which later advances in malaria research have developed. Thus, the subinoculation experiments at Cairns showed conclusively that there was an initial phase after the infective mosquito bite, in both vivax and falciparum malaria, during which the parasites were not present in the blood. This had a duration of about eight days in the case of *P. vivax* and around six days for *P. falciparum*. The precise timing of the first invasion of the blood supported the long-standing belief by malariologists that there was a tissue phase, or pre-erythrocytic phase, which followed sporozoite inoculation. Two British workers, Colonel H. E. Shortt and Professor P. C. C. Garnham, extended this line of investigation to observe parasite stages in the liver of a monkey infected with the primate malaria parasite *P. cynomolgi*. They found similar stages in liver sections of a human volunteer experimentally infected with vivax malaria by sporozoite inoculation.[31] Fairley acted in an advisory capacity in these groundbreaking experiments. The following year he played a more direct role in the confirmation of the liver stages of *P. falciparum* in a study where a human volunteer was exposed to the bites of infected mosquitoes on three successive days, and a liver biopsy was performed on the sixth day after the first bites. The sequential development of the pre-erythrocytic stages was observed in stained sections, thereby solving the last major problem of the malaria life cycle.[32]

A full account of the discovery of atebrin-resistant falciparum malaria during the Aitape–Wewak campaign was published by Fairley and the team at Cairns in the *Transactions of the Royal Society of Tropical Medicine and Hygiene*.[33] The test volunteers, who received parasites derived from individual malaria-infected soldiers flown to Cairns from the Wewak area, were classified into four separate categories from Class I (in which the suppressive dose of atebrin provided complete protection) to Class IV (indicating failure of suppressive atebrin and development of an overt attack of malaria). At the time of publication, in 1947, this work must have seemed to be solely of academic interest, but after the widespread emergence of drug resistance it became an important practical concern for malaria workers throughout the world. The World Health Organization monitors the global status of drug resistance. This is aided by a field test for chloroquine-resistant falciparum malaria in which the parasite response is graded from susceptible (parasites completely cleared) to three levels of resistance with the highest level corresponding to no marked reduction of parasite clearance.[34] This categorisation is based on parasite response to drug treatment rather than response to suppressive use of the drug (the basis for classification of the Aitape–Wewak isolates), but there is a close analogy between the two systems. Thus, the pioneering investigation of the Aitape–Wewak epidemic by the research team at Cairns not only provided the first evidence of drug resistance in the field but also recognised and documented the gradation in resistance levels 20 years before a similar system was adopted by the international scientific community.

From the vantage point of hindsight, the wisdom of Fairley's approach to the problem is particularly relevant at the present time when the inventory of effective antimalarial compounds has been progressively eroded by the seemingly inexorable increase of drug resistance. Despite advances in chemotherapy during the last 50 years, the stage has now been reached at which there is no single drug with sufficient reliability to guarantee long-term protection against the disease throughout all malarious areas of the world. The investigation of the Aitape–Wewak epidemic provided an ideal model for the application of careful field observations, together with complementary laboratory-based experiments, for thorough scientific scrutiny of suspected failures of malaria treatment and prophylaxis.

The subinoculation technique involving transfer of large quantities of blood from donors to volunteers could not be repeated nowadays because of the dangers of transmitting viral diseases such as hepatitis and AIDS, but novel molecular biology techniques now permit the detection of submicroscopic levels of parasites in small samples of blood. Australian researchers have recently used this approach for an assay method to follow the increase of *P. falciparum* parasites after the blood stages are released from the liver.[35] This involves the preparation of marker fragments of parasite DNA that are copied in very large numbers with the use of a specialised laboratory technique known as polymerised chain reaction (PCR). This method detected parasites in 3 ml of blood taken from an experimentally-infected volunteer five and a half days after the infective mosquito bite. This confirmed the Cairns findings on the timing of the pre-erythrocytic cycle of falciparum malaria more than 50 years after the original subinoculation experiments were performed.

It is unlikely that clinical experiments on malaria would be repeated on the scale of those undertaken at Cairns. Development costs and ethical restraints concerning the use of human volunteers are currently restricting the development of new antimalarial drugs. Studies in humans are now augmented by the use of *in vitro* cultivated parasites to monitor drug resistance and drug activity. For example, studies with *in vitro* cultured *P. falciparum* conducted at the Army Malaria Research Unit in the 1980s demonstrated strong synergistic antimalarial activity when cycloguanil (the active metabolite of paludrine) was combined with dapsone.[36] This provided a scientific explanation for the success of the paludrine–dapsone combination used by Australian troops in Vietnam 20 years previously.

Fairley did not live to see all these developments. His health became progressively impaired after his illness in 1948. He resigned from his professorial appointment and ceased active research, but he continued to act in an advisory capacity on various committees in England and overseas. He was knighted in 1950, and received many academic honours and scientific awards. He made several return visits to Australia, including in 1951 and 1952 when he also visited Singapore and Malaya to advise the British and Australian Armies on malaria prophylaxis.[37] In 1954 he provided advice to the Australian Army Medical Directorate on relapsing vivax malaria among Australian troops in Korea.[38] On his last visit to Melbourne in February 1956 he attended a meeting at Army Headquarters convened to seek his advice on malaria treatment and prophylaxis.[39] Fairley suffered an accelerated decline in health in his later years, and he died in April 1966.

In a memorial oration in 1969 Ted Ford (then Sir Edward Ford, Director of the School of Public Health and Tropical Medicine, University of Sydney) paid tribute to his 'tremendous service to Australia in the grim days of war. For this was perhaps the most valuable contribution ever made by an Australian doctor to his country'.[40] A commemorative monument was erected by the Australian Army, in association with co-workers and friends, at North Cairns Sports Ground in September 1972. In the mid-1990s the monument was relocated to the grounds of North Cairns State School. This was the original site of the unit, from June 1943 to May 1944, before the move to Jungara. The caption reads:

> This plaque commemorates the great work of Brigadier Sir Neil Hamilton Fairley KBE FRS and his devoted team of officers, men and women of the Australian Army Medical Corps and the army volunteers who made the work possible. Their studies at the LHQ Medical Research Unit, AIF, Cairns, provided a scientific basis for the control of malaria by drugs which has proved of immense value to Australia and to the world in war and peace.

Disclaimer

The nominal rolls in Appendixes 1–3 are reference documents only. Inclusion herein and the record of details for any person in no way confers evidence of eligibility for any award, medal, pension, health care entitlement or any other kind of benefit.

The Commonwealth of Australia, its officers, servants and agents, disclaim all liability for the consequences of anything done or omitted to be done by any person in reliance upon the nominal rolls or any information contained in the nominal rolls.

Appendix 1
Nominal Roll of Volunteers

This appendix lists soldiers, who had not previously been exposed to malaria, and volunteered to be experimentally infected with the disease. They were transferred to LHQ Medical Research Unit, and subsequently participated in the experiments at Cairns or Rocky Creek.

Name	Service no.	Rank	Unit
Abell, Ian Haywood	QX57130	Gnr	2/3 TANK A/BTY
Abramowicz, Maskymilian	VX95470	Pte	3 BOD
Adams, Colin Kevin	N482477	Pte	PW & I (HAY)
Adamson, Charles Hiles	NX505489	Pte	3 ARTB
Ahearn, Charles William	NX119560	Cpl	3 AUS ARM TNK Bn
Aird, Alexander McCord	QX57574	Pte	1 AUS HTTD
Allan, Mervyn William	NX174704	Pte	23 AITB
Allen, Frank Eikington	NX167170	Cpl	18 AUST INF
Allum, John Frank	WX18306	Cpl	1 ACDB
Allwright, Thomas Neville	TX12024	Sig	19 D/R SDC NGL of SIGS
Andersen, Oliver Keith	SX30597	Gnr	COAST ARTY LARGS BAY
Anderson, Allan Keith	NX137354	Tpr	15A MOTOR REGT
Anderson, Hector McLean	WX39071	Pte	1 PARA BN
Anderson, James	NX140704	Sgt	2/1 AUST DETN BKS
Anderson, Murray Harold	S114356	Pte	SANDY CK PW CAMP SA
Andrews, Frank Albert	NX162514	Pte	102 AGH
Andriske, Gordon Baron	VX105380	Spr	53 FD PK COY

Name	Service no.	Rank	Unit
Anning, Samuel Lanner	W5854	Cpl	66 DCRE
Appleby, Frank	NX85449	Tpr	2/4 ARMD REGT
Arbon, George Francis	SX24400	Pte	148 AGT COY
Archer, Alfred John	NX137819	Pte	140 AGT COY
Armistead, Percy Edward	VX71133	Pte	15 EMP COY
Armstrong, Alfred Keith	VX101388	Pte	1 BOD (MTS)
Armstrong, Edward George	VX65881	L/Cpl	147 AGT COY
Armstrong, George Harold	Q127878	Pte	2 ARTB
Ashdown, William Kenneth	Q125481	Pte	1 GAR
Ashton, Charles Harry	V187283	Pte	AUST REC TRG BN
Askew, William Philip	VX79742	Dvr	ADV LHQ
Astall, Joseph Charles	VX101595	L/Cpl	27 ASD COY
Austin, Ronald James	TX11792	Pte	1 ATB
Avery, William George	NX158030	Gnr	25 AUST A/A BTY
Bailey, Edward Charles	NX193565	Gnr	COAST ARTY
Bain, Alexander Ernest	SX19090	Cfn	2/4 AUST BSE W/SHOPS
Baker, Harold Austin	VX113288	Cfn	2/8 ADV WKSP
Baker, Neil	WX30453	Sgt	4 HVY AA BTY
Baldwin, Harold Clifford	VX80066	Pte	Q L of C ARME
Bampfield, John Godfrey	VX140642	Gnr	1 LT AA
Banks, Hector Roy	VX65353	Drv	10 DRSC
Bardon, Robert Frederick	WX37774	Tpr	10 LIGHT HORSE
Barker, Colin Leslie	SX19871	Pte	18 BN
Barnes, Dallas Henry	TX14372	Drv	4 ARMD BDE
Barnett, Kenneth Thomas	VX113677	Pte	1 AAMC
Barry, Graham	VX68923	Pte	121 AGH
Barsby, Andrew Edward	QX52120	Pte	16 AITB
Bartsch, Walter Reinold	S42314	Tpr	2 AUST TNK BN
Barwood, Leonard Alfred	V32631	Gnr	4 FD REGT
Bashford, Alfred Stephen	NX178401	Gnr	2 ARTY TRG REGT
Batchelor, Arthur Ronald	SX21563	Cpl	4 REMOUNT SQN
Batten, Frederick Charles	V175224	Sgt	3 MOTOR TPT TRG DEPOT
Baulch, Eric Fulton	VX81398	Sgt	4 MOTOR REGT
Baxter, Paul	VX129143	Pte	6 AUST MP COY
Beacham, Ronald Stephen	VX67057	Cpl	140 AG TPT COY
Beaton, Alan John	N252499	Pte	18 AUST EMP COY
Beattie, Leslie	NX48896	Sgt	16 AITB
Beckett, Cecil	QX42039	Pte	2 AUST CAV REGT
Beddoe, Leslie John	NX132704	L/Bdr	1 AUST BASE DEPOT
Beggs, William Charles	VX100975	Sig	AUST SPEC WIRELESS GP
Bell, Arthur Gordon	NX144175	Gnr	54 AA BTY
Bellamy, William Stanley	NX98364	Pte	AACC

274 Appendix 1

Name	Service no.	Rank	Unit
Bengtsson, Charles Henry	QX38503	Pte	COAST ARTY T' SVILLE
Bennett, Alfred James	VX129034	Sgt	116 BDE WKSHOPS AEME
Bennetto, Ian Maxwell	T14840	Cpl	6/30 GAR BN
Bentley, Thomas Arthur	W62346	Pte	9 ADV AMM DEPOT
Berger, Norman Bruce	NX152247	Tpr	12 A ARMD CARRIER
Berger, Stanley Clarence	NX122738	Cpl	21 TOFP
Bertrand, John William	VX137679	Sig	3 MOTOR TRADES TRG
Beutel, Frederick	Q106674	Pte	47 BN
Beveridge, Stanley Robert	NX174827	Tpr	17 PW CONT COY
Bevilaqua, Max Minford	WX34894	Dvr	BIPOD HOMEBUSH
Bird, Lloyd George	VX92826	Gnr	1 ANTI TK REGT
Blain, John Frederick	V83404	Sgt	33 AITB
Blanch, Samuel Roy	NX84780	Cpl	4 AO VEH PK
Blyth, Sydney Charles	VX97667	Pte	VIC ECH & REC
Boardman, Edward Winslow	VX105331	Tpr	20 AMR
Bodey, Gordon Ralph	SX14243	Cfn	2/4 ARMD REGT
Boehm, Frederick August	SX15825	Pte	3 WKS & PKS RAE
Bolton, Alwyn Rex	VX80633	Cfn	2/4 AUST W/S
Bolton, William Hammersly	VX96675	Pte	LTD (MELB)
Bones, William Edward	NX149093	L/Sgt	18 AUST FD REGT
Bonnett, Claude Charles	QX52542	Pte	33 AITB
Booth, John Francis	QX30458	Cpl	2/3 PROVO COY
Boxall, Edward William	N105153	Pte	3 AAOD
Boyling, Reginald William	NX203008	Pte	1 ARTB
Brace, Norman James	NX82975	Pte	HQ QLD L of C
Brain, Max	TX11147	Pte	123 AGT
Brannigan, William Matthew	N99014	Cpl	2 AUST BOD
Brennan, Michael John	NX178046	Pte	2 AUST ARMY TRG REGT
Brenton-Smith, Frederick	N335288	Pte	16 AUST POW CAMP HAY
Brindley, Francis Keith	VX150628	Pte	GDD VIC L of C
Brohman, William David	QX55792	Pte	1 FD ARMY TRG UNIT
Brown, Henry William	VX119799	Sgt	27 ASD COY
Brown, William Colin	V198208	Tpr	20 MOTOR REGT
Browne, Keith Charles	VX84510	Tpr	101 MOTOR REGT
Bryant, Kevin Charles	NX99994	Gnr	2 AUST FD ARTY TGR
Bubb, Raymond	WX33289	Pte	BIPOD HOMEBUSH
Buchanan, Neil Allan	VX60834	Pte	14/32 BN
Budd, Roy Stanley	N454740	Pte	8 RITB
Bungard, George Gordon	NX38390	Cpl	1 ARTB
Bunting, John Albert	S112292	Cfn	8 AAW/S
Burgess, Ronald George	NX149098	Pte	18 AUST FD REGT
Burke, George William	SX29446	Pte	48 MURCHISON PW
Burns, David John	V260031	Pte	20 SUPPLY DEPOT COY

Name	Service no.	Rank	Unit
Burns, George Robert	NX152695	Cpl	36 AUST COY ASC
Burrows, Charles Edward	NX94014	Pte	2 AITOF PARK
Butler, Peter Cedric	VX140335	L/Cpl	23 AUS SUP DEP COY
Butler, Richard John	WX31456	Cfn	2/1 ARMD TRP
Buzacott, John	SX24403	Pte	148 AGT COY
Byrne, Lawrence	V501934	Pte	1 LT A/A TRG REGT
Byrne, William Edward	VX127585	Cpl	107 CON DEPOT
Callaghan, James Francis	QX32048	L/Sgt	GDD QLD L of C
Callaghan, Martin	VX84454	Tpr	101 MOTOR REGT
Cameron, Clifford Frederick	VX41390	Cpl	147 AGT COY
Cameron, Ross	NX122846	Tpr	6 AATB
Campbell, Clayton Daniel	NX134357	Pte	23 ASD
Campbell, Colin Paris	NX105930	Gnr	COAST ARTY
Campbell, Kevin George	VX125295	Tpr	2/6 ANTI ARM REGT
Campbell, Richard Fremantle	QX61756	Gnr	1 AUST TNK AKK
Campesato, Giovanni	VX128626	Tpr	AATTB
Canham, Donald Frederick	S21478	Pte	27 BN
Carey, John	VX121385	Pte	25 AITB
Carlisle, Frederick Thomas	WX34913	Pte	BIPOD HOMEBUSH
Carra, Patrick Vincent	VX129289	Pte	2 TRADE TESTING DPT
Carroll, Christopher Arthur	S62990	Pte	2 ARTB
Carson, Wallace Colley	N265430	Pte	2A TTC
Casserley, Francis Norman	NX118284	Gnr	111 TNK ATT REGT
Castanelli, Kenworthy	VX60039	Pte	147 AGT COY
Cates, Russell Charles	NX200959	Gnr	COAST ARTY SYDNEY
Chalker, Cecil Charles	NX140881	Tpr	1 AATB
Charteris, Alan Frederick	VX147891	Pte	21 AITB
Chase, Leo Bernard	WX2923	Sgt	LOVEDAY INTERN CAMP
Chaseling, Jack Rowland	NX173331	Gnr	9 AUST FD REGT
Cheffirs, John Edward	SX21570	Sgt	4 REMOUNT SQN
Chislett, Peter James	VX97627	Pte	VIC ECH & REC
Chittleborough, Albert Ray	S7017	Pte	AUST CAMP STAFF
Christensen, Christian John	N91257	Pte	ARTB
Christianson, Kevin	NX177472	Pte	1 BOD
Clark, Jack	TX12011	Gnr	101 COMP AA REGT
Clark, Leslie Randle	VX84455	Tpr	101 MOTOR REGT
Clarke, Edward James	NX170633	Tpr	2/6 AUST ARMD REGT
Clarke, Ernest George	NX194632	Pte	5 AITB
Clarke, James Thomas	NX179481	Gnr	1 AUST TK/A REGT
Clarke, Victor Thomas	Q267524	Pte	FORT W/SHOPS
Cleaver, Gerald Harvey	VX91958	L/Cpl	1 AITB
Clelland, Donald Kenneth	NX121008	Pte	4 BN

Name	Service no.	Rank	Unit
Clemens, Frank	S60018	Pte	CAMP HQ WARRADALE
Clune, James Henry	NX142175	Cpl	19 ASDC
Coffey, Patrick Ambrose	V198118	Cpl	HQ VIC L of C
Colacino, Antonio	V506778	Pte	2/1 CON DEPOT
Cole, Frederick Richard	NX124837	Pte	35 TPT COY
Cole, Reginald Sydney	NX18225	Gnr	SYDNEY AREA WKSHOPS
Cole, Ronald	NX42134	Pte	SYDNEY AREA
Coleman, John William	VX66151	Tpr	2/9 AUST ARM REGT
Coleman, Russell Clifford	NX167596	Gnr	7 HVY A/A BTY
Collett, Alan Wesley	QX62088	Pte	7 AITB
Collier, Les James	VX105237	Pte	16 GAR BN
Connolly, Robert Edwin	NX96284	Dvr	4 AA BDE AASC
Considine, Bernard Joseph	Q113190	Pte	RRD
Cook, Harold Charles	NX180924	Pte	103 AUST CON DEP
Cook, Lawrence Charles	NX200013	Pte	17 AITB
Cooke, Kenneth George	VX84719	Gnr	106 TK AKK
Coombe, David	SX26850	Pte	148 AGT COY
Coombe, Roy Reginald	SX25648	Pte	148 AGT COY
Cooper, Ernest William	VX116096	Pte	140 AGT COY
Cooper, William	NX86593	Pte	31 AUST FD BAKING PL
Coote, Horace Norman	NX106629	Bdr	70 AUST ARTY TRG REGT
Cope, Gordon Joseph	NX195399	Pte	20 AUST PNR BN
Copping, Octave James	NX206510	Pte	SYDNEY AREA
Corbett, John William	NX137647	Pte	5 AUST PK TRNS COY
Cork, Maurice	QX40699	Gnr	56 A COMP A/A RGT
Cornish, Lionel Colin	WX42500	Gnr	25 AUST HVY AA REGT
Cowdroy, Frederick Allan	N461378	L/Cpl	8 BN
Cox, George Hastings	NX50145	Pte	1 PARA BN
Coy, Frederick Thomas	N250952	Pte	HQ JUNG TRG SCH
Craig, Christopher Robert	NX5653	Spr	2 CRE
Crane, Geoffrey David	NX137852	Dvr	148 AGT COY
Crane, Noel Robert	QX25848	Pte	1 BOD
Crawford, August Neil	SX22203	Sgt	LOVEDAY INTERN CAMP
Crockford, Harry Edward	NX66529	Tpr	2/4 AUST ARM REGT
Crombie, John Joseph	NX178026	Spr	103 ACD
Cross, Jack Leonard	NX97920	Tpr	1 ARMY TK BN
Croxton, Arnold	S57400	Sgt	SA L of C AREA
Crozier, Edward Peter	VX55265	Tpr	2/8 ARMD REGT
Cruden, Jack Neville	NX178813	Pte	30 AITB
Csintalan, Frank William	NX78427	Cfn	2/1 AUST BASE WKSHOPS
Cullen, Donald Wallace	TX12103	Gnr	6 FLD REGT
Cummings, Alan Francis	VX96065	Pte	LTD (MELB)
Cummings, Colin Wando	Q138413	Pte	1 COAST ARTY

Name	Service no.	Rank	Unit
Cummings, Reginald George	NX1693790	Pte	71 AASL
Cunningham, William Noel	NX202217	Pte	13/33 BN
Curran, Kevin	V66974	Gnr	1 ARTY TRG REGT
Curtis, Lloyd Henry	WX37068	Sgt	10 GAR BN
Dadson, Harry George	TX13838	Tpr	4 AUST ARM BDE
Daniel, Arthur Joseph	NX206170	Pte	101 CON DEPOT
Davidson, John	WX29530	Pte	5 GAR BN
Davies, Robert Perrie	VX151779	Pte	4 AITB
Davis, John William	NX109125	Pte	129 AGH
Day, Horace Anthony	NX168396	Pte	9 FD REGT
De La Rue, Alfred John	VX77766	Pte	2 ARTB
Deece, Stanley Osborne	N437017	Pte	12 L of C SIGS
Delbridge, Thomas Arthur	NX175304	Pte	23 AITB
Deller, Robert Mark	QX52083	Pte	31 AITB
Docking, Bernard Alfred	SX37228	Pte	43 AIB
Doecke, Henrich Herbert	SX35202	Pte	121 AGH
Doherty, Lenard Matthew	SX15034	Tpr	4 A A BDE HQ
Dolan, John Joseph	WX28028	Spr	HQ 4 DIV RAE
Dolphin, Selwyn Noble	NX160791	Gnr	25 AA BTY
Donnelly, Geoffrey Ivan	TX12200	Sgt	123 AGT COY
Donovan, Cyril, Joseph	NX138061	Sig	33 LINE SEC
Doornbusch, Johannes Nicolaas	VX57277	Tpr	2/4 ARMD REGT
Douglas, Leo Clarence	N451145	Pte	4 ARTB
Dowie, William John	VX93342	Pte	13/33 BN
Dowling, Bruce Sydney	S1165	Cpl	SA ECH & REC
Dowling, Victor Albert	V270641	Sgt	ELECT MECH ENG
Downs, Frank Warneford	SX16484	Gnr	2/9 AUST ARM REGT
Drayton, Benjamin	QX268365	Pte	1 COY ASC
Drew, John Athol	NX141492	Gnr	AUST B DEPT L' PL
Driscoll, George	WX39206	Pte	16 AITB
Drucker, Heinz	VX151786	Pte	12 EMP COY
Duddell, Cyril Spooner	Q151166	Cpl	ARTC
Duffield, Llewellyn	SX29604	L/Cpl	64 ACH
Duggan, Edmund Henry	WX40719	Gnr	7 AV HVY ARTY
Duncombe, Donald Victor	VX125518	Tpr	2/6 AUS ARMY AMD NT
Dunham, Lewis John	WX25285	Cpl	2/3 AUST KIT STORE
Dyer, Walter Horatio	Q137232	Spr	3 AUST W&P COY RAE
Eades, Arthur Edward	N237664	Pte	S AVST W/S
Earsman, Thomas Edward	N6356	Dvr	8 AAHT
Ebsworth, Keith	VX124776	Pte	2 AITB
Edelhofer, Fredrich	V377495	Pte	8 AUST EMP COY

278   Appendix 1

Name	Service no.	Rank	Unit
Edwards, Clifford John	NX175858	Pte	8 AITB
Egan, Keith Havelock	NX174742	Pte	13/33 BN
Egan, Ronald John	QX36080	Pte	2/2 AGH
Ellis, Jack Frederick	N367374	Pte	LHQ SCHOLL ARTY
Ellis, John Charles	VX124031	Pte	1 AITB
Ellis, Noel Ernest	Q132018	Pte	11 AITB
Fahey, Peter Kevin	NX201820	Pte	3 AITB
Falla, Jonathan Stephens	VX102050	Dvr	20 AMR
Fallon, George	VX147942	Pte	196 ASD
Falvey, Neville Eugene	QX50261	Pte	1 PARA BN
Farnell, Edward	VX84439	Sgt	101 MOTOR REGT
Farrell, Edward Joseph	NX113312	Sgt	2 ATB WS
Feldman, Ronald Fredrick	QX49104	Pte	2 RRD
Feltham, Walter Rodrick	WX7351	Dvr	8 AUST AA GRP
Field, Edward Mathew	VX35939	L/Cpl	14 AGT COY
Fish, Raymond William	NX164017	Pte	2 AUST BSE AMM DEP
Flatau, Gert	V377591	Cpl	8 EMP COY
Fletcher, Donald Leslie	NX132422	Pte	2 AIT ORD FLD
Flint, Lawrence Edwin	WX35888	Dvr	BIPOD SYDNEY
Flohr, Herber	Q147747	Spr	RAE
Flowers, George Pavier	VX122480	Cpl	2/6 AAR
Flynn, Thomas Henry	VX145609	Cfn	VIC L of C WKSHP
Foley, Paul Kieran	NX98807	Tpr	2/6 ARMD REGT
Forbes, Arthur John	Q271503	Pte	4 AITB
Forbes, Ernest James	NX118406	Pte	2/4 IND COY
Ford, Stanley	NX203000	Pte	1 ARTB
Forrest, Harry Mervyn	SX19982	Pte	41/2 BN
Fowler, Roy	QX6738	Gnr	2/2 TK/A REGT
Foxlee, Edward Thomas	QX38523	Tpr	1 AAG BN
Franks, Robert Kenneth	QX60025	Pte	14 AITB
Fraser, Peter Charles	VX97460	Pte	3 BOD
Freeman, Ernest	NX180755	L/Cpl	103 ACD
French, Alan Douglas	NX201663	Pte	41/2 BN
Friend, Donald Stewart	NX96987	Gnr	2 AATR
Fuge, Bernard	NX121678	Cpl	13/33 BN
Fuller, Andrew Duncan	VX112783	Pte	148 AGT COY
Fullerton, Garth	NX139929	Cpl	18 AUST FLD REGT
Furber, J. F.	NX207260	Capt	116 AGH
Furner, Fredrick James	NX194418	Tpr	1 AMTR
Furse, Colin McDonald	Q268788	Pte	4 AITB
Gale, Richard William	N410700	Gnr	1 ART TRG BN
Gann, Patrick James	NX172850	Gnr	COAST ARTY

Name	Service no.	Rank	Unit
Gannon, Thomas Michael	VX126953	Spr	57 DCRE
Gara, Thomas Tibor	S83021	Pte	4 EMP COY
Gardiner, Albert	SX35263	Pte	SA L of C AREA
Gardner, Keith	QX41194	Pte	3/102 AGT COY
Gason, Edward William	VX86095	Tpr	13 AAR
Geddes, Harry Lyle	NX146864	Tpr	18 AITB
George, Malcolm Lewis	NX105060	Pte	249 AUST LAD
George, Stanley Thomas	NX193347	Gnr	2 AATR
Gibson, Allan Roy	NX145799	Dvr	4 AUST ARMD BDE
Gibson, Thomas Robertson	NX99810	Spr	2 BN RAE
Giddy, Francis George	QX24727	Pte	3 AUST MOTOR BDE
Gilbert, Ronald Byers	NX98898	Cfn	CAIRNS AREA WKSHOPS
Gill, George Douglas	VX83938	Sgt	3 MOTOR BDE
Gillies, Donald Lewis	VX111895	Tpr	13 AAR
Gilmore, Colin William	NX101423	Tpr	2/6 ARMD REGT
Gimm, Edward	Q147527	Pte	1 GAR BN
Girling, James Grant	Q266458	Pte	HQ WARWICK
Glanville, Albert Edward	NX49922	Tpr	2/6 ARMD REGT.
Gleeson, Harold Thomas	NX127495	Cpl	2/2 AUST GD BN
Glover, Kenneth George	NX109133	Pte	129 AGH
Goble, Robert Thomas	SX35679	L/Sgt	SANDY CK PW CAMP
Godson, Thomas Pascoe	NX43251	Sig	HQ 1 COY AA FORT SGS
Golding, William George	NX98512	Pte	16 AITB
Goldsack, Kenneth Osmond	SX26704	Spr	1 AUST SPARE PARTS
Gooch, Ronald Henry	WX31385	Cpl	10 GAR BN
Good, Frederick Ross	VX119446	Sgt	AAPC VIC L of C
Good, John Patrick	SX19776	Pte	2 RSD
Goodlich, Peter	W53930	Pte	21 AITB
Goodwin, William John	Q269700	Pte	GDD HACKETT
Gould, Leslie William	NX32132	Cfn	2 BSE TNK W/SHP
Gowan, John Proudlock	N274987	Cpl	10 WKSHOPS PACK
Gowley, Ernest Edward	N71427	WO2	103 CON DEPOT
Graham, Ronald Brumley	VX78395	Cpl	MGO BN DESGIN DIV
Gray, Neville John	NX124472	Cpl	20 BN
Green, Ernest Edward	V377499	Pte	8 EMP COY
Green, Leslie	T14744	Pte	123 AGT COY
Green, Stanley Edward	Q269594	Pte	4 BN
Green, William Francis	NX134924	Pte	140 AGT COY
Greenland, John	VX128915	Pte	2 ORD AMM REPAIR
Gregurke, Hugo Albert	SX28989	Pte	INSPECT BR SA L of C
Grieger, Ronald Murry	SX25314	Pte	142 AGT COY
Griffiths, Andrew Aaron	346123	Pte	2/1 BSE WKSHOPS
Gross, John	NX176966	Spr	8 AITB

Name	Service no.	Rank	Unit
Grubb, Malcolm Charles	SX7498	Cpl	SA ECH & REC
Guerin, Maxwell Rolan	QX58424	Tpr	2 PACK TPT COY
Guest, Robert Roy	VX127406	Cfn	2/8 ADV WKSHOPS
Gully, Ronald	VX113176	Pte	23 ATTB
Gunn, Trevor Robert	VX146387	Gnr	1 AF ATR
Guthrie, Ronald Rawson	NX100619	Sgt	LTD NSW L of C AREA
Gwatkin, John Hatton	V175728	Cfn	VIC L of C WKSHOPS
Hagan, Bernard Ian	Q271123	Pte	13/33 BN
Hale, Ronald Cecil	NX177172	Pte	13/33 BN
Hall, Allan George	T102622	Pte	1 AITB
Hall, Bruce	QX62593	Gnr	3 ARTB
Hall, Irvan St Clair	TX15930	Pte	28 AITB
Halliday, Denis John	NX152554	Bdr	21 FD REGT
Halton, Mervyn Dennis	WX39466	Spr	22 FD COY RAE
Hames, Abraham Charles	VX69964	Gnr	2 FD REGT
Hamil, John Gilmore	N104083	Pte	7 GAR BN
Hampton, Leonard Keith	TX13760	Gnr	101 COMP AA REGT
Hansell, Charles Edward	NX178435	Pte	BIPOD
Harben, Peter Ross	VX124772	Pte	2 AITB
Harding, Reginald Ralph	Q266469	Pte	1 GAR BN
Hardisty, William George	NX174847	Pte	21 AITB
Hardy, William Kevin	NX169713	Pte	14 AI B
Harnden, Harry	VX91782	Pte	17 AITB
Harrison, Donal Gordon	VX96094	Pte	41/2 BN
Harrison, Edward George	NX134109	Cpl	4 ARMD BDE
Harrison, James	NX98666	Pte	18 AITB
Harrop, Roy James	S57499	Pte	1 AARD
Harvey, Rueben Vincent	VX65268	Tpr	2/9 ARMD REGT
Hatfield, Alan Richard	VX121653	Cpl	3 A POD
Hayden, Victor Joseph	N464946	Pte	RRD
Haydon, Ronald Arthur	VX141356	Pte	4 ARTB
Hayes, Cyril Joseph	NX99951	Cfn	4 L/C WKSHOPS
Hayes, William Francis	NX90477	Pte	30 BN
Hayne, Harry	NX126863	Pte	4 A ARMD BDE
Hayter, Edward George	N166692	Pte	102 AGH
Hayward, John William	V160795	Bdr	1 LT AA TRG REGT
Heapy, Raymond John	NX157356	Gnr	69 AUST SH BTY
Hearne, Keith	VX93355	Pte	11 AITB
Heaslip, Maxwell Benjamin	NX191169	Pte	106 AGH
Heathcote, George Ward	V5833	Sgt	2 O/ PATIENTS DEPOT
Heeps, Frank Keith	QX43034	Tpr	CAV TRG SQN
Hempsall, John	QX62992	Cpl	11 AITB

Name	Service no.	Rank	Unit
Hemsley, Frederick Joseph	WX16668	Gnr	3 FLD RGT
Henderson, Alexander Munro	NX90881	Pte	LHQ JUNGLE WARFARE
Henderson, Leslie Thomas	VX17086	Pte	1 ORD VEH PK
Henwood, John James	NX73729	Pte	2/3 MG BN
Hermes, Wallace Lindsay	S61995	Lsgt	64 DIST CASH OFFICE
Herrick, Geoffrey William	N351906	Gnr	1 ARTY TRG REGT
Herringe, Raymond Alfred	NX96873	Spr	115 AUST BD WKSHOPS
Highet, George Frederick	SX17999	Pte	4 REMOUNT SQN
Hill, Colin George	WX32282	Pte	16 AITB
Hill, George Henry	VX100108	Pte	LHQ DEP MED & VET
Hill, Harold Joseph	TX11239	Pte	123 AGT COY
Hill, Hector McDonald	Q119712	Dvr	1 AART COY
Hill, William Richard	VX89300	Spr	5 AUST DOCK OP COY
Hillier, Mervyn John	NX161328	Pte	121 AGH
Himstedt, Herbert Walter	Q107688	Pte	161 GEN TPT COY
Hipwood, William Arthur	Q144491	Pte	33 AITB
Hirsch, Walter Manfred	V377950	Pte	AACC
Hitchcock, Reginald George	V1481	Wo1	VIC ECH & REC
Hoad, Bede Joseph	NX125676	Cpl	1 AUST TK BN
Hobbs, Alfred Jacob	QX35452	Cpl	1 AUST PROVO COY
Hodge, George Percy	NX505546	Spr	WATER TPT RAE
Hodges, Dudley Henry	V515298	Pte	14 AITB
Hoey, Louis Gerald	WX17282	Pte	16 PW CAMP
Hogan, Francis Joseph	V165903	Pte	2 AUST TECH TRG SCH
Holder, Bryce Frederick	QX501063	Pte	1 MOTOR TPT TRG DEPT
Holland, John Anthony	NX171333	Sgt	112 CON DEPOT
Hollis, Lisle William	NX131153	Pte	6 LT FLD AMB
Holmes, Alan William	VX124730	Pte	1 AUST GEN ORD DEP
Holmesby, Roy Davis	SX23438	Cfn	SA AREA WKSHOPS
Homel, William James	QX52123	Pte	25 AITB
Hooker, William Albert	VX95370	Spr	AEME W/S SA L of C AREA
Hope, Douglas Haig	V67358	Pte	1 AUST ORTHO HOSP
Hopkins, Gordon William	SX33429	Pte	19 AITB
Hopkins, Norman Henry	NX170056	Pte	3 COY 25 L of C SIGS
Horne, Eric Norman	VX148657	Pte	15 FLD AMB
Horsley, Harry Lefevre	NX146645	Lcpl	BIPOD
Horwood, Wilfred	VX110945	Lcpl	20 SUP DEPOT
Hoskin, Raymond William	QX58696	Gnr	1 FLD ARTY TRG
Hoskin, Thomas Reginald	VX119846	Sgt	20 SUP DEPOT
Hosking, Ernest Beauchamp	V311810	Pte	18 AITB
Hourigan, Harold Atherton	V315738	Pte	TATURA INT GRP
Howard, Gilbert Victor	SX149	Pte	HQ SA L of C
Howard, Peter John	V377976	Pte	8 EMP COY

Name	Service no.	Rank	Unit
Hughes, Donald Walter	NX7154	Pte	2 BASE AMM DEPOT
Hughes, Francis James	VX94767	Spr	2 FLD SQN
Hughes, Llewelyn Edward	Q146477	Pte	7 AITB
Hughes, William Thomas	VX42434	Sgt	2/24 BN
Hunter, Norman Leslie	VX77019	Gnr	44 AUST LT BTY
Hutchins, Joseph Baden	VX146479	Pte	19 AITB
Hutson, Lewis Grant	QX53937	Pte	11 AITB
Hynes, Bernard Roy	W49998	Sig	10 LT HRSE REGT
Iannelli, Carmelo	NX111020	Gnr	9 AUST FLD REGT
Ingamells, Fred Harold	VX117530	Pte	STAFF SCHOOL
Ireland, Donald Rodger	NX144502	Pte	18 AITB
Irwin, John William	NX168195	Sig	SIG TRG BN
Izzard, Robert Jonas	NX98654	Pte	1 ATK ARTY TRG REGT
Jack, Edgar John	W15118	Spr	66 DCRE
Jackson, John Bryant	VX97709	Pte	TATURA PW GRP
Jackson, Thomas Arthur	NX2682	Sgt	2 BASE AMM DEPOT
Janke, John Francis	QX46586	Gnr	1 AUST ARMY BDE
Jasperson, Hans William	TX11055	Gnr	TATURA INT GRP
Jelliff, John Sydney	VX71191	Gnr	2 FLD REGT
Jenkin, Ian Berriman	N236550	Pte	JUN LEADER SCHOOL
Jenkins, Henry Mervyn	SX15348	Cpl	AUST TRANS LAND CFT
Jenyns, Ronald Arthur	WX26232	Cpl	16 AITB
Johnson, William Thomas	VX66317	Lcpl	148 AGT COY
Johnston, Marshall Ray	NX49748	Pte	15 ACH
Johnston, Ronald Clive	VX94106	Lcpl	13/32 BN
Johnstone, Norman Gerald	VX84032	Dvr	1 AUST ORTHO HOSP
Johnstone, Ronald Lang	QX32457	Tpr	1 AUST CAV COM
Jones, Albert Stewart	SX35384	Sgt	SA L of C INT SEC
Jones, David Owen	VX80498	Tpr	2/6 ARMD REGT
Jones, Frank	VX38390	Cpl	17 PW COY
Jones, Jack Uwins	V143580	Pte	QLD L of C BIPOD
Jones, Thomas Charles	WX37364	Pte	3 MOTOR BDE COY
Jordan, Edward Cecil	QX64393	Pte	18 BN
Jorgensen, William Desmond	V513203	Pte	28 AITB
Keightley, Ashley Baden	N454682	Gnr	1 AUST HVY AA ARTY
Kelly, James Lindsay	N378855	Gnr	SYD FORT NTH BTY
Kelly, Kenneth Lindsay	VX106709	Pte	13 AAR
Kelly, Maxwell Phillip	NX170556	Gnr	2 AATR
Kelly, Thomas Joseph	NX141557	Bdr	18 AUST FLD REGT
Kemp, Albert Ernest	N286005	Pte	AMBPH TRG CON
Kenneth, Ronald	VX93189	Pte	11 AITB

Name	Service no.	Rank	Unit
Kennett, Alexander William	SX26156	Spr	5 FLD SQN RAE
Kenny, Kevin Leopold	SX20051	Sgt	GDD SA
Kent, Harold Sydney	VX149057	Cpl	WKSHOPS
Kenyon, Keith Maxwell	SX19715	Pte	41/2 BN
Kessell, Sydney Ernest	SX28119	Cpl	148 AGT COY
Keyser, David Edward	V513204	Pte	23 AITB
Kiernan, Jack Vivian	T23228	Cpl	GDD HOBART
Kilday, Stanley	VX108956	Gnr	106 TK ATK REGT
King, Allan George	VX122649	Tpr	2/6 ARMD RRGT
Kingdom, Leslie William	VX94264	Pte	1 ARTB
Kingston, Robert	QX62546	Pte	12 EMP COY
Kirkman, Arthur George	NX93429	Pte	19 GAR BN
Knight, Ward Edward	VX119146	Gnr	67 AM S/L BTY
Knothe, Hans Walter	V377520	Pte	8 EMP COY
Knott, Keith Victor	N223717	Dvr	2 SUP COY
Kopp, John Fredrick	NX134802	L/Sgt	NEWCASTLE AREA WKS
Laird, Bruce Eccleston	N80438	L/Cpl	12 AAC REGT
Lamaro, Felix Richard	VX131172	Tpr	3 MOTOR BDE
Landford, Harold	NX147621	Tpr	3 TANK BDE
Lane, James Desmond	VX148437	Pte	103 ACD
Lane, William Walter	NX175912	Pte	RAA
Lange, Stanley George	WX19360	Pte	AIT 1 AUST BSE L'POOL
Langley, Harold Edward	NX81726	Dvr	3 ARTB (JW)
Langsford, Peter Paxton	SX16381	L/Cpl	121 AGH
Larsen, Norman Robert	SX18588	Pte	112 AGT COY
Laughton, Herbert James	S77416	Cpl	64 ACH
Lawler, Kevin Peter	NX117752	Sgt	RAA
Lawlor, Alfred Matthew	SX19449	Pte	1 ARTB
Lawrence, Alfred Ernest	NX138241	Cpl	16 AUST HVY A/A TP
Le Lievre, William Edward	NX170548	Gnr	2 AITB
Leane, William Albert	SX18678	Pte	WATER TPT TRG CENT
Learmonth, Jack Benjamin	VX114474	Pte	147 AGT COY
Lenton, Donald William	NX207224	Pte	BIPOD
Leo, Bruce Brown	SX16064	Spr	5 FLD SQN RAE
Letwin, Leonard Victor	VX128103	Pte	13 AAOD
Lewins, Aubury Harold	VX125380	Cfn	2/4 BASE WKSHOPS
Lewis, Jackson William	SX24618	Tpr	2 ARMD BDE
Lewis, Kenneth George	TX16788	Pte	23 AITB
Liddicut, Raymond Ernest	VX124141	Pte	1 ARTY TRG REGT
Liddy, Lancelot Michael	SX17058	Pte	11 GSH BN
Light, Lawrence John	VX93244	Pte	41/2 AIB
Littlejohn, Ronald James	NX104982	Cpl	3 AAHT

284 Appendix 1

Name	Service no.	Rank	Unit
Lohmeyer, Donald Fredrick	SX32031	Gnr	2/27 LT AA BTY
Longbottom, Victor Donald	SX26610	Pte	8 HORSE TPT COY
Lonsdale, Eric Albert	VX119674	Pte	197 ASD
Lowry, John James	QX45194	Pte	AUST ENG REGT
Luff, Leonard	W3144	Pte	10 GAR BN
Luke, Derek Harold	WX25921	Cfn	2/93 LAD
Lynch, Kevin Francis	VX93556	Pte	11 AITB
Lyons, Edwin Clegg	W38235	Cpl	BIPOD W COMD
McCabe, Patrick Joseph	NX160248	Pte	121 AGH
McCracken, Percy William	NX122866	Tpr	1 AUST TK BN
McDiarmid, Keith William	VX96775	Pte	VIC ECH & REC
McDonald, Andrew	N157170	Pte	11 GAR BN
McGavin, Leslie Octimus	NX119365	Tpr	AA TK BN
McGaw, Ronald	VX92716	Pte	GDD ROYAL PARK
McGrath, Gregory William	QX57591	Gnr	1 AATR
McGregor, Kenneth Clive	NX200627	Pte	JUNGLE WARFARE
McGuire, Eric	NX177648	Pte	21 AITB
McGuire, Milton Francis	NX180982	Pte	101 CON DEPOT
McGuren, John Thomas	NX137361	Tpr	15 MOTOR REGT
Mackay, Norwood George	VX95425	Pte	1 BASE AMM DEPOT
Mackay, William Bruce	NX131159	Pte	17 BN
Mackechnie, Alexander Patrick	N35885	Pte	11 GAR BN
Mackenzie, Alexander Douglas	WX34147	Pte	BIPOD
Mackie, Donald	VX96304	Pte	13/33 BN
McKlaren, Colin James	NX201390	Gnr	1 AUST LIGHT A/A
Maclaine, Malcolm Hugh	TX9087	Pte	13/33 BN
McLean, Douglas Robert	TX8366	Cpl	2/2 A TK TPT COY
McLean, Gordon Murdoch	VX77824	Tpr	20 AUST MOT TPT
McLeay, Roderick	VX115823	Tpr	AAC
Macleod, Peter	Q54627	Pte	13 AAOD
McMillan, Norman Alexander	N291631	Pte	230 AITB
McPherson, Alan Alfred	VX129199	Pte	GDD VIC L of C AREA
McPherson, Percival Keith	TX8840	Pte	TAS ECH & REC
McQueen, James Alexander	NX117353	L/Cpl	15 MOTOR REGT
McQuillan, John Alexander	W29243	Cpl	PW CAMP MARRINUP
Maidment, Lexil George	S41228	S/Sgt	HQ SA L of C AREA
Makinen, Alan Richard	NX168321	Sig	25 L of C SIGS
Mann, Lionel Stanley	Q144107	Pte	9 WKSHOP COY
Mannheim, Hans	V377957	Pte	8 EMP COY
Manning, Roydon Stanley	N462119	Pte	8 AITB
Mansel, John George	NX140837	Pte	16 A SUB DEP COY
Manteufel, Herbert Henry	QX36667	Sgt	1 SERV TRG BN

Appendix 1 285

Name	Service no.	Rank	Unit
Mapley, Bryan Allan	TX4966	Pte	3 TRG CAMP RAE
Marks, Clarence William	NX172205	Spr	1 BN RAE
Marsh, Samuel Joseph	WX34552	Pte	1 PARA BN
Marshall, Richard James	VX11684	Gnr	2/2 FLD REGT
Martin, Fredrick George	NX201864	Pte	1 ARTB
Martin, Henry Charles	WX38765	Pte	AACC
Martin, Ronald Bruce	V28488	Pte	5 AUST TNK TPT COY
Martin, William	NX200957	Pte	2 ARTB
Mason, Frank Joseph	T102842	Gnr	5/2 A/A TRG REGT
Matich, Frank Tony	WX15599	Pte	124 AGT COY
Matthews, Arnold William	SX31944	Pte	32 AITB
Matthews, Robert Cecil	NX195280	Pte	30 AITB
Maughan, Bernard William	T14963	Pte	10 AUX HORSE TPT
Mavromatis, Nicholas Angelo	SX25392	Pte	123 AUST SPEC HOSP
Meares, Rochford Devenish	QX62799	Gnr	33 AITB
Medhurst, Lindsay John	TX14054	Pte	40 BN
Melville, James Joseph	VX83201	Dvr	4 FLD REGT
Melville, Vincent Clifford	N211442	Pte	AACTR PUCKAPUNYAL
Menck, Eric Alan	VX119130	Pte	146 AGT COY
Miguel, Roy	DX875	Sig	25 L of C SIGS
Miles, Francis James	Q106044	Pte	11 AITB
Milkins, Alfred Leslie	SX24816	Cpl	123 AUST SPEC HOSP
Miller, James Herbert	VX84203	Pte	AAPC VIC L of C AREA
Miller, John Francis	V211957	Gnr	105 TNK AH
Milligan, Robert Francis	WX22241	Spr	RAE
Milton, Walter Ernest	W61940	L/Sgt	AEME WA AREA
Milton-Scoyne, Leonard Sidney	VX97321	Pte	2/4 BASE WKSHOPS
Minns, Charles	VX45329	Tpr	1 ARM TK BN
Mitchell, Keith Desmond	VX146032	Pte	41/2 BN
Mitchell, Norbert Sylvester	NX161218	Gnr	22 HVY AA BTY
Mitchell, Stanley William	QX1421	Pte	9 WKSHOP COY
Mitchell, William Duncan	VX145809	Pte	2/4 BASE WKSHOPS
Moeller, Robert Douglas	SX30325	Pte	1 ORD VEH PK
Moffatt, Robert Alfred	VX64583	Pte	27 SUP DEPOT COY
Mollross, Herbert Barry	TX8719	Pte	2/9 ARMD REGT
Moore, Edgar Allan	WX26372	Cpl	5 MOTOR AMB
Moore, Robert Matthew	WX33215	Sgt	4 ARMD BDE
Morgan, Bruce Rawland	NX204986	Pte	DFO SYDNEY
Morgan, Hugh Boyd	VX65264	Pte	3 ABSD
Moroney, Dennis Brendon	VX117805	Tpr	20 MOTOR REGT
Morris, Charles Hopeton	N393588	Pte	31 GAR BN
Morris, Walter William	NX178115	Pte	8 HOSP LAUNDRY

Appendix 1

Name	Service no.	Rank	Unit
Morrison, Archibald Hugh	QX41408	Sgt	CDD STAFF REDBANK
Morrison, Donald Edward	VX76064	Sig	SIGS 2 AUST ARMY
Morrison, George Rogers	QX49557	Sgt	7 A/A BTY
Morrissey, Vincent Edward	VX94348	Pte	19 AITB
Mott, Keith Frederick	WX19457	Pte	10 GAR BN
Moy, Wilfred Selwyn	NX99247	Pte	1 BDE MOTOR TPT
Muir, Harold Lionel	V75705	Pte	1 AASC
Murdoch, Norman William	NX44699	Cfn	5 WKSHOPS AEME
Murfett, Cedric Charles	VX121819	Lsgt	AAPC VIC L of C AREA
Murray, Colin Arthur	SX16854	Tpr	HQ 3 MOTOR BDE
Murray, Herbert George	NX174511	Sgt	28 AITB
Murrell, Kenneth Cameron	VX84343	Pte	4 ARMD BDE WKSHOPS
Murton, William Richard	NX95611	Tpr	2/4 ARMD REGT
Nash, Ross John	SX29426	Pte	18 BN
Neave, Stanley	VX116696	Pte	3 AAOD
Neilson, Alan Joseph	QX42325	Gnr	1 AA TRG REGT
Nettlefold, Francis Frederick	VX125227	Pte	13 PW GP
Neville, John	NX141181	A/Cpl	5 ARMY TK BN
Newlyn, Francis John	N267661	Pte	6 TK TPT COY
Newton, Robert John	VX89460	Dvr	13 ARMD REGT
Nicholas, John Henry	QX33021	Pte	1 AASC TD
Nicholls, Leonard Ernest	WX31208	L/Sgt	3 AUST CORPS PROVO
Nienaber, Maxwell Edward	NX180311	Pte	DPO SYDNEY
Normington, John Francis	WX37033	Pte	1 AITB
Norris, Douglas Ross	N443609	Gnr	21 AE COY
Northey, Douglas Arnold	NX105933	Bdr	COAST ARTY
Norton, Miles Edward	QX55725	Gnr	1 ARTB
Noskoff, Alex	QX26532	Pte	KIT STORE IPSWITCH
O' Brien, Thomas	Q271316	Gnr	1 LT AA TRG REGT
O' Donnell, Richard	WX41438	Pte	HAY POW CAMP
O' Kell, Reginald George	NX1029	L/Sgt	HQ 17 A L/C
O' Neale, Charles Joseph	NX201130	Gnr	1 AATR
O' Neill, James	Q266165	Pte	1 AUST SUC TRG BN
O' Rance, Robert Bede	N260555	Pte	133 AGC
O' Shaughnessy, Kevin John	NX169332	L/Cpl	2 FLD SQN
Osmond, Keith	NX93736	Pte	3 TANK BASE WKHSOPS
Owens, Frank Jordan	WX30446	Gnr	2/7 CDO SQN
Owens, Thomas Raymond	NX156091	Pte	30 BN
Page, Bernard Graham	QX44281	Gnr	1 AATR
Parker, Douglas James	TX15409	Dvr	4 ARMD BDE
Parker, John Thomas	TX15410	Tpr	4 ARMD BDE

Name	Service no.	Rank	Unit
Parker-Smith, Harold	S41570	Cpl	SA ECH & REC
Parry, Ronald William	SX13617	Tpr	2/4 AAR
Parsons, Arthur Dudley	NX177421	Pte	8/8 W/S AEME
Pascoe, Francis James	NX201532	Gnr	1 A/TK REGT
Paton, Norman	Q268339	Pte	29 AITB
Patrikeos, Engenios	V501567	Pte	23 AITB
Patton, Malcolm Charles	VX88069	Dvr	2/3 TP WKSHOPS
Paulin, John Lawrence	NX137824	Dvr	148 AGT COY
Pavletich, George William	VX97769	Pte	LTD MELBOURNE
Peck, Morrison Harold	VX148835	A/Cpl	JUNGLE WARFARE
Penhall, Fredrick Joseph	VX81414	Cpl	3 BOD
Pennell, John	NX68598	Pte	HQ 2 AUST ARMY
Peterson, Alfred	VX51946	Dvr	9 MOTOR AMB
Picton, Joseph Arthur	QX32902	Pte	21 AITB
Pirois, Raymond Claude	VX151795	Pte	30 AITB
Platt, Ronald Andrew	NX170553	Gnr	2 ARTY ENG REGT
Plumridge, Robert Hamilton	VX93973	Pte	1 BOD
Pointon, Sidney	NX157996	Pte	2/142 AGT COY
Polsen, William George	NX157541	Tpr	15 MOTOR REGT
Pope, Stewart William	VX97687	Pte	VIC ECH & REC
Popp, Stanley Allan	QX62959	Pte	2 ARTB
Porteous, Charles Francis	QX51970	Pte	15 AITB
Posluszny, Osluszny Kazinnerz	N480735	Pte	1 BOD
Poulsen, Harold Lund	WX35558	L/Cpl	25 MECH EQUIP PARK
Powell, John Richard	VX92699	Pte	4 ARTB
Powell, Thomas Henry	NX115698	L/Cpl	4 AIB
Pozzi, Archie	Q115743	Pte	9 WORKS COY
Price, Frederick Bruce	VX92365	Pte	11 AITB
Prince, Reginald Arthur	W96856	Pte	110 PERTH MIL HOSP
Proleta, Joseph James	SX20878	Spr	5 FLD SQN RAE
Protopopoff, Serg Nicholas	NX122204	Sgt	1 BOD
Purdon, Albert James	VX110125	Pte	147 AGT COY
Pyle, Robert Alfred	VX62869	Pte	148 AGT COY
Quaill, Lance Maurice	QX62509	Pte	5 DIV REC CAMP
Queripel, Harold George	VX88048	Tpr	24 WORKS COY
Quinlan, Fredrick James	VX31637	Cpl	148 AGT COY
Rawlings, Ronald Arthur	WX13248	Pte	138 AGT COY
Rawson, George	V511620	Pte	GDD
Rayward, Leslie Victor	N191937	Pte	BEXLEY CAMP STAFF
Rea, James Robert	SX25316	Pte	140 AGT COY
Real, James Henry	QX37101	Gnr	1 AA TRG REGT

Appendix 1

Name	Service no.	Rank	Unit
Rech, Alexander	VX151822	Pte	28 AITB
Reed, Charles Rowland	VX55251	Gnr	VIC L of C ACS/OFFICE
Reed, Leonard Ronald	VX62658	Pte	148 AGT COY
Rees, John Phillip	NX194781	Pte	JUNGLE WAR SCH
Reeves, Joseph	QX61388	Pte	1 ARTB
Reeves, Percival Ernest	VX96551	Pte	120 TPT COY
Regan, Vernon John	VX145864	Pte	41 BN
Reid, Noel Forrester	VX150559	Gnr	1 ARTY TRG REGT
Reid, Robert Edward	Q136552	Pte	33 BN
Richards, Gavin	NX124028	Gnr	16 MOTOR REGT
Richards, Stanley James	NX201283	Pte	21 AITB
Richardson, Brian Laurence	VX141257	L/Cpl	18 BN
Richardson, John Henry	V18560	Cpl	VIC L of C AEME WKS
Riddell, Arthur Charles	VX145781	Pte	4 ARTB
Rigby, Harold Stanley	VX46624	Cpl	2 AA BDE WKSHOPS
Rigney, Trentham Castleton	TX15961	Dvr	123 AGT COY
Rimington, Francis Charles	VX84297	Cpl	2 AUST FLD SQN RAE
Ritter, Ronald Keith	S40686	Pte	HQ SA L of C AREA
Rivers, Douglas Walker	QX56137	Pte	2/11 KIT STORE
Rixon, Gordon	NX98149	Pte	23 AITB
Roberts, Roy	VX114908	Pte	148 AGT COY
Roberts, Roy William	VX65601	Pte	148 AGT COY
Robertson, George Cummings	WX39258	Pte	1 ENG BASE STORE
Robinson, Jack Finlay	VX90278	Cpl	VIC L of C AREA
Robinson, James Henry	NX148722	Pte	HAY PW GRP
Robran, William Lancelot	SX21434	Gnr	HVY ARTY LARGS BAY
Rodda, Arnold Henry	VX66824	Dvr	1 ARD
Rogers, William John	VX63417	Pte	147 AGT COY
Ross, Arthur John	SX29438	Pte	18 BN
Ross, John	SX30121	Wo2	2 ARMD TNK BN
Ross, Kenneth Robertson	VX68902	Gnr	HQ RAA 4 AUST DIV
Ross, Laurence Robert	NX201863	Pte	1 MG TRG BN
Ross, Norman Keith	N445200	Pte	1 ARTB
Rossington, Cecil Willis	VX122639	Cfn	2/1 BASE WKSP
Rothenberger, Kevin	VX93363	Pte	41/2 BN
Rowlinson, William Joseph	237661	Cpl	1 PARA BN
Rowse, William Peter	VX138333	Tpr	20 AMR
Rule, Albert Henry	VX82738	Gnr	2 MED REGT
Rumsey, Arthur Ross	NX86981	Pte	2/93 LAD
Russ, Adelbert Edward	NX124542	Pte	2/2 MG BN
Russell, Eric James	QX52732	Pte	21 AITB
Ryan, John Edward	NX25783	Spr	A WATER TPT TRG

Appendix 1   289

Name	Service no.	Rank	Unit
Sabien, Eric Svaul	QX11421	Pte	2 AITB
Salisbury, Joseph Nile	Q269051	Gnr	1 AATR
Salomon, Ernest Gunther	SX38257	Pte	6 EMP COY
Sandbek, Allan Benjamin	QX58341	Pte	33 AITB
Saunders, Percy Eli	N108158	Sgt	HQ CAMP GLEN INNIS
Saunders, Tasman Vere	TX14371	Pte	4 ARMD BDE
Scheiner, Frank	V377770	Pte	6 EMP COY
Schuberth, John Thomas	N226546	Cpl	SA L of C AREA
Scott, Herbert (Jr)	Q131704	Pte	111 AGT COY
Scown, Ernest Albert	VX124365	Sig	HQ ASWG
Seary, Brian	QX58675	Pte	21 AITB
Seaton, Gilbert Rowland	WX22004	Gnr	4 HVY AA BTY
Sewell, Keith Jethro	NX168061	Pte	2 ORD TK DEP
Sexton, Walton Stanley	VX124260	Pte	148 AGT COY
Shaw, Edwin Hastings	VX112615	Pte	2 BOD
Shillinglaw, Gordon Robert	VX124975	Pte	13 PW GRP
Shippick, Joseph Patrick	VX93554	Gnr	651 LT AA BTY
Sines, Maurice William	WX21138	Pte	BIPOD
Slater, Arthur Charles	TX14483	Dvr	123 AGT COY
Smedley, John	NX77765	Spr	2/3 IND FLD SQN
Smith, Albert Percival	TX15965	Cpl	123 AGT COY
Smith, Alfred Frederick	NX114080	Pte	5 PACK COY
Smith, Cedric David	QX40368	Pte	2/6 ARMD REGT
Smith, Ernest Yarwood	QX32515	Pte	QLD L of C AEME
Smith, Jeffrey Martin	NX168613	Gnr	3 AUST HVY AA BTY
Smith, John Henry	QX42149	Pte	LHQ JWS
Smith, John Ronald	NX143137	Pte	2 AAOD
Smith, Kenneth	Q270835	Pte	1 ASTB
Smith, Leonard Clive	SX11539	Pte	LTD WAYVILLE SA
Smith, Noel Ernest	QX62845	Pte	7 AITB
Smith, Owen Thomas	S42153	Pte	CHQ WOODSIDE
Smith, Vincent Herbert	QX32591	Gnr	1 ARTY TRG REGT
Smoje, Pasko	WX42355	Pte	10 GAR BN
Somers, Harry Walter	V377871	Pte	12 EMP COY
Somers, John Stephen	NX196502	Spr	2/5 A FD COY
Sommerville, Harold Richard	NX171246	Gnr	9 FLD REGT
Sommerville, Thomas Colin	SX23263	Tpr	13 ARMD REGT
Sorenson, Albert Edward	QX31946	Pte	2 MG BN
Sorfleet, Horace Charles	WX26923	Gnr	7 HVY AA BTY
Spencer, Henry James	NX141464	Cpl	1 AITB
Sprake, Albert Edward	QX62814	Pte	2 AASC
Spratt, Lionel William	TX14656	Pte	GDD SYDNEY
Spriggs, Robert Edward	V145701	L/Sgt	56 DCRE

Appendix 1

Name	Service no.	Rank	Unit
Stacey, Colin Milroe	SX20088	Dvr	22 FLD REGT
Stafford, William Arthur	NX99336	Gnr	2 ARTY TRG REGT
Stapp, Albert Henry	VX110811	Sig	34 AITB
Starr, Stanley George	NX173225		657 LT AA BTY
State, Alan Arthur	N43605	Sgt	18 WORKS COY
Stead, Leonard Sydney	NX81359	Gnr	1 BASE STAGING CAMP
Stedman, James Rodney	NX157097	Pte	101 CON DEPOT
Stephenson, John Philippe	Q125127	Pte	3 ARTB
Stephenson, Wifred Henry	S42620	Cpl	SA L of C AREA
Sterling, Allan Frank	N297909	Cfn	4 ARTB
Stevens, John Walter	VX97327	Pte	2/4 BASE WkSHOPS
Stevenson, Eric William	VX33139	Cpl	147 AGT COY
Stewart, James Leslie	VX73354	Dvr	159 AGT COY
Stewart, Keith William	VX146444	Pte	2 ARTB
Stewart, Kenneth Reginald	NX117406	Sgt	15 MOTOR REGT
Stewart, Leslie Edward	NX28985	Cpl	2 BASE AMM DEPOT
Stewart, R. N.	V514850		2 ARTB
Stewart, William Francis	Q147141	Pte	7 AITB
Stibbs, Lenard Robert	QX34559	Tpr	5 MOTOR REGT
Stinson, William	WX38081	Tpr	65 DEPOT CASH OFFICE
Stolliznow, Werner Alexander	Q143739	Pte	ATTD
Stone, Stirling Macdonald	SX14933	Pte	148 AGT COY
Stone, William George	TX2388	Pte	111 AGH
Stoneham, Ernest Vaughan	WX30474	Sgt	4 HVY AA BTY
Stonham, Norman Stanley	N130371	Pte	18 WORKS COY
Sturrock, Greigh William	WX17523	Cpl	3 MOTOR BDE
Summers, Stanley Robert	NX134774	L/Cpl	140 AGT COY
Swan, James Claude	VX58225	Pte	147 AGT COY
Swiney, Norman William	NX142691	Pte	140 AGT COY
Talbot, Colin Roy	WX34184	Gnr	112 TK/ATK REGT
Talbot, William Richard	VX75331	LCpl	2 APSD
Tann, Robert Henry	QX49129	Gnr	111 TK/ATK REGT
Targett, Athol Creswick	VX78739	Gnr	2 FLD REGT
Tatum, William	NX97103	Pte	12 FLD BAKERY
Taylor, Albert	VX150033	Pte	33 AITB
Taylor, Earnest	VX140478	Dvr	2 PACK TPT COY
Taylor, Ernest Edward	W26818	Pte	1 PW GD COY
Theodorofski, Alexander	V377247	Pte	6 EMP COY
Therkelson, Peter	Q137485	Gnr	1 ARMY TRG
Thomas, Ronald	VX86691	Cpl	SIGS AD LHQ
Thomas, Walter Allan	W5882	Sgt	3 CRE
Thompson, Gordon Herbert	WX19918	Gnr	4 HVY AA BTY

Name	Service no.	Rank	Unit
Thompson, James William	VX122439	Pte	2 ARTB
Thompson, Leonard William	VX124779	Pte	32 AITB
Thompson, Lloyd Francis	VX94991	Pte	24 AUSTWORKS COY
Thompson, William Charles	N464402	Pte	23 AITB
Thurgood, Leslie Elijah	N291654	Pte	28 AITB
Tisher, Richard William	SX8332	Pte	AAMC
Tolliday, Alfred Noel	VX62442	Pte	1 AITB
Tonkin, James Anthony	NX153614	Sig	SPEC WIRLS GRP
Torpy, Leslie Patrick	13986	Tpr	15 MOTOR REGT
Tossell, Brien Garth	SX25796	Tpr	2 TK BN
Tout, William Henry	W59810	Pte	9 ADVAMM DEPOT
Trewren, Herbert James	NX147625	Tpr	2 TK BN
Trezise, Walter Steer	WX42226	Pte	BIPOD SYDNEY
Trinder, Edgar Ford	NX108081	Sgt	2/7 BN
Truscott, David	SX18462	Cfn	SA L of C AEME WKS
Tuck, Gilbert Arthur	VX126842	Pte	1 PARA BN
Tucker, Alec Francis	WX39836	Pte	BIPOD SYDNEY
Tudor, Kenneth Douglas	NX137983	Cpl	26 FLD COY RAE
Turnbull, Graham Henry	W10586	Pte	110 PERTH MIL HOSP
Turner, Alfred Edward	NX169203	Pte	8 ADV WKSHOPS AEME
Turner, John Albert	NX80878	Tpr	2/4 ARMD REGT
Turner, Leonard Harold	VX100950	Pte	148 AGT COY
Turner, Phillip Benjiman	W16427	Pte	110 PERTH MIL HOSP
Turner, Raymond Douglas	SX17276	Tpr	2/9 ARMD REGT
Tustain, Cyril Edmund	NX168168	Pte	7 HVY A/A BTY
Tuxford, Raymond John	NX154337	Sgt	AMEN HQ NGF
Twentyman, Mervyn William	VX141265	Pte	18 BN
Twist, John James	33300	Pte	18 AITB
Tyler, Roy	SX8117	Pte	140 AGT COY
Utz, Colin, Lindsay	QX50279	Pte	17 AE COY
Vail, John Athy	3103337	Pte	101 CON DEPOT
Vance, Robert Edmund	NX205980	Pte	PW CAMP HAY
Varian, Keith Percival	WX40236	Pte	19 GAR BN
Vears, Anthony Joseph	SX20097	Tpr	2/4 ARMD REGT
Venardos, William Emmaniol	QX59967	Cpl	42 BN
Viant, Edward Evans	S3093	Cpl	SA L of C INT SEC
Vidler, Gilbert Edward	VX92835	Pte	32 BN
Vince, Stanley Cyril	W58950	Pte	110 PERTH MIL HOSP
Viner Smith, Gavin	SX9261	Maj	116 AGH
Vogelsang, Arthur Ernest	SX27812	Cfn	2/4 BASE WKSHOPS AEME

Name	Service no.	Rank	Unit
Von Hoff, Herman Albert	Q270897	Pte	11 AITB
Voss, Leonard Rex	T23232	Pte	HQ TRG L of C
Wakely, William Henry	VX136727	Pte	147 AGT COY
Walker, Charles Maxwell	VX97468	L/Cpl	VIC ECH & REC
Walker, Kevin George	VX97174	Pte	VIC ECH & REC
Wallace, Kenneth Melville	NX175172	Gnr	1 A/A REGT
Wallace, William Leslie	VX93216	Pte	11 AITB
Wallace, Zane	VX112780	Pte	148 AGT COY
Wallis, William Arthur	VX145708	Pte	32 BN
Walsh, Reginald Joseph	N451006	Pte	28 AITB
Walter, Ernest George	NX124253	Pte	8 ADV WKSHOPS
Ward, Graham Albert	Q128733	Tpr	3 AAD
Warford, Thomas Leslie	VX125471	Pte	15 COY AASC
Waters, Donald Edward	QX51818	Pte	4 AITB
Watkins, William Edison	T22854	Pte	111 GEN HOSP
Watson, Claude Henry	SX33077	Cpl	21 AITB
Watson, John Alan	QX23590	Tpr	2/5 ARMD REGT
Watters, Allan James	WX22714	Pte	21 AITB
Webb, Derwent John	T26173	Dvr	123 AGT COY
Weightman, Robin James	11040	Pte	11 AITB
Wells, Raymond Edwin	TX9057	Pte	32 AITB
Wendland, Norman William	QX63238	Pte	4 AITB
West, Paul	NX12979	S/Sgt	VIC L of C AEME WKS
West, William Francis	VX73571	Cfn	2/4 BASE WKSHOPS
Westley, Cyril George	VX90620	Pte	18 BN
Weston, Frank Edward	WX33054	Tpr	16 BN
Weston, Harvey	VX111404	Cfn	173 LGH AAWS
Westphal, William Ernest	QX49125	Gnr	1 TK ATK REGT
Wheatley, Alfred	Q140363	Bdr	1 TK ATK REGT
White, Fredrick Alexander	NX162198	Tpr	1 CAV REGT
White, Stanley Mills	V144228	Pte	1 BOD
Whiteley, Raymond William	NX109137	Cpl	129 AGH
Whiteman, Albert Henry	NX94083	Dvr	103 ACD
Whitfield, Adam Alderson	N464548	Pte	2 INF SPEC GP
Whitton, Maxwell Douglas	NX142990	Pte	21 AITB
Wicks, Vincent Cyril	NX128798	Tpr	55/53 BN
Wight, Kelvin William	SX23455	Cpl	6 LT FLD AMB
Wilkins, Benjamin	QX44373	Pte	116 TPT PL
Wilkinson, Ritchie Lockhart	SX24889	Tpr	2/4 ARMD REGT
Williams, Edward Charlton	QX23857	Pte	2 BASE POSTAL UNIT
Williams, Raymond Alfred	V517972	Pte	VIC ECH & REC
Williams, Trevor Jack	NX194176	Sig	2/1 AA BDE SIGS

Name	Service no.	Rank	Unit
Williamson, Albert Francis	NX116637	Pte	FAR EAST LIASON
Wills, Cecil Arthur	NX169345	Tpr	65 DENT UNIT
Wilson, Ernest Albert	SX7781	Pte	4 RES & VEH SEC INT TPT
Wilson, George Anselm	QX53886	Pte	41/2 BN
Wilson, James Roland	NX180449	Pte	101 ACD
Wilson, John Francis	QX54000	Dvr	7 ORD VEH PARK
Wilson, Stanley James	VX132600	Sgt	29 WORKS COY
Wilton, Edward Alfred	Q269627	Pte	3 AUST ENG
Winchester, Vincent Roy	QX51388	Pte	3 AOD
Winkworth, John Henry	V280871	Pte	31 WORKS COY
Winter, Edmund Deslande	S33553	Cpl	86 ASD
Wirth, George Alfred	N255077	Pte	AREA WKSHOPS
Wolff, Alfred	V377489	Pte	8 EMP COY
Wolter, Victor Robert	SX1319	Cfn	SA L of C AEME
Wolters, Henry Fredrick	NX72307	Cfn	2/93 LAD
Wood, Allen Arthur	NX176505	Dvr	2/4 BASE WKSHOPS
Wood, Harold Doland	VX97249	Pte	TATURA INT GRP
Wood, Reginald John	QX52165	Gnr	1 ARTY TRG REGT
Woodgate, John Leonard	NX149097	Sgt	18 FLD REGT
Woods, Sydney William	TX13073	Pte	1 ARTB
Woolcock, Ernest Alexander	VX100960	Pte	148 AGT COY
Wootton, Francis Joseph	VX146249	Pte	13/33 BN
Worboys, Neville Raymond	N388888	Cpl	103 AC DP
Wright, Richard Luscombe	SX26316	Cfn	147 AGT COY
Wright, Warrick James	VX125519	Pte	2/6 ARMD REGT
Wright, William J.	VX100528	Pte	LHQ
Wurf, John Clement	VX96994	Pte	2 AAMC TRG BN
Yarrow, Byron Ross	SX26235	Pte	121 AGH
Yates, Colin Edward	SX16679	Spr	5 FLD SQN
Yeates, Robert Edward	SX38534	Gnr	22 FLD REGT
Young, Alick Kitchener	NX106609	Gnr	NEWCASTLE AA GRP
Yuke, Edward William	QX39526	Pte	2 PACK TPT COY
Zurvas, William	QX58509	Pte	1 AITB

Appendix 2
Nominal Roll of Donors

This appendix lists soldiers with malaria acquired on active service in New Guinea, who were transferred to LHQ Medical Research Unit to provide a source of infection for the volunteers at Cairns or Rocky Creek. Most were 'gametocyte carriers' whose blood contained the malaria stages that were infective to mosquitoes. Some were admitted for special investigation of their parasites.

Name	Service no.	Rank	Unit
Agnew, Craig Winnan	VX118338	Pte	2/5 BN
Alley, Frank Underwood	N180026	Pte	39 BN
Altmann, Erven Carl	VX45836	Pte	14 AEC
Ambler, Leslie Albert	VX68672	Pte	2/14 BN
Ambrose, Ronald Ernest	N21970	Pte	7 AUST MG BN
Anderson, Leslie John	NX56733	Pte	125 BDE W/SHOPS
Anderson, Ernest Arthur	QX27649	Pte	2/7 BN
Anstiss, Hector George	NX81513	Cpl	14 AUST FD BTY
Arnold, H. G.	NX54162	Spr	2/7 FD COY
Arnott, Malcolm Roger	NX21679	Sgt	2/13 BN
Ashley, Laurence Joseph	NX19451	L/Bdr	2/1 TK A REGT
Ashton, Mervyn Sidney	NX151518	Sgt	2/20 AUST SUP DEPOT
Avery, James Thomas	QX26600	Pte	2/1 BN
Ayres, Leonard	TX4666	Pte	2/6 BN
Bailey, John Henry	NX21673	Pte	2/17 BN
Ballard, Albert Edward	NX55471	Pte	2/2 BN
Bassula, William Raphael	WX14930	Pte	1/8 BN
Begley, Leo Austin	VX48531	Cpl	2/8 BN
Bell, William Gorton	TX5734	Pte	2/1 PNR BN
Benson, Allan Thomas	NX111507	Pte	2/6 BN
Beyer, Frederick Edward	VX19853	Pte	26 AITB
Biddle, William Elwood	NX40903	Sgt	2/3 BN
Birkett, Clair	NX73652	Pte	33 EMP COY
Blackburn, Oliver Joseph	QX19728	Pte	49 BN

Name	Service no.	Rank	Unit
Blackstock, Allan Roy	NX151482	Spr	39 BN
Blair, William	VX15372	Sgt	2/14 BN
Bland, Archibald Alexander	NX37159	Pte	AUST NG ADM UNIT
Bonner, Keith John	TX816	Cpl	9 DIV PRO COY
Boulton, William Sheridan	QX4436	Wo2	2/9 BN
Bowers, William Robert	QX11786	Pte	49 BN
Boyce, Ronald Cedric	NX125566	Pte	2/22 SUP DEP PL
Bramley, Charles William	NX39774	Pte	2/1 BN
Brennan, Gordon Cecil	VX131977	Spr	15 FD COY
Bridson, Frank Matthew	QX25158	Pte	2/2 MG BN
Briggs, Thomas Henry	N22358	Cpl	53 BN
Brown, William David	VX16322	Sgt	2/6 BN
Browne, Stanley Robert	QX28399	Pte	2/9 BN
Byrne, Stansaluis Thomas	NX116557	Pte	2/6BN
Cahill, John Joseph	SX2746	Pte	2/9 BN
Callaghan, John Page	VX14945	Sgt	2/14 BN
Cambridge, Percy Reuben	NX9305	Cpl	ADCS LHQ
Cannings, Leslie Ralph	NX68452	Pte	2/1 BN
Capararo, Kenneth Andrew	NX105184	Pte	2/9 BN
Carrol, Patrick Vincent	NX10950	Pte	2/3 BN
Carter, George Henry	QX3184	Pte	14 AUST EMP CO
Carter, Sidney Charles	NX116247	Sgt	18 AUST FD COY
Casey, John Vincent	VX43695	Cpl	2/7 AITB
Cavanagh, Jack Holbrook	WX11269	Pte	2/96 ATP PL
Cavanagh, Stanley Gordon	QX20899	Cpl	2/5 A TPT PL
Cawthorne, Atholl Bruce	NX71904	Pte	2/1 BN
Chadwick, George Leslie	QX24521	Pte	21 HQ B BN
Chapman, Alfred	QX27507	Pte	42 BN
Chardon, Royl Francis	SX30740	Pte	2/17 BN
Christensen, Bevan	QX10890	Lt	7 DIV SIGS
Christian, Julius Ruben	NX94390	Pte	2/7 BN
Clewer, Walter Eric	VX3839	Pte	2/6 BN
Collins, Archibald	SX17515	Pte	2/10 BN
Collis, Ernest Ward	VX48774	Pte	2/14 BN
Connell, Maurice Ednie	NX42057	Pte	2/2 BN
Coote, Cyril Jack	NX49314	Spr	1 AUST WATER TPT GP
Cowie, Alexander Bruce	NX111794	Pte	2/7 BN
Cramp, Ernest Earl	QX37434	Cpl	2/15 FD COY RAE
Cranston, Frederick Hugh	QX43393	Wo2	2/11 BN
Creed, Albert William	NX89177	Cpl	HQ 25 AUST INF BN
Creswick, Cecil Roy	NX72177	Cpl	2/2 BN
Cross, John Raymond	NX109420	Bdr	C HVY BTY CAM

Name	Service no.	Rank	Unit
Cunningham, Russell Maxwell	VX137630	Sig	3 DIV SIGS
Dann, Francis Oswin	QX62054	Pte	5 RD
Davis, George Edward	QX36796	Pte	2/1 BN
Davis, Norman Leslie	VX25662	Pte	2/7 BN
Dawson, Claude Harold	QX63634	Pte	25 BN
Dean, George	VX17763	Pte	14 EMP COY
Deed, Darcy	VX19780	Pte	2/12 BN
Denton, Laurence Samuel	VX105948	Sig	2/5 CAV COM SGTN
Derwin, Charles Lindsay	NX84897	L/Cpl	2/9 COMMS SQN
Dixon, Alexander Murdoch	QX16720	Cpl	2/12 AID
Donlan, Kenneth James	NX3430	Gnr	2/1 A FD REGT
Donnelly, Bernard Edward	NX113219	Pte	2/22 BN
Doust, Arthur Herbert	NX150163	Wo1	GEN REINF INF
Dowling, Alan Andrew	NX18612	Tpr	2/7 COM CAR REGT
Doyle, William Peter	VX63422	Pte	2/8 BN
Draffen, Thomas Malcolm	VX50180	Pte	2/24 BN
Drummond, James Lance	VX5329	Sgt	2/5 BN
Drysdale, Alexander Stuart	DX881	Pte	2/17 BN
Earl, James Henry	QX3895	Spr	2/13 FD COY RAE
East, Donald Matthew	SX4014	Pte	2/6/A FD AMB
Eggins, Keith Victor	NX130226	Pte	2/9 BN
Elsworthy, Herbert	NX89113	Pte	5 IND COY
Farrelly, Bernard Francis	NX106938	Pte	27 BN
Faucett, Harold Charles	NX57696	Gnr	2/5 FD REGT
Ferguson, Edward Alexander	NX58069	Cpl	13 FD BAKERY
Ferguson, Sydney John	VX46852	Pte	2/23 BN
Finlay, Laurence William	VX44267	Cpl	2/6 BN
Fleay, John Vernon	WX14768	Pte	2/11 BN
Francis, David Henry	QX15270	Cpl	2/15 BN
Frawley, Thomas	VX17556	Pte	2/7 BN
Freeguard, Norman Frederick	WX13388	Pte	2/7 BN
Friend, Percy John	NX87971	L/Sgt	2/5 BN
Frost, Stanley	QX36787	Pte	2/1 BN
Gardiner, Jonathon Stuart	NX57928	Pte	2/102 AUST GEN TPT COY
Gee, William Frederick	NX82481	Pte	2/5 BN
Gemmell, James William	VX25095	Pte	2/5 BN
Golding, Myles	Q31561	Pte	49 BN
Gonsal, Eric William	VX120727	Pte	2/5 BN
Govan, William Alexander	VX59093	Pte	2/7 BN
Grant, Allan	NX84604	Pte	2/1 ATB

Name	Service no.	Rank	Unit
Gray, Edward	QX38296	Spr	2 AUST CPS RCPT CMP
Greco, Vincenzo	NX163951	Pte	32 AUST HYAA BTY
Greer, Leonard Collins	NX23765	Cpl	2/7 AC SQN
Greer, Athol Eden	N268231	Pte	36 BN
Groom, Horace	QX20573	Pte	GD BN
Gunn, John William	VX115454	Pte	2/6 ATB
Handsaker, Thomas Samuel	NX85913	Cpl	2/7 BN
Hards, William Henry	VX17696	Pte	2/14 BN
Harkness, Albert Ernest	SX5766	L/Sgt	2/43 BN
Harris, Donald Murray	SX30871	Gnr	13 FD REGT
Harrison, Henry Joseph	VX33391	Spr	2/8 FLD COY
Harvey, Clarence Edgar	VX136024	Cpl	2/2 AUST INF BTN
Herbert, Eardley John	VX53160	Bdr	2/2 A FLD REGT
Hickey, Kenneth Thomas	NX97812	Pte	2/7 BN
Hills, Norman John	NX9870	Cpl	2/2 BN
Hinman, Arthur Harry	TX768	Sgt	2/1 TK/A REGT
Hocking, Leslie Henry	SX32084	Cpl	17 AUST INDEP PROV PL
Hodge, Stanley Robert	NX51884	Cpl	2/4 ARMD REGT
Hogben, John Rae	NX86030	Pte	2/7 COM SQN
Hopkins, Arthur Vincent	QX1890	Sgt	2/9 BN
Hopper, Ross Wallace	NX30846	Bdr	2/1 AUST AITK REGT
Horlock, Leslie	QX38350	Sgt	49 BN
Huggins, Brian Arthur	NX5411	Pte	2/3 BN
Jansson, William	WX20342	Pte	2/28 BN
Johnston, Merton Douglas	NX194094	Pte	55/53 BN
Jones, William Alexander	VX8423	Gnr	16 A PERS STAG CAMP
Jones, Ernest Edgar	NX141438	Lt	3/22 NGF
Jubb, Frederick Edwin	NX97272	Pte	2/12 BN
Kay, Albert Ernest	NX113973	Gnr	73 AASH
Keaney, Patrick	VX37043	Pte	7 DIV HQ
Kelly, Philip Francis	QX44896	Pte	2/5 SUP PL
Kemp, Harold	VX52215	Sgt	2/7 BN
Kemp, Horace Banksie	NX40296	Sgt	2/3 BN
Kendrick, Edward Ernest	QX27449	Pte	2/5 BN
Kenny, Jack	WX4138	L/Cpl	2/3 MC BN
Kidner, Edgar Benedict	QX41567	Pte	2/3 BN
Knight, Eric	QX16556	Pte	2/9 BN
Knoblock, Leslie Frederick	V65251	Pte	39 BN
Krome, Henry	QX52319	Cpl	7 DIV PREV COY
Lee, Victor Colin	QX26994	Pte	2 AUST CORP RcPT CMP
Leese, John Vincent	WX15405	Pte	2/11 BN

Name	Service no.	Rank	Unit
Lehfeldt, Rudolph Ludwig	QX32325	Sgt	23 AMGU
Leighton, Erle Roy	VX11385	Sgt	6 DIV HQ SIGS
Luckie, Leolin Alfred	NX155459	Pte	2/5 BN
Lyons, Edward John	VX103126	Pte	2/2 BN
Lyons, Oswalt Alfred	V250434	Spr	15 FD CO RAE
McBride, John	NX20928	Sig	K SEC SIG HQ 21 BDE
McBurnie, Robert Colin	SX31200	Cpl	1 AUST PACK CO
McCafferty, Donald James	VX46927	Pte	2/14 BN
McCaffery, Leo David	VX53530	L/Cpl	2/8 A FD COY
McCarthy, John Joseph	QX6935	Sgt	2/15 BN
MacCarthy, Thornton Edward	QX2653	Wo2	2/9 BN
McClelland, Edward William	NX58281	Pte	2/13 BN
McCurry, Harry Malcolm	VX56727	Pte	2/7 BN
McDonald, Jack Clarence	WX11984	Pte	2/7 BN
McEvoy, Wallis Rex	NX83080	Pte	6 DIV REG CAMP
McEwan, Laurence John	SX30940	Cpl	3/14 AUST FD AMB
McGrath, Gordon Charles	NX39820	Pte	2/1 BN
McGregor, Albert George	QX5268	Spr	2/7 FD COY
McKeon, Charles	VX62564	Pte	2/7 BN
McKinnon, William Syme	VX5251	Pte	2/11 AGH
McLennan, John Henry	NX128978	Pte	2/7 BN
McNamara, Francis	NX127330	Sig	NG AIRWING W/T COY
McPherson, Thomas Eric	VX120042	Pte	2/5 BN
McPherson, Frederick Grand	VX19086	Pte	2/6 BN
Malone, John Patrick	QX17524	Pte	2/2 MG BN
Marriage, Albert Roy	VX92147	Pte	2/1 AUST FD AMB
Marsh, Ronald	NX24794	Pte	16 BOC HQ
Mason, John Gerald	NX92761	Pte	2/31 AI BN
Mawer, Victor Henry	TX2416	Dvr	2/4 ASC
Maye, Keith Thomas	VX53863		2/7 BN
Meakins, Douglas	WX11968	Cpl	2/28 BN
Menz, John Arthur	SX8158	S/Sgt	2/8 FD AMB
Millington, James Clarence	N16646	Gnr	13 FD REG RAA
Mingramm, Jack Albert	NX28699	Pte	2/1 AID
Mitchell, Athol Thomas	TX14244	Pte	S FD BAKERY PL
Mitchell, Edward John	VX117547	Sgt	2/8 BN
Moir, George Deans	QX18742	Pte	2/1 A GRD BN
Moon, Arnold	VX71586	Pte	2/2 A PAR BN
Moore, Charles Richard	QX15065	Pte	7 DIV W/SHPS
Morrison, Alan Frederick	QX31722	Pte	2/7 BN
Mosley, Alfred Andrew	NX157583	Pte	4 BN
Muirhead, Graham Aitken	VX54097	Pte	2/7 BN

Name	Service no.	Rank	Unit
Mulholland, Hector James	NX47738	Pte	2/1 BN
Murdock, Robert Andrew	N17207	Pte	ZES
Murphy, Allan Charles	N21621	Cpl	36 BN
Murphy, Patrick Aloysius	NX89796	Pte	2/3 AMG BN
Murphy, Sidney	NX29155	Gnr	2/6 FD REGT
Neale, Stanley Gains	QX11098	Pte	2/25 BN
Newman, Ronald Archibald	NX19148	Pte	AC SIGS
Nichols, Raymond Albert	TX14687	Pte	2/5 BN
Norcott, Ronald Charles	NX116130	Cpl	1 AUST PCK COY
Oliver, Lewis William	QX29217	Pte	2/10 BN
O'Neill, Clement Hugh	NX77927	Cpl	2/3 BN
Outteridge, Percy Maxwell	NX149692	Pte	2/6 BN
Overall, Neil William	VX141618	L/Cpl	2/2 BN
Palmer, Norman William	V19552	Dvr	1 A PCK TPT COY
Pannell, Edwin Gordon	SX12625	Lcpl	2/27 BN
Parker, Allan James	QX22680	Pte	2/12 BN
Partridge, Allen Leonard	QX32392	Cpl	2/9 BN
Paul, Claude Hamilton	WX14780	Pte	HQ 19 BDE
Paul, Gorgon Graham	QX15256	Sig	16 BN
Pendle, Alfred McIntire	VX141621	Cpl	39 BN
Peoples, John Archibald	VX116778	Sig	SIGS 6 A DIV
Perram, James John	NX203088	Tpr	2/10 COMM SQN
Perry, Allan Alexander	NX41931	Pte	2/3 PNR BN
Perry, Atholl Hunter	NX48052	Sig	25 BDE HQ
Perry, Clifton Wallace	NX105536	Gnr	157 AUST CAS & D
Phillips, Leonard John	VX29399	Pte	2/7 BN
Pimblot, George Herbert	VX6751	Cpl	2/6 BN
Pinson, James George	NX151224	Sig	GL SIGS
Piper, Edwin Ronald	WX1404	Pte	2/5 ASD COY
Plew, Errol Gordon	QX22424	Cpl	2/11 BN
Porter, William John	QX6509	Sgt	2/9 BN
Prendergast, John	WX29194	Tpr	2/7 A COMMS SQN
Preston, Joseph	NX85458	Pte	2/22 FD PARK
Primrose, Stanley Walter	NX122835	Pte	2/9 BN
Pringle, Alexander	NX98387	Spr	2/22 FD PARK
Pulbrook, Cyril	N197607	Cpl	53/53 BN
Pye, Cornelius John	VX53781	Pte	2/5 BN
Quinn, John Patrick	NX4609	Wo2	2/3 AGT COY
Radnell, Ernest	VX70115	Spr	2/15 FD COY RAE
Rees, Thomas	QX20000	L/Cpl	GEN REIN ASC

Appendix 2

Name	Service no.	Rank	Unit
Remilton, George Alfred	QX3510	Cpl	2/12 BN
Rewbridge, William Andrew	VX89863	Pte	2/3 CAV COM SQN
Reynolds, John Edward	VX45500	Pte	2/5 BN
Riches, Harold Thomas	QX17483	Gnr	2/1 TK/A REGT
Riseley, Lenard Albert	VX136235	Pte	5 AAW AEME
Ritchie, Richard Oswald	VX23509	Sgt	2/16 BN
Robertson, Alan McArthur	NX79283	Pte	2/4 FD AMB
Robson, James Alexander	VX86958	Dvr	1 AUST PACK TPT COY
Rodwell, John Robert	NX21777	Pte	2/3 BN
Rudd, John William	NX72786	Pte	2/2 BN
Russell, Emerald Ernest	QX9105	Pte	2/2 MG BN
Rutherford, John Allen	QX60686	Gnr	1 A MOUNT BTY
Salter, Gavin Alexander	NX69011	Pte	6 DIV REC CAMP
Sanders, Robert George	QX28870	Pte	2/7 BN
Scott, Gavin Jones	NX16316	Tpr	2/5 FIELD COY
Semple, William	QX3884	Gnr	2/1 FD REGT
Shepherd, Geoffrey	Q143551	Pte	A SUB HQ AUST KIT STORE
Shoesmith, John McLean	N152501	Pte	36 BN
Sim, John Lewis	VX103147	Sgt	2/2 BN
Simpson, W. C.	NX8129	Pte	2/1 AFD RGT
Sligar, Allan Patrick	NX93847	Sig	1 AUST CORPS SIGS
Sloan, Harold Charles	NX68697	Pte	2/3 BN
Smith, Ray Joseph	VX54941	Pte	2/5 ATB
Smith, Reginald David	WX16930	Pte	24 BDE HQ
Smith, A. E.	NX87786	Spr	2/102 AGT COY
Speers, James Alexander	NX46136	Cpl	2/1 BN
Spinks, Victor George	NX107141	L/Cpl	2/1 BN
Stack, Walter Charles	VX21863	Pte	2/5 FD AMB
Stagg, Frank Gordon	TX872	Pte	2/12 BN
Stanton, Pierre Alfred	QX44151	Sgt	49 BN
Stephen, Maxwell Leslie	VX137550	L/Cpl	39 BN
Sterritt, Neil Joseph	VX117331	Spr	2/15 FD COY RAE
Stewart, Norman John	WX13682	Pte	2/11 BN
Taylor, Colin McNeil	VX50861	Pte	2/6 BN
Taylor, William Ernest	NX19384	Sgt	2/17 BN
Teasdale, David James	NX79754	Pte	2/3 MG BN
Thompson, John Henry	WX15778	Pte	2/11 BN
Thorpe, Donald Albert	NX67936	L/Cpl	2/105 AG TPT COY
Tighe, Robert Charles	NX66463	L/Cpl	2/3 BN
Townsend, Donald Malville	VX3319	L/Cpl	2/5 BN
Traill, Victor George	QX8552	Sgt	2/15 BN
Trapp, William Joseph	QX1087	Dvr	2/5 SUP DEPOT

Name	Service no.	Rank	Unit
Trethowan, William Howard	NX66602	Sgt	2/2 BN
Turnbull, Reginald	NX170562	Gnr	2/2 A FLD REGT
Turner, Ronald Edward	NX41034	Pte	2/3 BN
Turner, William Henry	SX580	Pte	2/10 BN
Twomey, Francis John	N247535	Pte	55/53 BN
Ullyatt, Geoffrey Harold	VX46671	L/Cpl	2/3 A MOB BAC AB
Walker, Alfred Edward	QX31426	Pte	2/2 PNR BN
Walker, Bruce Alfred	NX104943	Pte	36 BN
Walker, Ernest Harry	QX33388	Pte	2/7 BN
Wallbank, Robert Arthur	NX47497	Pte	2/1 BN
Warhurst, Dudley Arthur	VX15317	Sgt	2/14 BN
Watters, Harold	QX3595	Pte	2/12 BN
Wearing, Thomas Arthur	SX6355	Dvr	2/43 BN
Webb, John	TX8063	Pte	1 AUST CAV REGT
Webster, Stuart Stanley	NX6047	Pte	2/4 BN
Weise, Edward Paul	VX109500	Sig	3 A DIV
Wells, Robert Francis	QX28975	Pte	2/7 BN
Westbury, Maxwell	SX6365	Cpl	2/2 BN
Whitmore, Alfred	QX3104	Cpl	HQ 2/9 BN
Wilkinson, Howard Richard	VX132163	Pte	39 BN
Williams, Albert Ernest	VX11866		2/5 BN
Williams, Wilfred Edwin	WX15396	Pte	2/1 BN
Wills, David Francis	WX32395	Sig	FRT SIGS MED
Wilson, Andrew	WX13009	Pte	2/11 BN
Winton, Herbert John	QX4229	Ssgt	49 BN
Wood, Edwin Earle	NX863	Pte	2/1 AUST TPT PE
Worrall, William Howard	QX36901	Pte	49 AUST INF BN
Yates, Francis Patrick	NX112251	Pte	13APSC
Yelland, Reginald Charles	QX33377	Pte	2/7 BN
Zillfleish, Herbert	QX18942	Pte	2/10 BN

Appendix 3
Nominal Roll of Staff

This appendix lists staff of LHQ Medical Research Unit, Cairns, as well as members of the Malaria Experimental Group attached to 5 Australian Camp Hospital and personnel detached from other units to assist with the work.

* Indicates staff members who volunteered as subjects during the last phase of the work in 1946.

Name	Service no.	Rank	Remarks
Akhurst, Thomas Adrian	NX84842	Lt	
Allmann, Stuart Leo	NX97239	Capt	Detached 6 AMES
Anderson, J.	NX37564	Cpl	Detached 6 AMES
Andrew, Richard Roderick	WX29	Maj	
Astill, Gladys	QF273509	Pte	
Backhouse, Thomas Clive	VX48607	Maj	
Banks, Grace Eileen	QF119729	Lt	
Barry, Iris Joan	NFX152922	Cpl	
Barry, Lorna Olga	NFX152923	Cpl	
Bellert, Mary Brown	QFX40989	Lt	
*Birch, Albert Roy	QX53106	Pte	
*Black, Robert Hughes	QX36074	Capt	
*Blackburn, Charles Ruthven	NX12614	LtCol	
*Bladon, Dudley Ivo	NX136261	Pte	
Brockhurst, John Henry	QX38395	Sgt	
Bullock, Joyce Millicent	QFX60675	Pte	
Burbidge, Beryl Emma	QFX43171	Capt	
Cameron, Douglas Archibald	NX87606	Sgt	Detached 6 AMES
Carberry, Annie Josephine	QFX56775	Pte	
Challinor, Ernest William	Q267226	Pte	
Clancy, Rita Margaret	QFX59199	Pte	
Clarke, Alexia Emily	QF273511	Pte	née Alcorn
*Clarke, Kenneth Roy	NX149002	Pte	
Cockfield, Bernard Joseph	QX63647	Pte	
Colless, Donald H.	NX99144	Cpl	Detached 6 AMES

Appendix 3   303

Name	Service no.	Rank	Remarks
Connors, John Blandford	TX5543	Pte	
Curlewis, Nancy	QF119851	L/Cpl	
Cusack, Eric Daniel	Q138309	Pte	
Daly, Ellen Angela	QF119946	Lt	
Dann, Eva Jean	QFX62085	Pte	
Davies, Dawn Dove	QFX56052	Pte	
*Davies, Howard Edwin	NX26496	S/Sgt	
Duff, James Thomas	N165180	Pte	
*Dunn, Stancy Raymond	VX85813	Lt	
Dwyer, Charles Max	Q128724	Pte	
Dymock, Margery	NFX148843	Cpl	
Ercole, Quinto Noel	NX87345	Lt	
Farthing, Gladys Jean	NFX76449	Capt	
Fenner, Ellen Margaret	WFX1536	Capt	née Roberts
Ferns, Francis Henry	VX58522	Pte	
Findlayson, James Leighton	NX133599	S/Sgt	
Fitzherbert, Henry Patrick	VX18230	Cpl	
Foster, Walter William	N200685	Pte	
Francis, Arthur Edwin	QX62095	Pte	
Gilbert, Robert William	NX81573	Pte	
Gilmore, Lydia Grace	QF119783	Lt	née McPherson
Goodger, Gladys Lilywhite	QFX48903	Lt	
Gore, Rosemary Ella	QFX52404	Cpl	
Gregory, Thomas Screen	VX38159	Maj	
Griffin, Leila	QF141550	Pte	
Harper, Harry	VX85817	Pte	
Hayes, Patricia Marie	QFX48919	Lt	
Holmes, Jessie Ellen	QFX54954	Lt	
Hunter, Lorna Rae	VFX97204	Pte	
Johnson, Patricia Beatrice	QFX61122	Pte	
Jones, Arthur Breinl	QX42293	WO2	
Jose, Ronald Albert	VX9920	Pte	Detached 2/2 AGH
Keddie, Isabelle Cynthia	QFX64363	Pte	
Kinsman, Constance Mona	QFX56537	Pte	
Kretschmer, Frederick Melville	QX62842	Pte	
Lembcke, Reginald John	VX98612	Pte	
Lemerle, Thomas Hodges	NX99874	Lt	
Lohmeyer, Donald Frederick	SX32031	Pte	
Lugge, Hazel Elizabeth	QFX51318	Pte	

Name	Service no.	Rank	Remarks
McCullough, Jessie Margaret	QFX40762	Pte	
Macdonald, Colin Ferguson	VX72842	Cpl	
Macdonald, Ian Campbell	VX102759	Maj	
McDonough, John Michael	VX117552	Pte	
Mackerras, Mabel Josephine	NFX137899	Maj	
McNamara, John William	VX40337	S/Sgt	
Mantell, Alma	QF273510	Pte	
Merritt, George Clifford	NX171496	Cpl	
Nickel, Frederick William	WX19147	Cpl	
O'Sullivan, P.		S/Sgt	Detached 2 AMES
Pitts, Alice Mary	QFX54303	Pte	
Pope, Joyce Abbott	QFX63568	Pte	née Birt
*Pope, Kenneth Geoffrey	SX28400	Lt	
Quinlan, Allan	WX15184	Pte	
Redwood, Maurice Charles	QX37310	S/Sgt	
Ricketts, Edith Maud	QFX40982	Lt	
Rixon, Joyce Claudine	QFX49310	Pte	
Roberts, Frederick Hugh	QX39262	Capt	Detached 2 AMES
Rudan, Thomas	Q151831	Pte	
Scott, Eric James	VX122026	Pte	
Shaw, Joan Towart	QF269337	Pte	
Sheridan, Corrie Ella	QFX48906	Lt	
Simpson, Jean	QFX50887	Pte	
Star, Nancy	QFX61344	Pte	
Stretch, Margaret	VFX80824	Lt	
Swan, Maxwell Stuart	VX38828	Lt	
Taylor, Kay Glasson	NF409413	Pte	
Tindale, Daryl Kathleen	QF142106	Lt	
*Tonge, John Iredale	NX13847	Maj	
Vines, Reginald	VX16515	Pte	
Walsh, Leonard Francis	QX20603	Pte	
Wild, Betty Jean	QX58100	Pte	
Williams, B.		Cpl	Detached 6 AMES
Williams, Helen Margaret	QFX46800	Pte	
*Winterbottom, William James	NX120699	WO2	
Wouda, William George	VX53476	Pte	
Young, Leslie Aurel	Q145289	Pte	

Appendix 4
Summary of Findings from Repatriation Medical Authority Workshop, July 1999

Background

The potential health effects for Australian troops involved in the malaria drug tests undertaken during World War II form the basis of this report. The conduct and carriage of the antimalarial trials undertaken in north Queensland during World War II received adverse media attention in April 1999. Subsequently, the Minister for Veterans' Affairs, Hon. Mr Bruce Scott announced that the issue of 'the health effects of these experiments' was to be referred to the Repatriation Medical Authority.

Workshop

On 12–13 July 1999 the Repatriation Medical Authority held a workshop to help its members clarify and consider the short and long-term side effects of the specified antimalarial agents and the Australian Army malarial experiments testing those agents. The accurate presentation of the history and carriage of the trials was also considered. Workshop participants included a volunteer and representatives involved in the World War II experiments; individuals who have researched the experiments; individuals who have past or current involvement with ethics in medical research; past and current staff of the Australian Malaria Institute and representatives from a number of ex-service organisations; staff of the Department of Veterans' Affairs, and members and staff of the Repatriation Medical Authority.

Outcomes of the workshop

Identify all of the drugs used in the malaria trials

The antimalarial drugs used in the trials were atebrin, paludrine, quinine, chloroquine, santochin, stilbamidine, plasmochin (plasmoquine), neostam, and the sulphonamides sulphadiazine, sulphamethazine and sulphamerazine.

Were there adverse health effects on the soldiers involved in the trials that could now affect the Repatriation Medical Authority's determination of Statements of Principles?

The Statements of Principles are developed by examining the sound medical-scientific evidence in relation to the causes of a particular disease, injury or death and not by the consideration of any 'class, type or group' of veterans. Information on antimalarial agents and other therapeutic drugs is currently considered in the development of the Statements of Principles.

The antimalarial drugs used in the trials were agents (e.g. quinine and atebrin) which had either been established for some time in the management of malaria or other infectious diseases, or they had received pharmacological and toxicological assessment in the USA and/or UK before use by the Australian volunteers.

The experiments in question were of short duration, the dosage regimen was monitored and clearly documented, the medical supervision accorded to the volunteers was vigilant and of a high standard, and high quality medical records were maintained and kept for each individual volunteer and are still available.

There was no identified sound medical-scientific evidence concerning the possible adverse health effects in the soldiers involved in the trials which could now alter the Repatriation Medical Authority's determination of existing Statements of Principles. Current Statements of Principles have, where applicable, factors to cover exposure to drugs which include those agents used in the Malaria Trials.

What are the positive and negative outcomes of the trials/experiments?

The experiments were considered a remarkable piece of Australian history with overwhelming positive outcomes for the nation and the Allied forces in general. The advances in malaria prophylaxis and treatment contributed to the Allies success in the Pacific theatre in World War II and the lives of many Allied troops were saved.

The evidence presented to the workshop showed that the men infected with malaria and treated during the antimalarial trials were informed military volunteers and that no ethnic bias of any sort operated. The ethical processes of the World War II experiments were considered to be best practice setting for the time and by current standards, even allowing for the substantial developments of research ethics in recent years, were well conducted.

The antimalarial trials were widely and accurately reported in the media of the day with sensible non-biased reporting. The trials appear to have been widely known of and understood by the Australian population of the time. The trials demonstrated Australians' support for 'volunteerism' and clinical research, and had positive impacts for morale for the men involved, the military forces and the wider Australian community. The experiments played a significant role in the war effort and contributed to the saving of thousands of Allied troops by allowing the maintenance of troop strength in the face of enemy attack.

Continuing public health and scientific benefits achieved by the trials include:
- the first evidence that the sulphonamide group of drugs did not act as causal prophylactics in human malaria.
- confirmation that 100 mg of atebrin per day suppresses both vivax and falciparum malaria.
- comprehensive evaluation of the antimalarial activity of paludrine (proguanil) and the discovery of the stages it affects in the parasite life cycle in the mosquito and human.
- Determination of the time that sporozoites of *Plasmodium vivax* and *Plasmodium falciparum* remain in the peripheral circulation after being bitten by infected mosquitoes.
- determination of the duration of the pre-erythrocytic cycle of *P. vivax* and *P. falciparum*.
- first documentation of drug resistance in human malaria, through field observations and laboratory experiments.
- discovery that the 4-aminoquinolines sontoquine and chloroquine act only on the blood stages of human malaria and are not causal prophylactics.

These issues and the conduct of the trials were subsequently published widely in scientific journals and in textbooks.

One of the volunteers, Private Chittleborough, died from acute appendicitis and peritonitis, a condition not caused by the experiments. He received appropriate and skilled medical and surgical intervention however it is not possible to exclude a hypothesis that the early diagnosis of his appendicitis may have been delayed by the circumstances of his participation in the trials.

What are the implications and/or lessons that can be learnt from the experiments?

The experiments were well designed, with high ethical, clinical and scientific values. They were vital to Allied troop strength maintenance and the lessons learnt from the experiments were concisely and quickly conveyed to military commanders for implementation.

With regard to the World War II malaria trials the workshop participants suggested:
- the publication of a nominal roll identifying individuals involved in the experiments;
- follow-up of 'grievance' cases to assess specific concerns;
- that no scientifically valid follow-up cohort study on the volunteers could be done; given that the total number in the cohort was small and that the members were exposed to different antimalarial agents often for relatively short periods of time.

Some issues remain current for modern armed forces and general populations and need to be addressed, for example, that large population data bases and available literature would be appropriate sources to address such issues as long-term risk of uncomplicated malaria, long-term risk of antimalarials and other drugs, and long-term risk of blood transfusion.

The Repatriation Medical Authority, as part of the process of Statements of Principles development, has already considered these issues as potential factors with regard to disease causation where sound medical-scientific evidence is available.

In addition, the workshop participants supported the establishment of a prospective register of current antimalarial usage in Defence force personnel. They considered that any future adverse effects following the use of antimalarials or other drugs in military personnel should be studied prospectively. This would be achieved by a surveillance system established by the Department of Veterans' Affairs and/or Department of Defence, preferably at the Army Malaria Institute, to monitor long-term health effects after exposure, prophylaxis and/or treatment of military personnel for malaria and other vector-borne diseases. All prophylactic therapy given should also be specifically noted on the military medical record so that appropriate monitoring can occur.

The workshop participants were saddened that media reports earlier this year were inaccurate and incomplete in their reporting and served to denigrate the role of the volunteers in this important contribution to Australia's military effort in World War II and to world public health knowledge. The participants support any ministerial actions to correct this, including a parliamentary record of the facts.

Glossary

atebrin/atebrine	An antimalarial drug, also known as mepacrine (UK) or quinacrine (USA).
benign tertian malaria	Malaria infection (also known as BT malaria) caused by *Plasmodium vivax*. A common term in use until the end of World War II when it was replaced by the term ***vivax malaria***.
breakthrough	An attack of malaria caused by failure of the drug to prevent parasites from invading (breaking through into) the blood.
BT malaria	See ***benign tertian malaria***.
causal prophylaxis	Complete prevention of malaria infection by drugs that destroy the sporozoites or the pre-erythrocytic forms.
chemoprophylaxis	Protection from or prevention of malaria by administration of drugs; also known as prophylaxis.
chloroquine	An antimalarial drug, also known as SN-7618, resochin, resoquine or nivaquine.
drug parade	A military term for administration of antimalarial drugs in which the men of a unit line up and take their drugs under the supervision of an NCO or officer.
erythrocytes	Red blood cells.
erythrocytic stages	Forms of malaria parasites that develop in humans within the red blood cells.
exoerythrocytic stages	Forms of malaria parasites that develop in humans outside the red blood cells. See ***tissue stages***.

falciparum malaria	Infection caused by the malaria parasite *Plasmodium falciparum*. If not properly treated it may develop to cerebral malaria, a potentially lethal form of the disease. It does not relapse after the initial attack is cured. See ***malignant tertian malaria***.
gametocytes	The sexual stages of malaria parasites that develop in red blood cells. Very young gametocytes are difficult to distinguish from trophozoites. Malaria-infected humans with gametocytes in their blood are infectious to mosquitoes.
gametocyte carriers	Malaria-infected humans with gametocytes in their blood. Such gametocyte carriers among Australian soldiers with malaria infections acquired in New Guinea were used as 'donors' to infect mosquitoes for the experiments at Cairns.
hyperendemic area	An area in which the prevalence of malaria is very high.
in vitro	The growth of micro-organisms in artificial culture (test tubes).
in vivo	The growth of parasitic organisms in a living host. In the case of malaria this is the growth of the malaria parasite in humans.
larium	See ***mefloquine***.
latent malaria	Stage during which malarial infection is not evident clinically by any symptoms of disease, and/or by the inability to detect parasites by microscopic examination. There is a period of latency preceding the initial attack of malaria and between relapses of vivax malaria when the erythrocytic stages have disappeared from the blood but the infection persists in the tissue stages in the liver.
M.4888	See ***paludrine***.
malarious area	An area in which transmission of malaria is taking place.
malignant tertian malaria	Malaria infection (also known as ***MT malaria***) caused by *Plasmodium falciparum*. A common term in use until the end of World War II, when it was replaced by the term ***falciparum malaria***.
mefloquine	An antimalarial drug, also known as larium.

mepacrine	See *atebrin*
merozoites	The product of schizonts, which are released into the blood stream on rupture of the infected erythrocyte. The merozoites invade fresh blood cells to start another cycle of erythrocytic infection.
nivaquine	See *chloroquine*.
oocysts	Spherical stages on the gut wall of infected mosquitoes within which sporozoites develop.
ookinete	The first stage of development of malaria parasites in the mosquito following sexual fusion of gametocytes in the mosquito gut. The motile ookinetes penetrate the gut wall where they develop into oocysts.
overt attack	Clinical symptoms of malaria due to invasion of the blood by malaria parasites.
paludrine	An antimalarial drug which is also known as M.4888 or proguanil.
pamaquine	See *plasmoquine*.
parasitaemia	The presence of malaria parasites in the blood of a patient, confirmed by microscopic examination of a blood slide.
plasmochin	See *plasmoquine*.
plasmoquine	An antimalarial drug, also known as plasmochin or pamaquine.
pre-erythrocytic stages	Forms of malaria parasites that occur in humans before the invasion of the red blood cells. See *tissue stages*.
primaquine	An antimalarial drug with activity against the tissue stages of vivax malaria.
prophylaxis	See *chemoprophylaxis*.
quartan malaria	Infection caused by the malaria parasite *Plasmodium malariae*. It is rare in comparison to vivax malaria and falciparum malaria.
quinacrine	See *atebrin*.

312 Glossary

quinine	The first antimalarial drug derived from the bark of the cinchona tree.
radical cure	Complete elimination of malaria parasites so that relapses cannot occur. See *radical treatment*.
radical treatment	Treatment adequate to achieve radical cure of malaria. In vivax malaria this implies the use of drugs that eliminate the tissue stages.
recrudescence	Renewed manifestation of malaria infection (clinical symptoms and/or parasitaemia) due to survival of the erythrocytic stages.
relapse	Renewed manifestation of malaria infection (clinical symptoms and/or parasitaemia) after the primary attack is cured. See *vivax malaria*.
resochin	See *chloroquine*.
resoquine	See *chloroquine*.
schizonts	Mature forms of malaria parasites growing in the red blood cells. The schizonts undergo segmentation to form merozoites.
SN-6911	See *sontochin*.
SN-7618	See *chloroquine*.
sontochin	An antimalarial drug, also known as SN-6911 or sontoquine.
sontoquine	See *sontochin*.
sporozoite	The final stage of the malaria parasite in the mosquito. These motile thread-like forms migrate to the salivary glands after rupture of the oocysts. They are injected with the saliva when the mosquito takes a blood meal to begin the cycle of development in humans.
subinoculation	Experimental procedure used at LHQ Medical Research Unit in which blood (usually 200 or 500 ml) was transfused from an infected volunteer (the donor) to an uninfected volunteer (the recipient) with a compatible blood group.

This technique was one thousand times more sensitive than microscopic blood examination in detecting the erythrocytic stages of malaria parasites. The development of malaria in the recipient confirmed the presence of parasites in the blood of the donor; conversely, the failure of the recipient to develop malaria indicated the absence of parasites in the donor's blood at the time of subinoculation.

sulphadiazine See *sulphonamides*.

sulphamerazine See *sulphonamides*.

sulphamezathine See *sulphonamides*.

sulphonamides A group of drugs, some of which have antimalarial properties. Those tested at Cairns were sulphamerazine (code named A-S I), sulphamezathine (code named A-S II), and sulphadiazine (code named A-S III).

suppressive treatment Treatment aimed at preventing or eliminating clinical symptoms and/or parasitaemia by early destruction of the malaria parasites in the red blood cells.

tissue stages Forms of malaria parasites occurring in cells other than the red blood cells. It was discovered after World War II that these stages develop in the liver. See also *exoerythrocytic stages* and *pre-erythrocytic stages*.

trophozoites Early forms of malaria parasites growing in the red blood cells.

vivax malaria Infection caused by the malaria parasite *Plasmodium vivax*. It is not usually lethal, but may relapse in humans for three to four years after the initial attack is cured. See *benign tertian malaria*.

Abbreviations

AA (ACT)	Australian Archives, Australian Capital Territory
AA (Vic)	Australian Archives, Victoria
AAMC	Australian Army Medical Corps
AAMCU	Australian Army Malaria Control Units
AAMWS	Australian Army Medical Women's Service
AAS	Australian Academy of Science, Basser Library, Canberra
ACD	Australian Convalescent Depot
ACH	Australian Camp Hospital
A/Cpl	Acting Corporal
ADGMS	Assistant Director General of Medical Services
AGH	Australian General Hospital
AHQ	Army Headquarters
AIF	Australian Imperial Force
AMES	Australian Mobile Entomological Section
AMF	Australian Military Forces
ANZAC	Australia New Zealand Army Corps
AWM	Australian War Memorial
Bdr	Bombardier
BMR	Bulletin on Malaria Research, National Academy of Sciences Archives, Washington, DC
BN	Battalion
Board	Board for the Coordination of Malarial Studies (USA)
Brig	Brigadier
BT	Benign tertian malaria
Capt	Captain
CCS	Casualty Clearing Station
Cfn	Craftsman
CIC	Commander-in-Chief
CO	Commanding Officer
Col	Colonel
COY	Company
Cpl	Corporal
CRS	Commonwealth Record Series

Abbreviations

CSIR	Council for Scientific and Industrial Research
CSIRO	Commonwealth Scientific and Industrial Research Organization
CSM	Company Sergeant Major
DDGMS	Deputy Director General of Medical Services
DDMS	Deputy Director of Medical Services
DDT	Dichloro-diphenyl-trichloro-ethane (insecticide)
DGMS	Director General of Medical Services
DMS	Director of Medical Services
DVA	Department of Veterans' Affairs
Dvr	Driver
GHQ	General Headquarters
Gnr	Gunner
GOC	General Officer Commanding
HQ	Headquarters
ICI	Imperial Chemical Industries
L/Bdr	Lance Bombardier
L of C	Lines of Communication
L/Cpl	Lance Corporal
LHQ	Land Headquarters
L/Sgt	Lance Sergeant
Lt	Lieutenant
LtCol	Lieutenant Colonel
Maj	Major
MBBS	Bachelor of Medicine Bachelor of Surgery
MO	Medical Officer
MRC	Medical Research Council (UK)
MRU	Medical Research Unit
NAS	National Academy of Sciences Archives, Washington, DC
NCO	Non-Commissioned Officer
NIH	National Institutes of Health (USA)
NRC	National Research Council (USA)
NSW	New South Wales
OC	Officer Commanding
OSRD	Office of Scientific Research and Development (USA)
Pte	Private
QAP	Quinine, atebrin, plasmoquine therapy
RAAF	Royal Australian Air Force
RAP	Regimental Aid Post
RMA	Repatriation Medical Authority
RMO	Regimental Medical Officer
SEAC	South East Asia Command
Sgt	Sergeant
Sig	Signaller
Spr	Sapper
S/Sgt	Staff Sergeant

SWP	South West Pacific
SWPA	South West Pacific Area
Tpr	Trooper
UK	United Kingdom
US	United States
USA	United States of America
WO1	Warrant Officer, First Class
WO2	Warrant Officer, Second Class
WHO	World Health Organization

Notes

Foreword
[1] Schmid, 'History of viral hepatitis', pp. 718–22.

Prologue
[1] Works consulted on military operations in this chapter include Wigmore, *The Japanese Thrust*, and Keogh, *South West Pacific 1941–1945*.
[2] AAS 65/11/19, 'Medical aspects of the evacuation from the south coast of New Britain', report by Lieutenant Colonel Palmer, 8 July 1943.
[3] ibid.
[4] Selby, *Hell and High Fever*, p. 100.
[5] AAS 65/11/19, 'Medical aspects of the evacuation from the south coast of New Britain', report by Lieutenant Colonel Palmer, 8 July 1943.
[6] Selby, *Hell and High Fever*, p. 133.
[7] AAS 65/11/19, 'Medical aspects of the evacuation from the south coast of New Britain', report by Lieutenant Colonel Palmer, 8 July 1943.
[8] ibid.
[9] ibid.

1 War and Malaria
[1] Macpherson et al., *History of the Great War*, pp. 227–46.
[2] Falls, *History of the Great War*, p. 294.
[3] Downes, *The Australian Army Medical Services in the War of 1914–1918*, p. 736.
[4] ibid., p. 742.
[5] ibid., p. 747.
[6] ibid.
[7] Bean, *Anzac to Amiens*, p. 502.
[8] Schulemann, 'Synthetic anti-malarial preparations', pp. 897–904.
[9] Sinton et al., 'Studies in malaria', pp. 793–814.
[10] Schulemann, 'Retrospectives and perspectives of chemotherapy of malaria'.
[11] Malaria Commission, 'Fourth General Report, Therapeutics of Malaria', pp. 897–1017.
[12] ibid.
[13] AAS 65/9/3, notes in War Diary of Col N. H. Fairley, 1940.
[14] AAS 65/19/1, Memorandum of the danger of malaria in south east Europe and Asia Minor, by Col N. Hamilton Fairley and Col J. S. K. Boyd, 22 January 1941.
[15] AAS 65/19/1, Minutes extracted from B.M/100 M, para. 5, signed by General A. Wavell, 10 February 1941.

2 Critical Shortages of Antimalarial Supplies

16 ibid., para. 8, signed by Col R. G. Shaw for DGMS, 14 February 1941.
17 ibid., para. 9, signed by General A. Wavell, 15 February 1941.

1 Fairley's movement details derived from AAS 65/29/6, personal diary, January–June 1942.
2 'Proceedings of conference on certain aspects of prevention of disease in tropical warfare', AWM printed records.
3 AA (Vic), MP742/1, Dept of Defence (111) Army Headquarters files, multiple number series 1943–51, file no. 220/21/31.
4 AAS 65/11/22, document entitled 'Quinine: Conservation of supplies'.
5 AAS 65/11/22, notice to pharmaceutical chemists from Pharmaceutical Association of Australia and New Zealand, 16 July 1942.
6 'The war, quinine and the medical profession in Australia', p. 83.
7 AAS 65/11/22, handwritten notes headed 'Stocks in Australia', in Fairley's handwriting, indicate that the Army had around 8 500 000 quinine tablets (approximately 2760 kg) and a further 2000 kg untabletted quinine.
8 AAS 65/11/6, An appreciation of the present grave position regarding antimalarial drugs and other supplies essential for troops operating in highly malarious area, Report no. 1, 23 October 1942.
9 AAS 65/19/1, diary notes headed 'Tour of NSW and Brisbane L of C area, Aug 2–11 1942'.
10 AAS 65/19/1, letter, Fairley to DGMS, 12 August 1942.
11 AAS 65/11/22, letter, Professor Earle to Sir Alan Newton, 14 August 1942.
12 Details from AAS 65/29/6, Fairley's personal diary 1942, and AA (ACT), CRS A2670/1, War Cabinet Agendum 14/1943, Report by Colonel N. Hamilton Fairley on results of mission to USA and UK regarding malaria, antimalarial drugs, and other essential supplies for the control of malaria, 13 March 1943.
13 Details from AAS 65/11/6, An appreciation of the present grave position regarding antimalarial drugs and other supplies essential for troops operating in highly malarious area, Report no. 1, 23 October 1942, and Report on anti-malarial drugs and other supplies, no. 2, 26 November 1942.
14 AAS 65/11/6, Report on anti-malarial drugs and other supplies, no. 2, 26 November 1942.
15 AAS 65/11/6, An appreciation of the present grave position regarding anti-malarial drugs and other supplies essential for troops operating in highly malarious area, Report no. 1, 23 October 1942.
16 ibid.
17 ibid.
18 ibid.
19 ibid.
20 AAS 65/29/7, Fairley personal diary, October–December 1942.
21 Details from AAS 65/11/6, Note of a meeting held in Portland House on 17 Nov 1942.
22 AAS 65/11/6, Report on anti-malarial drugs and other supplies, no. 2, 26 November 1942.
23 AAS 65/11/6, letter, Aust Army Representative London to Allied Land Forces, Melbourne, 30 November 1942.

3 Our Worst Enemy

1 AAS 65/9/26, itinerary of tour to Port Moresby, New Guinea Force, 26/6/42–3/7/42.
2 ibid.
3 AAS 65/9/8, War Cabinet Agendum 14/1943, 20 February 1943, E: Medical appreciation of malaria casualties in troops fighting in hyperendemic areas of malaria in the S. W. Pacific.
4 Australian College of Physicians Library, Sydney, Ford papers, undated report, Malaria, New Guinea Operations: Report of subject of interview ordered by the Commander-in-Chief by A.D. of Pathology, NGF.

5 AAS 65/32/11, letter, Keogh to DGMS, 18 December 1942.
6 ibid.
7 Walker, *Clinical Problems of War*, p. 91.
8 AA (Vic), MP742/1, Dept of Defence (111) Army Headquarters files, multiple number series 1943–51, file no. 211/6/118, letter, A. D. Path to DDMS, NGF, 3 March 1943, subject: malaria—discipline and organisation.
9 AAS 65/32/11, letter, Keogh to DGMS, 18 December 1942.
10 Australian College of Physicians Library, Sydney, Ford Papers, undated report, Malaria, New Guinea Operations: Report of subject of interview ordered by the Commander-in-Chief by A.D. of Pathology, NGF.
11 Australian College of Physicians Library, Sydney, Ford papers, article on malaria in *Guinea Gold*, 20 December 1942, annotated in Ford's hand 'by C in C'.
12 AAS 65/11/4, interview with Captain Brown, re malaria casualties in US Marines, 12 February 1943.
13 AAS 65/32/11, 'Malaria in New Guinea', four-page secret document annotated in Fairley's hand 'Report for Prime Minister', undated but probably written in January 1943.
14 AA (ACT), CRS A2670/1, War Cabinet Agendum 106/1943, 13 March 1943.
15 AA (ACT), CRS A2670/1, War Cabinet Agendum 14/1943, Part Two, Review from the Manpower Aspect, 22 February 1943.
16 AA (ACT), CRS A2670/1, minute by Defence Committee, no. 39/1943, 4 March 1943.
17 AAS 65/9/39, minutes of 7th meeting of Tropical Diseases Advisory Committee, 10 March 1943.
18 Walker, *Clinical Problems of War*, p. 99.
19 AA (Vic), MP742/1, Dept of Defence (111) Army Headquarters files, no. 211/6/92, letter, Blamey to GHQ SWPA, 19 February 1943.
20 ibid., letter, GHQ SWPA, 2 March 1943.
21 AAS 65/13/7, Combined Advisory Committee, activities to 30 June 1944, p. 4.
22 ibid., p. 5.
23 Manchester, *American Caesar*, p. 77.
24 Page, *Truant Surgeon*, p. 368.
25 AAS 65/11/16, report on malaria to Prime Minister by Sir Earle Page, 3 June 1943.
26 AAS 65/11/12, letter, Page to Curtin, 3 June 1943.
27 AAS 65/13/9, letter, Macarthur to Curtin, 27 July 1943.
28 Allied Land Forces in SWP Area, General Routine Order A.404, 24 May 1943.

4 Anti Sweat

1 AAS 65/19/1, Tour of NSW and Brisbane 2–11 August 1942, Appendix 5, Objects of mission.
2 Shute, 'Thirty years of malaria therapy', pp. 57–61.
3 Yorke and Macfie, 'Observations of malaria made during treatment of general paralysis', pp. 13–44.
4 James, 'Some general results of a study of induced malaria in England', pp. 477–538.
5 James and Tate, 'New knowledge on the life cycle of the malaria parasite', pp. 545–6.
6 Ciuca et al., 'On drug prophylaxis in therapeutic malaria', pp. 241–4.
7 AAS 65/19/1, Tour of NSW and Brisbane 2–11 August 1942, Appendix 5, Objects of mission.
8 Coatney and Cooper, 'The prophylactic effect of sulfadiazine and sulfaguanidine against mosquito-borne *Plasmodium gallinaceum* in the domestic fowl', pp. 1455–8.
9 Coggleshall et al., 'The effectiveness of two new types of chemotherapeutic agents in malaria', pp. 1077–81.
10 AAS 65/11/6, Results of mission to USA & UK, Research organisations for synthesising and testing possible new anti-malarials.
11 Findlay, 'Investigations in the chemotherapy of malaria in West Africa', pp. 1–3.
12 Proceedings of conference on certain aspects of prevention of disease in tropical warfare, AWM printed records.

[13] Walker, *Clinical Problems of War*, p. 104.
[14] AAS 65/13/7, Combined Advisory Committee, Review of activities to 30 June 1944, p. 4.
[15] AAS 65/32/11, Queensland Tour 27 April–12 May 1943.
[16] Australian College of Physicians Library, Sydney, Ford Papers, letter, Keogh to Ford, 31 May 1943.
[17] Australian College of Physicians Library, Sydney, Ford Papers, letter, Keogh to Ford, undated but probably June 1943.
[18] AAS 65/9/26, Sydney tour, 1–6 June 1943.
[19] ibid.
[20] AAS 65/29/8, Meeting at GHQ re programme for Cairns and Atherton. Andrew, Wood, Keogh and Mackerras present, Fairley personal diary, Sunday, 20 June 1943.
[21] AA (Vic), MP742/1, Dept of Defence (111) Army Headquarters files, multiple number series 1943–51, file no. 211/6/1114, letter, DGMS to DDMS Queensland, 22 June 1943.
[22] AAS 65/11/9, Handwritten note on cover page of report on the blood inoculation experiments at Rocky Creek (probably written by Ian Wood): '"AS" was coined in the Barracks, Melbourne by Fairley and Keogh (at the suggestion of I.J.W.) for "anti sweat"'.

5 Priority Neill

[1] AWM 54, item 267/6/7, also AAS 65/11/8, Malaria Experiment, Cairns, under direction of Col N. Hamilton Fairley D of M., undated. AAS copy of this document has the following text added in Fairley's hand: 'This was the preliminary set up. It has been modified with the progress of time in the light of experience', signed NHF.
[2] AA (Vic), MP742/1, Dept of Defence (111) Army Headquarters files multiple number series 1943–51, file no. 211/6/1114, letter, Malaria experiment, 5 Aust Camp Hosp., DGMS to DDMS Queensland, 22 June 1943.
[3] AA (Vic), MP742/1, Dept of Defence (111) Army Headquarters files, multiple number series 1943–51, file no. 211/6/118, letter, A. D. Path to DDMS, NGF, 3 March 1943, subject: malaria—discipline and organisation.
[4] R. R. Andrew, pers. comm., 13 April 1992.
[5] Australian College of Physicians Library, Sydney, Ford Papers, letter, Keogh to Ford, undated but probably June 1943.
[6] AA (Vic), MP742/1, Dept of Defence (111) Army Headquarters files, multiple number series 1943–51, file no. 211/6/1114, letter, Malaria experiment, Cairns, DGMS to DDMS Queensland, 22 June 1943.
[7] AAS 65/32/20, audiotape provided by Dr M. S. A. Swan.
[8] AAS 65/9/26, Tour to Queensland and Papua, Col N. H. Fairley, 23 June–9 July 1943.
[9] AAS 65/9/35, typescript ms entitled 'Introduction', undated.
[10] AAS 65/9/26, Tour to Queensland and Papua, Col N. H. Fairley, 23 June–9 July 1943.
[11] R. R. Andrew, pers. comm., October 1990.
[12] AAS 65/9/26, Tour to Queensland and Papua, Col N. H. Fairley, 23 June–9 July 1943, 8 July: 'Saw Col Dawkins and Major General Berryman and arranged code word for Cairns experiment'.
[13] Mackerras, 'Australia's contribution to our knowledge of insect-borne disease', pp. 157–67.
[14] AAS 65/9/35, information in this and subsequent para. from typescript report entitled 'Entomological Laboratory', undated and unsigned but presumably written by M. J. Mackerras in 1945.
[15] AWM 54, item 267/6/7, also AAS 65/11/8, Malaria experiment, Cairns, under direction of Col N. Hamilton Fairley D. of M., undated.
[16] AAS 65/9/17, tabulated typescript document: list of gametocyte carriers and summary of infection experiments, undated, annotation on title page in hand of C. R. Blackburn: 'This file contains Major Josephine Mackerras's records of gametocyte dates, carriers used . . .'
[17] AAS 65/32/6, war diary, Maj R. R. Andrew, 5 July 1943.
[18] AAS 65/9/26, Tour to Queensland and Papua, Col N. H. Fairley, 23 June–9 July 1943.

[19] AAS 65/9/17, tabulated typescript document: list of gametocyte carriers and summary of infection experiments, undated. It appears that these mosquitoes, pooled from batches 3 and 4, were used for the first sulphonamide experiment on 17 July.
[20] AAS 65/32/6, war diary, Maj R. R. Andrew, 15 July 1943.
[21] ibid., 17 July 1943.
[22] ibid.
[23] AAS 65/9/35, typescript report entitled Entomological laboratory, undated.

6 Neil Desperandum

[1] AAS 65/32/6, war diary, Maj R. R. Andrew, 15 July 1943.
[2] AAS65/11/9, typescript report entitled 'A study of the relative values of the drugs AS 1, AS 2, and AS 3 and atebrin in the cure or control of malaria produced by blood inoculation'.
[3] AAS 65/9/17, tabulated typescript document: list of gametocyte carriers and summary of infection experiments, undated.
[4] AAS 65/32/6, war diary, Maj R. R. Andrew, 23 August 1943.
[5] AAS 65/9/39, minutes of 10th Meeting of Tropical Diseases Advisory Committee, 23 August 1943.
[6] Professor R. R. Andrew, pers. comm., October 1990.
[7] AAS 65/9/39, minutes of 10th Meeting of Tropical Diseases Advisory Committee, 23 August 1943.
[8] AAS 65/32/6, war diary, Maj R. R. Andrew, 29 August 1943.
[9] ibid., 25 September 1943.
[10] Details of Fairley's movements from AAS 65/29/8, personal diary, July–December 1943.
[11] AAS 65/11/8, Report, as at 15 October 1943, by R. R. Andrew.
[12] AAS 65/11/8, Fourth Interim Report from the Malarial Experimental Group 5 Aust Camp Hospital, as at 31 October 1943, by R. R. Andrew.
[13] AAS 65/11/9, typescript report entitled 'A study of the relative values of the drugs AS 1, AS 2, and AS 3 and atebrin in the cure or control of malaria produced by blood inoculation'.
[14] AAS 65/32/6, war diary, Maj R. R. Andrew, 3 and 7 November 1943.
[15] AAS 65/9/33, letter, Andrew to Fairley, 16 November 1943.
[16] AAS 65/11/8, Fifth Interim Report from the Malarial Experimental Group, 26 November 1943, by R. R. Andrew.
[17] ibid.
[18] NAS, Bulletin on Malaria Research, 12 April 1943, p. 86.
[19] ibid.
[20] ibid.
[21] NAS, Bulletin on Malaria Research, 7 October 1943, p. 137.
[22] ibid., p. 136.
[23] AAS 65/13/1, minutes of 6th meeting of Combined Advisory Committee on Tropical Medicine, Hygiene and Sanitation, 18 March 1943.
[24] ibid., minutes of 16th meeting, 17 August 1943.
[25] ibid., minutes of 20th meeting, 3 November 1943.
[26] NAS, Bulletin on Malaria Research, 22 December 1943, p. 187.
[27] Coatney et al., 'Studies in Human Malaria. I. The protective action of sulfadiazine and sulfapyrazine against sporozoite-induced falciparum malaria', pp. 84–104.
[28] NAS, Bulletin on Malaria Research, 31 January 1944, p. 232.
[29] AAS 65/9/35, typescript report entitled Entomological Laboratory, undated and unsigned but presumably written by M. J. Mackerras in 1945.
[30] AA (Vic), MP742/1, Dept of Defence (111) Army Headquarters files, multiple number series 1943–51, file no. 211/7/202, Report on visits to various areas in N.G. 2 September–14 November 1943, by Maj. F. N. Ratcliffe.
[31] AAS 65/9/35, typescript report entitled Entomological Laboratory, undated and unsigned, but presumably written by M. J. Mackerras in 1945.

322   *Notes (Chapters 6–7)*

[32] AAS 65/32/6, war diary, Maj R. R. Andrew, 19 July 1943.
[33] AAS 65/32/11, LHQ Medical Research Unit, War Establishment, 17 November 1943.
[34] AWM 11/1/2, war diary, LHQ MRU, 29 June 1944.

7 Atebrin

[1] AAS 65/9/39, minutes of 6th meeting of Anti-Malaria Advisory Committee, 19 January 1943.
[2] NAS, Bulletin on Malaria Research, 3 June 1943, p. 100.
[3] ibid.
[4] W. Trager, pers. comm., 30 June 1992.
[5] ibid.
[6] AAS 65/32/10, report of the malaria unit on temporary duty at 42nd General Hospital, by Lt F. B. Bang, 15 July 1943.
[7] AAS 65/29/8 and AAS 65/29/9, personal diaries of Col N. H. Fairley, 17 July 1943.
[8] AAS 65/32/10, typescript copy of Bang's first report has handwritten annotations in pencil: 'N. Hamilton Fairley (Maj R. Andrew)'.
[9] AAS 65/32/6, war diary, Maj R. R. Andrew, 25 August 1943.
[10] AAS 65/11/8, Fifth Interim Report from the Malarial Experimental Group, 26 November 1943.
[11] AAS 65/9/33, attachment to letter, Andrew to Fairley, 16 November 1943.
[12] Page, *Truant Surgeon*, p. 368.
[13] AAS 65/11/12, letter, Page to Curtin, 3 June 1943.
[14] AAS 65/9/26, Sydney tour, 1–6 June 1943.
[15] AAS 65/32/6, war diary, Maj R. R. Andrew, 2 and 8 February 1944.
[16] AAS 65/11/20, Progress notes on experimental work, 6 March 1944.
[17] AAS 65/9/44, Interim report of LHQ Medical Research Unit, 16 February 1944.
[18] Australian College of Physicians Library, Sydney, Ford Papers, letter, Fairley to Ford, 28 February 1944.
[19] AWM 52 11/1/2, war diary, LHQ MRU. Notes in this paragraph from Appendix 5, quartering, undated but probably written by C. R. Blackburn in May 1944.
[20] ibid.
[21] AWM 52 11/1/2, war diary, LHQ MRU, Movement Order, 15 May 1944.
[22] AAS 65/9/34, letter, Blackburn to Fairley, 24 May 1944.
[23] C. R. Blackburn, pers. comm., April 1993.
[24] Circular letter no. 153, The drug treatment of malaria, suppressive and clinical, pp. 205–8.
[25] AWM 52 11/1/2, war diary, LHQ MRU, 17 March 1944.
[26] AWM 52 11/1/2, war diary, LHQ MRU, Appendix 3, Summary of experiments proposed by Brigadier Fairley, 17–20 March 1944.
[27] AAS 65/11/20, Progress Notes, 16 April 1944.
[28] AAS 65/11/20, Progress Notes, 6 March 1944.
[29] AAS 65/11/20, Progress Notes, 16 April 1944.
[30] ibid.
[31] AAS 65/32/20, audiotape, M. S. A. Swan.
[32] AAS 65/9/34, letter, Blackburn to Fairley, 5 May 1944.
[33] AAS 65/32/5, Investigation of the effects of activity and environment on atebrin therapy, Report from Armored Medical Research Laboratory, Project no. 18, 23 December 1943.
[34] AAS 65/13/9, letter, Bayne-Jones to Fairley, 27 January 1944.
[35] AAS 65/13/9, letter, Fairley to Bayne-Jones, 17 April 1944.
[36] AAS 65/9/35, letter, Blackburn to Fairley, 6 July 1944.
[37] AAS 65/8/3, report on plasma atebrin levels, undated.
[38] AAS 65/11/20, Progress Notes, 16 April 1944.
[39] AAS 65/9/33, letter, Blackburn to Fairley, 6 July 1944.
[40] AAS 65/11/20, Progress Notes, 16 April 1944.
[41] AA (ACT), CRS A2670/1, 106/1943, RAAF report of malaria and other tropical diseases, supporting document for Defence Committee meeting, 4 March 1943.

Notes (Chapters 7–9)   323

[42] AAS 65/13/1, minutes of 3rd meeting of Combined Advisory Committee on Tropical Medicine, Hygiene and Sanitation, 15 March 1943.
[43] AWM 52 11/1/2, war diary, LHQ Medical Research Unit, 25 May 1944.
[44] AAS 65/32/11, report on decompression chamber runs conducted by No. 1 Flying Personnel Research Unit, June 1944.
[45] AWM 52 11/1/2, war diary, LHQ MRU, Appendix 3, Summary of experiments proposed by Brigadier Fairley, 17–20 March 1944.
[46] AAS 65/9/41, Experiment XVI, Summary of first group having quinine suppressive treatment, undated but probably on or after 10 May 1944.
[47] AAS 65/9/35, typescript report entitled The value of quinine as a suppressive drug in volunteers exposed to experimental mosquito-transmitted malaria (New Guinea Strains) from the LHQ Medical Research Unit Cairns, undated.
[48] Australian College of Physicians Library, Sydney, Ford papers, letter, Fairley to Ford, 28 February 1944.
[49] AAS 65/32/11, letter, Fairley to Steigrad, 6 July 1944.
[50] AAS 65/32/11, Australian Military Mission, Washington, letter, 19 October, probably 1944.
[51] AAS 65/32/11, letter, Steigrad to DGMS, 17 June 1944.
[52] AAS 65/32/11, letter, Fairley to Steigrad, 6 July 1944.
[53] Fairley et al., *Recent Advances in Tropical Medicine*, p. 101.
[54] Russell et al., *Practical Malariology*, pp. 433–9.
[55] AAS 65/9/35, Blackwater fever in volunteers, title handwritten (presumably by Fairley), undated.

8 The Atherton Conference

[1] AAS 65/9/26, Tour to Queensland and Papua, Col N. H. Fairley, 23 June–9 July 1943.
[2] Proceedings of conference on certain aspects of prevention of disease in tropical warfare, AWM printed records.
[3] ibid.
[4] AWM 52 11/1/2, war diary, LHQ MRU, 10 June 1944.
[5] Proceedings of conference on certain aspects of prevention of disease in tropical warfare, AWM printed records, p. 4.
[6] ibid., p. 7.
[7] ibid., p. 9.
[8] ibid.
[9] ibid., p. 11.
[10] ibid.
[11] ibid., p. 12.
[12] ibid., pp. 12–13.
[13] ibid., p. 13.
[14] ibid., pp. 14 and 23.
[15] ibid., pp. 24–6.
[16] ibid., p. 27.
[17] AAS 65/13/1, minutes of Combined Advisory Committee meeting, 20 June 1944.
[18] ibid.
[19] 'This was our longest and dearest campaign', *Salt*, pp. 10–14.
[20] Fairley et al., 'Malaria in the South-West Pacific, with special reference to its chemotherapeutic control', pp. 147–62.

9 Subinoculation

[1] Ciuca et al., 'On drug prophylaxis in therapeutic malaria', pp. 241–4.
[2] James and Tate, 'New knowledge on the life cycle of the malaria parasite', pp. 545–6.
[3] Smith, 'The transfusion of whole blood', pp. 384–92.

4 AAS 65/11/20, Progress Notes, 6 March 1944.
5 ibid.
6 Fairley et al., 'Sidelights on malaria in man obtained by subinoculation experiments', pp. 621–76.
7 AWM 52 11/1/2, war diary, LHQ MRU, Appendix 3, Summary of experiments proposed by Brigadier Fairley, 17–20 March 1944.
8 Fairley et al., 'Sidelights on malaria in man obtained by subinoculation experiments', pp. 621–76.
9 AAS 65/11/8, Fifth Interim Report from the Malaria Experimental Group by Maj R. R. Andrew, 26 November 1943.
10 AAS 65/32/11, addendum, 16 March 1944.
11 AAS 65/11/20, letter, Blackburn to Fairley, 4 April 1944.
12 AAS 65/11/20, progress notes, 16 April 1944.
13 Fairley et al., 'Sidelights on malaria in man obtained by subinoculation experiments', pp. 621–76.
14 James, 'Some general results of a study of induced malaria in England', pp. 477–538.
15 Yorke and Macfie, 'Observations of malaria made during treatment of general paralysis', pp. 13–44.
16 World Health Organization, *Terminology of Malaria and Malaria Eradication*, p. 15.
17 Fairley et al., 'Sidelights on malaria in man obtained by subinoculation experiments', pp. 621–76.

10 Setbacks and Dilemmas in the US Program

1 Dr E. K. Marshall, Memorandum on research in malarial chemotherapy, in NAS, Minutes of third meeting of Conference on Chemotherapy of Malaria, 13 October 1941.
2 NAS, Bulletin on Malaria Research, 20 June 1942, p. 41.
3 NAS, Bulletin on Malaria Research, 12 April 1943, p. 81.
4 NAS, Bulletin on Malaria Research, 25 August 1942, p. 46.
5 NAS, Bulletin on Malaria Research, 12 April 1943, p. 82.
6 NAS, Bulletin on Malaria Research, 20 January 1943, p. 53.
7 NAS, Bulletin on Malaria Research, 3 June 1943, p. 101.
8 NAS, Bulletin on Malaria Research, 22 December 1943, p. 184.
9 NAS, Bulletin on Malaria Research, 16 September 1944, p. 512.
10 NAS, Bulletin on Malaria Research, 20 January 1943, p. 59.
11 NAS, Bulletin on Malaria Research, 7 October 1943, p. 131.
12 NAS, Bulletin on Malaria Research, 29 April 1944, p. 277.
13 NAS, Bulletin on Malaria Research, 4 December 1943, pp. 182–3.
14 NAS, Bulletin on Malaria Research, 12 January 1944, p. 201.
15 NAS, Bulletin on Malaria Research, 10 November 1943, p. 163.
16 NAS, Bulletin on Malaria Research, 22 December 1943, p. 195.
17 ibid.
18 Coatney et al., 'Studies in human malaria. VI. The organisation of a program for testing potential antimalarial drugs in prisoner volunteers', pp. 113–19.
19 NAS, Bulletin on Malaria Research, 31 January 1944, p. 232.
20 Clark, 'History of the co-operative wartime program', in Wiselogle (ed.), *A Survey of Antimalarial Drugs, 1941–1945*, pp. 1–28.
21 NAS, Bulletin on Malaria Research, 27 October 1943, p. 148.
22 NAS, Bulletin on Malaria Research, 20 January 1944, p. 215.
23 ibid.
24 ibid.
25 NAS, Bulletin on Malaria Research, 21 January 1944, p. 220.
26 NAS, Bulletin on Malaria Research, 4 March 1944, p. 241.
27 NAS, Bulletin on Malaria Research, 'Minutes of the Conference for a Review of the Malaria Research Program', 29 March 1944, pp. 251–66.
28 NAS, Bulletin on Malaria Research, Exhibit 1, Report on a consideration of the rationale of the clinical testing program (antimalarials), 29 March 1944, p. 855.
29 ibid.

[30] NAS, Bulletin on Malaria Research, 'Minutes of the Conference for a Review of the Malaria Research Program', 29 March 1944, pp. 251–66.

11 Captured from the Enemy

[1] Clark, 'History of the co-operative wartime program', in Wiselogle (ed.), *A Survey of Antimalarial Drugs, 1941–1945*, pp. 1–28.
[2] NAS, Bulletin on Malaria Research, 29 June 1945, p. 1111.
[3] ibid.
[4] Coatney, 'Pitfalls in a discovery: The chronicle of chloroquine', pp. 121–8.
[5] ibid.
[6] NAS, file, testing centres, Army Field tests 1943–46, report on sontoquine by Dr Jean Schneider, 31 May 1943.
[7] NAS, Bulletin on Malaria Research, 2 September 1943, p. 122.
[8] NAS, Bulletin on Malaria Research, 16 September 1943, p. 127.
[9] NAS, Bulletin on Malaria Research, 4 November 1943, p. 155.
[10] Coatney, 'Pitfalls in a discovery: The chronicle of chloroquine', pp. 121–8.
[11] NAS, Bulletin on Malaria Research, 4 November 1943, p. 155.
[12] NAS, file, testing centres, Army Field tests 1943–46, report on sontoquine by Dr Jean Schneider, 31 May 1943.
[13] NAS, Bulletin on Malaria Research, 4 November 1943, p. 155.
[14] NAS, Bulletin on Malaria Research, 10 November 1943, pp. 165–6.
[15] NAS, Bulletin on Malaria Research, 4 March 1944, p. 246.
[16] NAS, Bulletin on Malaria Research, 18 April 1944, p. 281.
[17] NAS, Bulletin on Malaria Research, 29 April 1944, p. 268.
[18] ibid., p. 269.
[19] NAS, Malaria Report no. 67, '1. Cable from Colonel Fairley to Dr Burns summarising information on atebrin therapy. 2. Extract from letter from Colonel Fairley to Colonel Anderson', received 14 January 1944.
[20] NAS, Bulletin on Malaria Research, 4 November 1943, p. 154.
[21] NAS, Malaria Report no. 67, received 14 January 1944.
[22] NAS, Bulletin on Malaria Research, 29 March 1944, p. 258.
[23] NAS, Bulletin on Malaria Research, 29 April 1944, p. 270.
[24] AAS 65/6/4, Report of visit to UK and USA by Lieutenant Colonel I. Mackerras, undated.
[25] AAS 65/11/8, typescript entitled Malaria Research by I. M. Mackerras, undated but probably written in late 1943.
[26] Lee and Woodhill, *The Anopheline Mosquitoes of the Australasian Region*.
[27] NAS Panels, clinical testing, general, letter, K. T. Compton, Office of Field Service, OSRD, to Dr E. C. Andrus, Committee of Medical Research, Washington, 1 February 1944.
[28] NAS, Bulletin on Malaria Research, 22 December 1943, pp. 184–6.
[29] ibid., p. 186.
[30] AAS 65/6/4, report on visit to USA by Lt Col Mackerras, 22 March–4 November 1944.
[31] NAS, Bulletin on Malaria Research, 26 May 1944, p. 306.
[32] AAS 65/6/4, report from USA by Lt Col Mackerras, 22 May 1944.
[33] AAS 65/6/4, report on visit to USA by Lt Col Mackerras, 22 March–4 November 1944.
[34] NAS, Bulletin on Malaria Research, 31 May 1944, p. 322.
[35] NAS, Malaria Report no. 121, Researches in Malaria Therapy, report submitted by Brig. Kellaway from Brig. Hamilton Fairley, 27 May 1944.
[36] AAS 65/2/3, letter, Downie to Fairley, Appendix L, 1 June 1944.
[37] ibid.
[38] NAS, Bulletin on Malaria Research, 31 May 1944, p. 326.
[39] AAS 65/2/3, letter, Downie to Fairley, 1 June 1944.
[40] NAS, Bulletin on Malaria Research, 29 June 1944, p. 373.
[41] AAS 65/2/3, letter, Downie to Fairley, 1 June 1944.

326 *Notes (Chapters 11–12)*

42 AAS 65/9/37, Report on interview with Dr E. K. Marshall Jr, Baltimore, 6 June 1944.
43 AAS 65/9/37, serial letter, no. 2, Downie to Fairley, 7 June 1944.
44 AAS 65/9/37, Drug SN-6911, Proposed outline of studies, prepared for Colonel Downie by James A. Shannon, 8 June 1944.
45 NAS, Bulletin on Malaria Research, 9 June 1944, p. 365.

12 'SB'

1 AAS 65/9/34, letter, Fairley to Blackburn, 1 July 1944.
2 AAS 65/9/33, letter, Blackburn to Fairley, 6 July 1944.
3 NAS Panels, clinical testing, general, letter, K. T. Compton, Office of Scientific Research and Development, to Dr E. C. Andrus, Committee of Medical Research, Washington, 1 February 1944.
4 NAS, Bulletin on Malaria Research, 29 April 1944, pp. 272–3.
5 NAS, Malaria Report no. 254, Report of the Malaria Mission to the South West Pacific Area by F. C. Bishopp and R. B. Watson, 20 August 1944.
6 NAS, letter, Watson to Shannon, 21 July 1944.
7 AAS 65/2/3, letter, Downie to Fairley, 24 August 1944.
8 AAS 65/9/37, Drug SN-6911, Proposed outline of studies, prepared for Colonel Downie by James A. Shannon, 8 June 1944.
9 AAS 65/9/34, letter, Fairley to Blackburn,1 July 1944.
10 NAS, letter, Watson to Shannon, 21 July 1944.
11 ibid.
12 Clark, 'History of the co-operative wartime program', in Wiselogle (ed.), *A Survey of Antimalarial Drugs, 1941–1945*, p. 17.
13 AAS 65/2/3, letter, Shannon to Downie, 10 August 1944.
14 AAS 65/9/37, Drug SN-6911, Proposed outline of studies, prepared for Colonel Downie by James A. Shannon, 8 June 1944.
15 AAS 65/9/37, Report on interview with Dr E. K. Marshall Jr, Baltimore, 6 June 1944.
16 AAS 65/9/33, Future experiments, 21 July 1944.
17 ibid.
18 AAS 65/9/33, letter, Blackburn to Fairley, 28 July 1944.
19 AAS 65/32/5, Investigation of the effects of activity and environment on atebrin therapy, report from Armored Medical Research Laboratory, Project no. 18, 23 December 1943.
20 AAS 65/9/33, letter, Blackburn to Fairley, 28 July 1944.
21 AAS 65/9/33, Future experiments, 21 July 1944.
22 ibid.
23 AAS 65/9/34, Progress Notes, 21 August 1944.
24 AAS 65/9/34, letter, Blackburn to Fairley, 7 August 1944.
25 AAS 65/9/35, information in this and the subsequent paragraph from typescript report entitled Entomological Laboratory, undated and unsigned, but presumably written by M. J. Mackerras in 1945.
26 AWM 52 11/1/2, war diary, LHQ MRU, 22 August 1944.
27 ibid., 24 August 1944.
28 AAS 65/9/33, letter, Blackburn to Fairley, 6 September 1944.
29 AAS 65/12/1, Report on the supply of *Anopheles punctulatus* for LHQ Medical Research Unit by Lt T. H. Lemerle, 7 October 1944.
30 AAS 65/9/33, letter, Blackburn to Fairley, 13 September 1944.
31 AAS 65/12/1, Report on the supply of *Anopheles punctulatus* for LHQ Medical Research Unit by Lt T. H. Lemerle, 7 October 1944.
32 AAS 65/9/34, letter, Fairley to Blackburn, 14 October 1944.
33 ibid.
34 AAS 65/9/35, typescript entitled Entomology Laboratory.
35 AWM 52 11/1/2, war diary, LHQ MRU, 28 August 1944.

[36] AAS 65/9/33, letter, Blackburn to Fairley, 6 September 1944.
[37] AAS 65/9/34, letter, Fairley to Blackburn, 12 September 1944.
[38] AAS 65/9/34, signal, LHQ MRU to Fairley, 12 September 1944.
[39] AAS 65/9/33, signal, LHQ MRU to Fairley, 24 September 1944.
[40] AAS 65/9/37, Preliminary report on malaria-infected volunteers receiving SN-6911, covering letter, Blackburn to Fairley, 16 October 1944.
[41] ibid.
[42] AAS 65/9/34, letter, Fairley to Blackburn, 12 September 1944.
[43] AAS 65/9/37, Preliminary report on malaria-infected volunteers receiving SN-6911, covering letter, Blackburn to Fairley, 16 October 1944.
[44] AAS 65/9/41, Interim reports Experiment XX, 26 September 1944 and Experiment XXIB, 27 September 1944.
[45] AWM 52 11/1/2, war diary, LHQ MRU, 27 September to 4 October 1944.
[46] Mrs Rosemary Adams (née Gore), pers. comm., 8 October 1992.
[47] NAS, Bulletin on Malaria Research, 31 May 1944, pp. 325–6.
[48] AAS 65/9/37, report by I. M. Mackerras, recent developments in malarial drug research (2), 19 June 1944.
[49] AAS 65/9/37, letter, Blackburn to Fairley, 18 November 1944.
[50] AAS 65/9/34, letter, Fairley to Blackburn, 14 October 1944.
[51] NAS, RAAF message no. MW2908, Fairley to Downie, 11 October 1944.
[52] AAS 65/9/37, letter, Blackburn to Fairley, 20 October 1944.
[53] NAS, Malaria Report no. 260, Preliminary report on experiments carried out by L.H.Q. Medical Research Unit on malaria-infected volunteers receiving SN-6911, 31 October 1944.

13 The Birth of Chloroquine

[1] AAS 65/9/37, serial letter no. 2, Downie to Fairley, 7 June 1944.
[2] NAS, Malaria Report no. 222, Preliminary report on Drug SN-7618, 18 September 1944.
[3] NAS, Malaria Report no. 213, Observations on the pharmacology of SN-7618, by Leon H. Schmidt et al., 1 September 1944.
[4] NAS, Bulletin on Malaria Research, 31 May 1944, p. 336.
[5] AAS 65/9/37, Recent developments in malaria drug research (2), report by Lieutenant Colonel I. M. Mackerras, 19 June 1944.
[6] NAS, Bulletin on Malaria Research, 29 June 1944, p. 373.
[7] NAS, Bulletin on Malaria Research, 31 July 1944, p. 416.
[8] NAS, Bulletin on Malaria Research, 22 November 1944, pp. 569–73.
[9] NAS, Bulletin on Malaria Research, 22 December 1944, p. 635.
[10] NAS, Bulletin on Malaria Research, 29 June 1944, p. 373.
[11] NAS, Bulletin on Malaria Research, 4 August 1944, pp. 396–400.
[12] NAS, letter, Sebrell to Carden, 9 September 1944.
[13] NAS, Bulletin on Malaria Research, 18 September 1944, p. 421.
[14] NAS, Bulletin on Malaria Research, 21 September 1944, p. 474.
[15] AAS 65/2/3, letter, Shannon to Downie, 10 August 1944.
[16] AAS 65/2/3, signal, WM2198, Austmil Washington to Landforces Melbourne, 14 September 1944.
[17] AAS 65/2/3, letter, Downie to Fairley, 14 September 1944.
[18] AWM 52 11/1/2, war diary, LHQ MRU, 21 October 1944.
[19] AAS 65/9/37, Preliminary report on the value of SN-7618 as a suppressive in volunteers exposed to experimental mosquito-transmitted malaria (New Guinea strains of *P. vivax*), 18 November 1944.
[20] AAS 65/9/37, letter, Blackburn to Fairley, 18 November 1944.
[21] NAS, Klamath Falls Marine Base, Oregon, letter, Coggleshall to Shannon, 7 October 1944.
[22] NAS, Klamath Falls Marine Base, Oregon, letter, Shannon to Coggleshall, 14 October 1944.
[23] NAS, Klamath Falls Marine Base, Oregon, letter, Coggleshall to Shannon, 18 October 1944.

328   *Notes (Chapters 13–14)*

²⁴ NAS, Klamath Falls Marine Base, Oregon, letter, Shannon to Coggleshall, 1 November 1944.
²⁵ NAS, Bulletin on Malaria Research, 6 November 1944, pp. 527–39.
²⁶ NAS, Bulletin on Malaria Research, 22 December 1944, p. 631.
²⁷ AAS 65/9/37, Preliminary report on the value of SN-7618 as a suppressive in volunteers exposed to experimental mosquito-transmitted benign tertian malaria (New Guinea strain of *P. vivax*), 18 November 1944.
²⁸ AAS 65/9/35, The value of resochin (SN-7618) as a suppressive drug in volunteers exposed to mosquito-transmitted malaria (New Guinea strains), undated.
²⁹ AAS 65/9/37, The value of SN-7618 as a suppressive in volunteers exposed to experimental malignant tertian malaria (New Guinea strain of *P. falciparum*), 18 November 1944.
³⁰ AAS 65/9/35, The value of resochin (SN-7618) as a suppressive drug in volunteers exposed to mosquito-transmitted malaria (New Guinea strains), undated.
³¹ Council on Pharmacy and Chemistry, 'Chloroquine, non proprietary name for SN-7618', p. 787.

14 The Problem of Vivax

¹ NAS, Bulletin on Malaria Research, 29 March 1944, p. 256.
² NAS, Malaria Report no. 229, The action of quinine sulfate in protective tests against sporozoite-induced malaria (first report), 15 September 1944.
³ NAS, Malaria Report no. 227, The action of large doses of SN-6911 and of atebrine in protective tests against sporozoite-induced vivax malaria (first report), 17 September 1944.
⁴ NAS, Bulletin on Malaria Research, 29 March 1944, p. 856.
⁵ NAS, Bulletin on Malaria Research, 31 May 1944, p. 322.
⁶ AAS 65/11/8, Fifth interim report from the malaria experimental group by Major R. R. Andrew, 26 November 1943.
⁷ AAS 65/11/20, Progress Notes, 6 March 1944.
⁸ AAS 65/9/37, Relapses reported in the first 49 volunteers exposed to experimental mosquito-transmitted malaria, by Lieutenant Colonel C. R. Blackburn, 28 September 1944.
⁹ NAS, Malaria Report no. 191, Summary of research conducted in the Cairns area by the Director of Medicine, AAMC, Brig. N. H. Fairley, 3 August 1944.
¹⁰ NAS, letter, Watson to Shannon, 21 July 1944.
¹¹ NAS, Malaria Report no. 236, Interim report on researches in malaria suppressive therapy conducted by L.H.Q. Medical Research Unit and Medical Personnel 2/2 Australian General Hospital under the direction of Brigadier N. Hamilton Fairley, A.M.F., 20 August 1944.
¹² AAS 65/9/37, memorandum of interview with Dr James A. Shannon, by Colonel E. Downie, 7 September 1944.
¹³ NAS, Bulletin on Malaria Research, 21 September 1944, p. 476.
¹⁴ NAS, Bulletin on Malaria Research, 22 September 1944, pp. 483–4.
¹⁵ NAS, Malaria Report no. 39, Susceptibility of *Anopheles quadrimaculatus* from northern United States to *Plasmodium vivax* infections acquired in the South Pacific, by Raymond L. Laird, 27 December 1943.
¹⁶ NAS, Malaria Report no. A-57, Observations on the transmissibility of South Pacific strains of *Plasmodium vivax* by *Anopheles quadrimaculatus*, Robert Briggs Watson, 1 November 1943.
¹⁷ NAS, Bulletin on Malaria Research, undated but probably August 1944, p. 480.
¹⁸ NAS, Bulletin on Malaria Research, 31 August 1944, p. 482.
¹⁹ NAS, Malaria Report no. 254, Report of the malaria mission to the Southwest Pacific Area, by Fred C. Bishopp and Robert Briggs Watson, 20 August 1944.
²⁰ Blackburn, 'Observations on the development of resistance to vivax malaria', pp. 117–62.
²¹ NAS, Bulletin on Malaria Research, 18 September 1944, p. 427.
²² ibid.
²³ NAS, Bulletin on Malaria Research, 6 November 1944, p. 525.
²⁴ NAS, Bulletin on Malaria Research, 22 November 1944, pp. 563–4.

25 NAS, Bulletin on Malaria Research, undated but probably August 1944, p. 480.
26 NAS, Malaria Report no. 229, The action of quinine sulfate in protective tests against sporozoite-induced vivax malaria, (first report), 15 September 1944.
27 NAS, Malaria Report no. 236, Interim Report on researches in malaria suppressive therapy conducted by LHQ Medical Research Unit and 2/2 Australian General Hospital under the direction of Brigadier N. Hamilton Fairley, 20 August 1944.
28 Ehrman et al., '*Plasmodium vivax* Chesson strain', p. 377.

15 Reorientation of the US Program

1 NAS, Bulletin on Malaria Research, 6 November 1944, p. 521.
2 NAS, Malaria Report no. 260, Preliminary report on experiments carried out by LHQ Medical Research Unit on malaria-infected volunteers receiving SN-6911, 31 October 1944.
3 NAS, Bulletin on Malaria Research, 6 November 1944, p. 522.
4 NAS, Testing Centers, University of Tennessee, letter, Parker to Watson, 2 November 1944.
5 AAS 65/29/11, Fairley, personal diary, July–December 1944.
6 AAS 65/19/9, Fairley, notebook with diary notes of visit to United States, October–November 1944.
7 NAS, Testing Center, Klamath Falls Marine Base, Oregon, letter, Coggleshall to Shannon, 18 October 1944.
8 NAS, Testing Center, Klamath Falls Marine Base, Oregon, telegram, 4 November 1944.
9 NAS, Bulletin on Malaria Research, 20 November 1944, pp. 543–4.
10 AAS 65/19/9, Fairley, notebook with diary notes of visit to United States, October–November 1944.
11 ibid.
12 Sinton et al., 'Studies in Malaria, with special reference to treatment. Part XII', pp. 793–814.
13 Malaria Commission, Third General Report, Therapeutics of Malaria, pp. 185–285.
14 Malaria Commission, Fourth General Report, Therapeutics of Malaria, 1011–12.
15 Carson et al., 'Enzymatic deficiency in primaquine sensitive erythrocytes', pp. 484–5.
16 NAS, Bulletin on Malaria Research, 20 July 1943, p. 108.
17 NAS, Bulletin on Malaria Research, 22 December 1943, p. 188.
18 NAS, Bulletin on Malaria Research, 28 April 1944, p. 287.
19 NAS, Bulletin on Malaria Research, 29 March 1944, p. 849.
20 NAS, Bulletin on Malaria Research, 16 September 1944, pp. 513–14.
21 NAS, Goldwater Memorial Hospital, letter, Shannon to Packer, 9 August 1944.
22 NAS, Bulletin on Malaria Research, 20 November 1944, p. 542.
23 AAS 65/19/9, Fairley, notebook with diary notes of visit to United States, October–November 1944.
24 NAS, Bulletin on Malaria Research, 20 November 1944, p. 542.
25 NAS, Bulletin on Malaria Research, letter, Loeb to Downie, 24 November 1944, p. 568.
26 NAS, letter, Downie to Loeb, 27 November 1944.
27 AAS 65/9/37, letter, Blackburn to Fairley, 20 December 1944.
28 AAS 65/9/37, letter, Blackburn to Fairley, 28 December 1944.
29 AAS 65/32/11, Report: Plasmocidal activity of plasmoquine, 18 January 1945.
30 AAS 65/9/35, Studies in chemotherapy: The antimalarial activity of plasmoquine in volunteers exposed to experimental mosquito-transmitted malaria (New Guinea strains), undated.
31 ibid.
32 NAS, letter, Major Wheatland to Dr Carden, 13 February 1945.
33 NAS, Bulletin on Malaria Research, 5 March 1945, p. 820.
34 NAS, Malaria Report no. 442, Minutes of the ninth meeting of the therapy subcommittee, Malaria Committee of the Medical Research Council, England, 27 April 1945.
35 NAS, Bulletin on Malaria Research, 21 February 1945, p. 814.

330   Notes (Chapters 15–17)

36. NAS, Bulletin on Malaria Research, 25 May 1945, p. 985; Berliner et al., 'Pamaquin. 1. Curative antimalarial activity in vivax malaria', p. 165.

16 The Answer to the Maiden's Prayer

1. Greenwood, 'Conflicts of interest: The genesis of synthetic antimalarial agents in peace and war', pp. 857–72.
2. Curd, 'The activity of drugs in the malaria of man, monkeys and birds', pp. 115–43.
3. Curd et al., 'Studies on synthetic antimalarial drugs. II. General chemical considerations', pp. 157–64.
4. Curd et al., 'Studies on synthetic antimalarial drugs. I. Biological methods', pp. 139–56.
5. Adams and Sanderson, 'Studies on synthetic antimalarial drugs. V. Further investigation of the therapeutic action of 3349 on benign tertian and malignant tertian malaria infections', pp. 173–9.
6. AAS 65/12/1, M4430, Summary of information, ICI report, B.T. 1085, by D. G. Davey, 19 February 1945.
7. AAS 65/9/44, Minutes of the fourth meeting of the Malaria Committee of the Medical Research Council, 15 December 1944.
8. ibid.
9. Fairley, 'Chemotherapeutic suppression and prophylaxis in malaria: An experimental investigation undertaken by medical research teams in Australia', pp. 311–65.
10. ibid.
11. ibid.
12. AAS 65/9/44, official letter, Fairley to Burston, 24 February 1945.
13. AAS 65/9/44, personal letter, Fairley to Burston, 24 February 1945.
14. AAS 65/9/44, Serial letter, no. 109, from A/ADGMS London to DGMS Australia, undated.
15. ibid.
16. AAS 65/9/44, signal, AAS London to LHQ Melbourne, 20 February 1945.
17. AAS 65/9/44, official letter, Fairley to Burston, 24 February 1945.
18. AAS 65/32/11, letter, Fairley to Keogh, 24 February 1945.
19. AAS 65/12/1, letter, Davey to Fairley, 20 February 1945.
20. AAS 65/12/1, report, B.T. 1085, 19 February 1945.
21. AAS 65/12/1, letter, Adams to Fairley, 28 February 1945.
22. AAS 65/12/, report, B.T. 1085, 19 February 1945.
23. AAS 65/12/1, letter, Adams to Fairley, 28 February 1945.
24. AAS 65/32/11, letter, Fairley to Keogh, 24 February 1945.
25. AAS 65/12/1, letter, Fairley to Blackburn, 16 February 1945.
26. ibid.
27. AAS 65/12/1, folder 2, secret document entitled 'Experiments with M.4888 and M.4430', undated.
28. AA (Vic), MP742/1, Department of Defence Army Headquarters, file no. 211/6/1114, memo HQ QLD L of C to LHQ, 5 April 1945.
29. AAS 211/6/935, letter, DGMS to Blackburn, 9 April 1945.
30. The timing of experiments in the first M.4888 series was derived from AAS 65/32/15, Recipients and gametocyte carriers, notebook, commenced January 1945.
31. AAS 65/12/1, draft signal, Landforces Melbourne to Austarm London, 5 June 1945. It appears that this signal was actually sent as ML.3350 on 9 June 1945 (AAS 65/12/1, letter, Anderson to Fairley, 30 July 1945).

17 The Possibility of an 'X' Factor

1. AA (Vic), Department of Defence Army Headquarters, MP742/1, file no. 211/6/906, Secret Report 44/3121/23, 9 December 1944.

2. AA (Vic), MP742/1, Department of Defence Army Headquarters, file no. 211/6/934, Analysis of the incidence of malaria in 6 Australian Division by Major G. Read, 45/3121/41, Appendix B to 211/6/934, 8 February 1945.
3. ibid.
4. ibid.
5. AWM 52 11/12/11, Conference on Malaria, held at 6 Division Headquarters, Address by Major General Stevens, 31 January 1945.
6. AWM 52 11/12/11, war diary, 2/2 Australian Field Ambulance, 6 Australian Division Administrative Order no. 10, 31 January 1945.
7. ibid., letter, Stevens to ADMS, February 1945.
8. ibid., Malaria investigation, 2/7 Australian Infantry Battalion, ref. 45/3121/1, 25 January 1945.
9. AA (Vic), MP742/1, Department of Defence Army Headquarters, file no. 211/6/934, Memorandum Maitland to LHQ (for DGMS), MD45/3121/610, 8 February 1945.
10. Australian Army Special Technical Instruction no. 120, 'The efficacy of suppressive atebrin', issued 19/2/45, from Australian Medical Headquarters.
11. AWM 52 11/2/27, war diary, 3/14 Field Ambulance, December 1944.
12. ibid., 27 January 1945.
13. Fairley et al., 'Malaria in the South-West Pacific, with special reference to its chemotherapeutic control', pp. 145–62.
14. AWM 52 11/12/16, war diary, 2/7 Field Ambulance, 13 June 1945.
15. AAS 65/9/34, letter, Fenner to Blackburn, 5 May 1945.
16. C. R. Blackburn, pers. comm., 16 June 1993.
17. Clinical details of individual malaria cases and experimental results in this chapter are derived from notebooks and data sheets in the Fairley Papers as well as Fairley et al., 'Atebrin susceptibility of the Aitape–Wewak strains of *P. falciparum* and *P. vivax*—a field and experimental investigation by L.H.Q. Medical Research Unit', pp. 229–73.
18. AWM 54 267/6/7, part 127, Conference on Malaria, Address by Brigadier Fairley, 22 August 1945.
19. AWM 52 11/12/11, war diary, 2/2 Australian Field Ambulance, 31 May 1945.
20. Dates of Fairley's movements after his return to Australia are from file nos AAS 65/29/12 and AAS 65/29/13, personal diaries, 1945.
21. AAS 65/16/1, letter, Fairley to Sinton, 29 January 1945.
22. Long, *The Final Campaigns*, p. 353.
23. C. R. Blackburn, pers. comm., 23 March 1995.
24. AWM 52 11/12/27, war diary, 3/14 Australian Field Ambulance, 18 June 1945.
25. Fairley et al., 'Malaria in the South-West Pacific with special reference to its chemotherapeutic control', p. 156.
26. Walker, *The Island Campaigns*, pp. 345–70.
27. Fairley et al., 'Atebrin susceptibility of the Aitape–Wewak strains of *P. falciparum* and *P. vivax*—a field and experimental investigation by L.H.Q. Medical Research Unit', pp. 229–73.
28. Peters, *Chemotherapy and Drug Resistance in Malaria*, pp. 426–8.
29. AAS 65/9/26, notebook with writing in Fairley's hand, June 1945.
30. Mackerras and Aberdeen, 'A malaria survey at Wewak, New Guinea', pp. 763–71.
31. AWM 54 267/6/7, part 127, Conference on Malaria, Address by Brigadier Fairley, 22 August 1945.
32. Fairley et al., 'Malaria in the South-West Pacific with special reference to its chemotherapeutic control', pp. 145–62.
33. ibid.
34. Selby, 'Malaria in the South-West Pacific: Additional facts about malaria control in the Australian Military Forces', pp. 249–50.
35. Fairley et al., 'Malaria in the South-West Pacific with special reference to its chemotherapeutic control', pp. 145–62.

332   Notes (Chapters 17–18)

36 ibid. This is not strictly correct, as there was no suggestion that the first case who arrived at Cairns with atebrin-resistant parasites (case 620) avoided taking atebrin. Fairley is referring here to the first resistant case (case 2) he selected for evacuation to Cairns during his investigation of the epidemic.
37 Fairley et al., 'Atebrin susceptibility of the Aitape–Wewak strains of *P. falciparum* and *P. vivax*— a field and experimental investigation by L.H.Q. Medical Research Unit', pp. 229–73.
38 Mackerras, 'Malaria in the South-West Pacific', pp. 249–50.
39 AAS 65/11/13, Allied Translator and Interpreter Section, South West Pacific Area, Information Bulletin, Malaria in the Japanese Forces, 8 July 1944.
40 Peters, *Chemotherapy and Drug Resistance in Malaria*, p. 441.
41 Mackerras, 'Malaria in the South-West Pacific', pp. 249–50.
42 AA (Vic), MP742/1, Department of Defence Army Headquarters, file no. 211/6/906, Secret Report 44/3121/23, 9 December 1944.
43 NAS, Malaria Report no. 254, Report of the Malaria Mission to the South West Pacific Area by F. C. Bishopp and R. B. Watson, 20 August 1944.
44 Fairley et al., 'Atebrin susceptibility of the Aitape–Wewak strains of *P. falciparum* and *P. vivax*— a field and experimental investigation by L.H.Q. Medical Research Unit', pp. 229–73.

18 Paludrine

1 This report of 10 June 1945 and covering letter are not among the Fairley Papers. They are referred to in AAS 65/12/1, letter, Anderson to Fairley, 30 July 1945.
2 The report of 10 June 1945 was later circulated by the Board for the Co-ordination of Malarial Studies, NAS, Malaria Report no. 484, Part 1. Experiments with the compound ICI—M.4888, by Brigadier N. H. Fairley et al., received 9 August 1945.
3 The timing of experiments in the first M.4888 series was derived from AAS 65/32/15, Recipients and gametocyte carriers, notebook, commenced January 1945.
4 AAS 65/12/1, secret signal, Y36/LM1554, for Fairley from Goulston, undated.
5 AAS 65/12/1, notes taken at a meeting of the Therapeutic Sub-Committee of the M.R.C. Malaria Committee, 27 April 1945.
6 NAS Malaria Report no. 484, Part 2, protocol for further studies with M.4888, by Brigadier N. H. Fairley et al., received 9 August 1945.
7 The timing of all experiments in this series was derived from AAS 65/32/16, notebook, Recipients, June–October 1945.
8 Fairley et al., 'Researches on paludrine (M.4888) in malaria', pp. 105–51.
9 AAS 645/9/35, The value of M.4430 as a suppressive in volunteers exposed to experimental mosquito-transmitted malaria (*P. vivax*—New Guinea Strains), typescript report, undated.
10 AAS 65/12/1, letter, Fairley to Anderson, 4 December 1945.
11 NAS, letter, Blackburn to Keogh, 1 June 1945.
12 AAS 65/12/1, signal, ML 4927, Landforces Melbourne to Austarm London, undated.
13 AAS 65/12/1, folder 4, letter, Maegraith to Fairley, 24 September 1945.
14 AAS 65/12/1, folder 4, letter, Fairley to Maegraith, 5 December 1945.
15 AA (Vic), MP742/1, Department of Defence Army Headquarters, file no. 220/20/608, letter, DGMS (Burston) to ADGMS London (Anderson), 5 December 1945.
16 AAS 65/12/1, folder 5, letter, Fairley to Anderson, 4 December 1945.
17 AAS 65/12/1, folder 5, signal, LM5231/LW 1287, 6 November 1945.
18 AAS 65/12/1, folder 3, letter, Anderson to Fairley, 24 January 1946.
19 ibid.
20 ibid.
21 'Triumph against malaria', pp. 653–4.
22 ibid.
23 AAS 65/12/1, folder 5, Signal Landforces Melbourne to LHQ MRU Cairns, MD90936, 9 November 1945.

[24] AA (Vic), MP742/1, Department of Defence Army Headquarters, file no. 220/20/608, signal, Landforces Melbourne to London, ML 6501, 13 November 1945.
[25] AAS 65/12/1, folder 5, letter, Fairley to Anderson, 4 December 1945.
[26] AAS 65/12/1, folder 4, letter, Fairley to Maigraith, 5 December 1945.
[27] AA (Vic), MP742/1, Department of Defence Army Headquarters, file no. 220/20/608, letter, DGMS to ADGMS, London, OL 2749, 6 December 1945.
[28] AAS 65/12/1, folder 3, letter, Anderson to Lansborough Thompson, 11 January 1946.
[29] AAS 65/12/1, statement by D. G. Davey, undated.
[30] *Age*, 20 December 1945.
[31] *Daily Telegraph*, 20 December 1945.
[32] *Age*, 20 December 1945.
[33] Fairley et al., 'Researches on paludrine (M.4888) in Australia from the Land Headquarters Medical Research Unit, Cairns', pp. 234–6.
[34] 'Paludrine', p. 229.
[35] 'More about paludrine', pp. 919–20.
[36] Fairley et al., 'Researches on paludrine (M.4888) in malaria', pp. 105–51.

19 Mode of Action

[1] AAS 65/9/35, typescript ms entitled Introduction, undated.
[2] AWM 11/1/2, war diary, LHQ MRU, Appendix 1, for period May–July 1944, Unit staff meeting—Gametocytes, 1 June 1944.
[3] ibid.
[4] NAS, Testing Centers, Cairns Army Camp Australia, document entitled Gametocytes, by M. J. Mackerras, undated.
[5] Mackerras and Ercole, 'Observations on the action of quinine, atebrin, and plasmoquin on *Plasmodium vivax*', pp. 443–54.
[6] Mackerras and Ercole, 'Observations on the action of quinine, atebrin, and plasmoquin on *Plasmodium falciparum*', pp. 455–63.
[7] NAS, Malaria Report no. 484, Part 1, Experiments with the compound ICI M.4888 by Brigadier N. H. Fairley et al., received 9 August 1945.
[8] AAS 65/12/1, folder 5, letter, Fairley to Anderson, 4 December 1945.
[9] Black, 'A preliminary note on the cultivation in vitro of New Guinea strains of human malaria parasites', pp. 500–1.
[10] Mackie and McCartney, *Handbook of Practical Bacteriology*, p. 511.
[11] Black, Studies in Chemotherapy, p. 3.
[12] C. R. Blackburn, pers. comm., June 1994.
[13] Black, Studies in Chemotherapy, p. 4.
[14] Bass, 'Some observations on the effect of quinine upon growth of malaria plasmodia "in vitro"', p. 289.
[15] Black, 'The effect of anti-malarial drugs on *Plasmodium falciparum* (New Guinea strains) developing in vitro', pp. 163–70.
[16] AAS 65/9/17, table of mosquito dissections compiled by Maj M. J. Mackerras, with list of gametocyte carriers, undated.
[17] Mackerras and Ercole, 'Observations on the action of paludrine on malarial parasites', pp. 365–76. A graph showing the gametocyte wave in this volunteer is on p. 373.
[18] ibid.
[19] ibid.
[20] ibid.
[21] Mackerras and Ercole, 'Observations on the life cycle of *Plasmodium malariae*', pp. 515–19.
[22] Fairley et al., 'Researches on paludrine (M.4888) in malaria', pp. 105–51. The chronology of the individual experiments in this chapter was derived from individual case details in the Fairley Papers in notebooks: AAS 65/32/15 and AAS 65/32/16.
[23] AAS 65/12/1, folder 3, Precis of current work, 10 December 1945.

20 Tolerance and Immunity

1. Blackburn, 'Observations on the development of resistance to vivax malaria', pp. 117–62. This case is described in Experiment 7 of this article.
2. C. R. Blackburn, pers. comm., 23 March 1995.
3. AAS 65/9/41, Experiment XVI, Summary of first group having quinine suppressive therapy, undated but probably 10 May 1944.
4. Blackburn, 'Observations on the development of resistance to vivax malaria', pp. 117–62. The chronology of the individual experiments in this chapter was derived from individual case reports in the Fairley Papers, particularly in AAS 65/32/14, notebook containing details of gametocyte carriers, 1944.
5. C. R. Blackburn, pers. comm., 23 March 1995.
6. AAS 65/9/34, letter, Fairley to Blackburn, 14 October 1944.
7. AAS 65/9/37, letter, Blackburn to Fairley, 18 November 1944.
8. AAS 65/9/7, report entitled An experiment designed to test subinoculation and subsequent inoculation of trophozoites as a criterion of cure in volunteers who have had experimental mosquito-transmitted benign tertian malaria, 18 December 1944.
9. ibid.
10. Blackburn, 'Observations on the development of resistance to vivax malaria', pp. 117–62. This man was volunteer 000030 in Experiment 3.
11. ibid, p. 127.
12. ibid, Experiment 6.
13. ibid, p. 140.
14. ibid, Experiment 8.
15. ibid, pp. 159–60.

21 Guinea Pigs

1. AA (Vic), MP742/1, file no. 211/6/1114, secret signal, XL/16344, from Andrew to Fairley, 17 July 1943.
2. AA (Vic), MP742/1, file no. 211/6/1114, minute from DGMS to Adjutant-General, 20 July 1943.
3. AA (Vic), MP742/1, file no. 211/6/281, memorandum from Adjutant General to Adv LHQ, First and Second Aust Army, L of C Qld., NSW, Vic., 29 July 1943.
4. ibid.
5. E. E. Viant, pers. comm., 29 September 1993.
6. AAS 65/9/44, Interim Report of LHQ Medical Research Unit, 16 February 1944.
7. AAS 65/9/33, letter, Blackburn to Fairley, 6 July 1944.
8. ibid.
9. AA (Vic), MP742/1, file no. 211/6/1114, Adjutant General memo 109331, 9 August 1944.
10. *Australian Women's Weekly*, 1 July 1944, p. 12.
11. C. R. Blackburn, pers. comm., 14 April 1993.
12. AAS 65/32/11, signal to Chief Publicity Censor, Canberra, from DGPR, 1 August 1944.
13. AAS 65/9/34, letter, Fairley to Blackburn, 7 August 1944.
14. AA (Vic), MP742/1, file no. 211/6/1114, letter, Blackburn to DGMS, 27 November 1944.
15. AA (Vic), MP742/1, file no. 211/6/1114, letter, NSW L of C area to LHQ, 3 December 1944.
16. AA (Vic), MP742/1, file no. 211/6/1114, letter, Private Sandbek to Fairley, 3 July 1944.
17. AA (Vic), MP742/1, file no. 211/6/1114, Adjutant General memo 179031, 22 December 1944.
18. AAS 65/9/37, report of death of S7017 Pte Chittleborough A. R., 16 December 1944.
19. ibid.
20. AA (Vic), MP742/1, file no. 211/6/1114, Adjutant General memo 20028, 12 February 1945.

21 AA (Vic), MP742/1, file no. 211/6/1114, minute from Adjutant General to LHQ, 16 May 1945. This minute refers to LHQ signal 13794 of 24 February 1945 [not seen], which doubles the quotas for March and April. This signal was sent just four days after the first information on the new British drugs was signalled from London (AAS 65/9/44, signal AAS London to LHQ Melbourne, 20 February 1945).
22 ibid.
23 ibid.
24 AA (Vic), MP742/1, file no. 211/6/1114, letter, Queensland L of C Area to LHQ, 5 April 1945.
25 AA (Vic), MP742/1, file no. 211/6/1114, letter, DGMS to Blackburn, 9 April 1945.
26 AA (Vic), MP742/1, file no. 211/6/1114, Secret report, Provision of volunteers for malaria experiments, signed by Fairley, 11 June 1945.
27 AA (Vic), MP742/1, file no. 211/6/1114, Adjutant General memo 86414, 29 June 1945.
28 AA (Vic), MP742/1, file no. 211/6/1114, signal, DGMS to Medical Research Unit Cairns, 13 July 1945.
29 AA (Vic), MP742/1, file no. 211/6/1114, signal, LHQ MRU to Landforces, 15 July 1945.
30 AA (Vic), MP742/1, file no. 211/6/1114, letter, Adjutant General to Air Member for Personnel, RAAF, 16 July 1945.
31 AA (Vic), MP742/1, file no. 211/6/1114, note for the file signed by Fairley, 8 September 1945.
32 AA (Vic), MP742/1, file no. 211/6/1114, Landforces signal 71503, 6 September 1945.
33 See Appendix 1.
34 See Appendix 2.
35 National Library of Australia Manuscript Collection, MS 5959, Diaries of Donald Friend, Item 16: 1 September–4 October 1943; Item 17: 5–30 October 1943; Item 18: 30 October–21 November 1943.
36 ibid., Item 16, diary, 2 September 1943.
37 ibid., diary, 10 September 1943.
38 ibid.
39 ibid., adjacent to diary entries for September 1943.
40 ibid., diary, 22 September 1943.
41 Fry and Fry, *Donald Friend: Australian War Artist 1945*, comment in Foreword by Donald Friend.
42 In 1953 she married Robert H. Black, who was then malariologist at the School of Public Health and Tropical Medicine, University of Sydney.
43 E. E. Viant, pers. comm., 29 September 1993.
44 ibid.; these comments are from an account of E. E. Viant's wartime experiences that he has compiled for his family.
45 K. G. Glover and R. W. Whiteley, pers. comm., 15 December 1992.
46 ibid.
47 AAS 65/32/11, letter, OIC 2nd Echelon LHQ to CO 2/1 Aust Convalescent Depot, undated but probably 24 March 1945.
48 AAS 65/32/11, Department of Veteran's Affairs Benefits Memorandum 1983/019, 14 June 1983.
49 AA (Vic), MP742/1, File no. 211/6/1114, Adjutant General memo 109331, 9 August 1944.
50 *Trials of War Criminals before the Nuremburg Military Tribunals*, pp. 181–2.
51 ibid.
52 AA (Vic), MP742/1, file no. 211/6/1114, Adjutant General memo 20028, 12 February 1945.
53 Carson et al., 'Enzymatic deficiency in primaquine sensitive erythrocytes', pp. 484–5.
54 AAS 65/9/33, letter, Blackburn to Fairley, 6 September 1944.
55 Fairley, 'Chemotherapeutic suppression and prophylaxis in malaria', pp. 311–65.
56 Address by Dr N. Hamilton Fairley accepting the Richard Pearson Strong Medal. University Club, New York, 26 November 1946, quoted in *New York Times*, 27 November 1946.
57 E. E. Viant, pers. comm., 17 June 1997.
58 J. Hardy, pers. comm., 26 September 2001.

22 The Military Value of the Cairns Research

[1] AAS 65/11/13, Malaria in the Japanese Forces, information bulletin from captured Japanese documents and statements of POWs, 8 July 1944.
[2] AAS 65/9/19, Japanese Medical Services in New Guinea, New Britain and the Solomon Islands, from General Staff Intelligence Advanced HQ Allied Land Forces SWPA, October 1944.
[3] AAS 65/15/1, Army pamphlet, CR/ME/3557/M, *The prevention of Malaria*.
[4] ibid.
[5] ibid.
[6] Proceedings of conference on certain aspects of prevention of disease in tropical warfare, AWM printed records.
[7] Routine Order no. 210 of 28 August 1944, by GOC New Guinea Force, quoted in AAS 65/9/4, Notes on a tour of Australia and New Guinea, Brigadier G. Covell, August–September 1944.
[8] Ford, 'Arthur E. Mills Memorial Oration', pp. 991–6.
[9] ibid.
[10] C. R. Blackburn, pers. comm., 30 June 1994.
[11] Blackburn, 'Sir Neil Hamilton Fairley', p. 6.
[12] Blackburn, 'Chemoprophylaxis of malaria—an exercise in problem solving'.
[13] Blackburn, 'Sir Neil Hamilton Fairley', p. 6.
[14] Boyd, 'Neil Hamilton Fairley 1891–1966', pp. 123–41.
[15] Blackburn, 'Sir Neil Hamilton Fairley', p. 6.
[16] AAS 65/9/34, letter, Fairley to Blackburn, 1 July 1944.
[17] Keogh, 'Obituary, Neil Hamilton Fairley', pp. 723–6.
[18] Covell, *Anti-mosquito Measures*.
[19] AAS 65/9/4, Notes on a tour of Australia and New Guinea, Brigadier G. Covell, August–September 1944.
[20] Public Records Office, Kew, England, file WO203/3230, Malaria in SWPA, 12 January 1945.
[21] ibid.
[22] Public Records Office, Kew, England, file WO 203/1942, DMS Brief for C in C, 20 February 1945.
[23] Sinton et al., 'Studies in malaria, with special reference to treatment. Part XII. Further research into the treatment of chronic benign tertian malaria with plasmoquine and quinine', pp. 793–814.
[24] Smythe, *The Story of the Victoria Cross*, p. 207.
[25] AAS 65/26/19, personal (handwritten) letter, Sinton to Fairley, 26 June 1945.
[26] Fairley et al., 'Malaria in the South-West Pacific with special reference to its chemotherapeutic control', pp. 145–62.
[27] AA (Vic), MP742/1, file no. 211/4/418, Post discharge malaria, GRO 237/45, 7 September 1945.
[28] AA (Vic), MP742/1, file no. 211/6/1114, signal, LM 139, Austarm London to Landforces for DGMS, 26 January 1946.
[29] AA (Vic), MP742/1, file no. 220/20/608, minute, Supply of paludrine, 24 June 1946.
[30] AA (Vic), MP742/1, file no. 220/20/608, letter, Davey to Fairley, 5 June 1946.
[31] AA (Vic), MP742/1, file no. 220/20/608, personal note, Davey to Fairley, 22 May 1946.
[32] AAS 65/9/35, The antimalarial activity of plasmoquine in volunteers exposed to experimental mosquito-transmitted malaria (New Guinea strains), undated.
[33] Fairley et al., 'Researches on paludrine (M.4888) in Australia', pp. 234–6.
[34] AAS 65/12/2, Progress notes on therapy of secondary vivax malaria, by Lieutenant Colonel C. R. Blackburn, 7 June 1946.
[35] ibid.
[36] AA (Vic), MP742/1, file no. 211/6/1956, DGMS Technical Instruction no. 134, Treatment of malaria in the AMF, 1 July 1946.
[37] AA (Vic), MP742/1, file no. 211/6/1956, letter, Wootton to DGMS, 4 February 1947.
[38] AA (Vic), MP742/1, file no. 211/6/1956, letter, ADGMS to Blackburn, 11 February 1947.

[39] AA (Vic), MP742/1, file no. 211/6/1966, memo G1638, Chairman Repatriation Commission to DGMS, 15 September 1947.
[40] AA (Vic), MP742/1, file no. 211/6/1956, letter, Fairley to DGMS, 9 April 1947.
[41] AAS 65/2/5, letter, Blackburn to Fairley, 15 May 1947.
[42] ibid.

23 A Glorious Gamble in Science

[1] NAS, Bulletin on Malaria Research, 5 March 1945, p. 821.
[2] NAS, Bulletin on Malaria Research, 29 June 1945, p. 1111.
[3] Council on Pharmacy and Chemistry, 'Chloroquine, non proprietary name for SN-7618', p. 787.
[4] Board for Co-ordination of Malarial Studies, 'Wartime research in malaria', pp. 8–9.
[5] NAS, letter, Marshall to Shannon, 21 June 1945.
[6] NAS, Bulletin on Malaria Research, 4 June 1946, pp. 1454–9.
[7] NAS, letter, Marshall to Shannon, 21 June 1945.
[8] NAS, letter, Shannon to Alving, 31 July 1945.
[9] NAS, Bulletin on Malaria Research, 16 October 1945, p. 1329.
[10] ibid.
[11] NAS, Bulletin on Malaria Research, 4 June 1946, p. 1444.
[12] NAS, Malaria Report no. 723, Clinical testing of antimalarial drugs, final report by A. S. Alving, 31 August 1946.
[13] Schmidt et al., 'Delineation of the potential of primaquine as a radical curative and prophylactic drug', pp. 666–80.
[14] Arnold et al., 'The effect of continuous and intermittent primaquine therapy on the relapse rate of Chesson strain vivax malaria', pp. 429–38.
[15] Coatney et al., 'Studies in human malaria. X. The protective and therapeutic action of chloroquine (SN 7618) against St Elizabeth strain vivax malaria', pp. 49–59.
[16] Fairley et al., 'Experiments with antimalarial drugs in man. VI. The value of chloroquine diphosphate as a suppressive drug in volunteers exposed to experimental mosquito-transmitted malaria (New Guinea strains)', pp. 493–501.
[17] Fairley, 'The chemotherapeutic control of malaria', pp. 925–32.
[18] Fairley et al., 'Sidelights on malaria in man obtained by subinoculation experiments', pp. 621–76.
[19] Clark, 'History of the co-operative wartime program', in Wiselogle (ed.), *A Survey of Antimalarial Drugs, 1941–1945*, pp. 1–28.
[20] Most, 'Clinical trials of antimalarial drugs', in Medical Department, United States Army, *Internal Medicine in World War II*, Vol. II, pp. 525–98.
[21] AAS 65/9/44, letter, NHF to DGMS, 24 February 1944.
[22] NAS, Bulletin on Malaria Research, 18 April 1944, p. 283.
[23] NAS, Bulletin on Malaria Research, 31 July 1944, p. 405.
[24] NAS, Bulletin on Malaria Research, 19 August 1944, p. 511.
[25] ibid.
[26] Macfarlane, *Howard Florey*, pp. 336–7.
[27] NAS, Bulletin on Malaria Research, 29 June 1944, p. 373.
[28] NAS, letter, Southworth to Carden, 8 August 1944.
[29] NAS, Report to the Committee on Medical Research on Malaria Mission to England, by James A. Shannon and Robert F. Loeb, 8 May 1945.
[30] NAS, letter, Southworth to Carden, 8 August 1944.
[31] ibid.
[32] NAS, Bulletin on Malaria Research, 22 December 1944, p. 630.
[33] ibid., p. 638.
[34] ibid., p. 633.
[35] ibid., p. 640.
[36] AAS 65/9/44, letter, NHF to DGMS, 24 February 1944.
[37] NAS, Bulletin on Malaria Research, 2 May 1945, p. 943.

24 Press Reports

1. *Telegraph*, '1000-bite-an-hour men in malaria test', 6 February 1944.
2. *Mail*, 'Troops well-bitten in war on mosquito', 6 February 1944; *Age*, 'Fight against malaria, army experiments', 7 February 1944.
3. *Worker*, 'Achievements in malaria control', 26 June 1944.
4. ibid.
5. ibid.; *Herald*, 'Malaria helps destroy Japanese but our losses are kept low', 7 June, 1944; *Adelaide Advertiser*, 'Low malaria death rate success of medical researches, 7 June 1944; *Bulletin*, 'A noble victory', 21 June 1944.
6. *News*, Adelaide, 'Secret report tells how malaria was beaten', 22 October, 1945; *News* (Perth), 'Australians lead malaria fight', 22 October 1945; *Age*, 'Control of malaria, new drugs effective', 23 October 1945; *Adelaide Advertiser*, 'Triumph over malaria, medical work in New Guinea', 24 October 1945.
7. *Argus*, editorial, 'Australia's thanks', 30 April 1946.
8. *Bulletin*, 'Malaria in the AMF', August 21 1946.
9. Fairley et al., 'Malaria in the South-West Pacific, with special reference to its chemotherapeutic control', pp. 145–62.
10. *Guardian Weekly*, 'How we won the war with malaria', 7 June 1992.
11. *Age*, 'Army used soldiers, Jews in experiments', 19 April 1999.
12. *Sydney Morning Herald*, 'Troops and refugees given malaria', 19 April 1999.
13. *Age*, editorial, 'War experiments shame Australia', 20 April 1999.
14. *Age*, 'Experiments a "scandal": Jews', 21 April 1999.
15. *Sydney Morning Herald*, editorial, 'Malaria tests fail the mark', 21 April 1999.
16. *Age*, editorial, 'War experiments shame Australia', 20 April 1999.
17. *Sydney Morning Herald*, letter, to editor, 'Malaria test volunteers not targeted', Henry Lippmann, Dover Heights, 26 April 1999.
18. 'Australian anti-malarial drug experimentation conducted during World War Two', pp. 7–9.

Epilogue

1. Fairley, 'The chemotherapeutic control of malaria', pp. 925–32.
2. Bishop and Birkett, 'Acquired resistance to paludrine in *Plasmodium gallinaceum*', pp. 884–5; Williamson et al., 'Effects of paludrine and other antimalarials', pp. 885–6.
3. Seaton and Lourie, 'Acquired resistance to proguanil (paludrine) in *Plasmodium vivax*', pp. 394–5.
4. ibid.
5. Edeson and Field, 'Proguanil-resistant falciparum malaria in Malaya', pp. 147–52; Field et al., 'Studies on the chemotherapy of malaria. II. The treatment of acute malaria with proguanil (paludrine)', pp. 303–17.
6. Coatney, 'Pitfalls in a discovery: The chronicle of chloroquine', pp. 121–8.
7. Moore and Lanier, 'Observations on two *Plasmodium falciparum* infections with an abnormal response to chloroquine', pp. 5–9.
8. Harinasuta et al., 'Chloroquine resistance in *Plasmodium falciparum* in Thailand', pp. 148–53.
9. O'Keefe, *Medicine at War*, pp. 18–21.
10. Wilson et al., 'Proguanil resistance in Malayan strains of *P. vivax*', pp. 564–8.
11. O'Keefe, *Medicine at War*, p. 30.
12. Black, 'Report on a visit made to Southeast Asia to advise on malaria', p. 15.
13. O'Keefe, *Medicine at War*, pp. 80–160.
14. Black, 'Report on a visit ... made to Southeast Asia to observe and advise on malaria and other health matters', pp. 22–3.
15. O'Keefe, *Medicine at War*, pp. 151–60.
16. ibid., pp. 155–6.
17. ibid., pp. 154–7.

18. Black, 'Malaria as a military problem', pp. 1–15.
19. ibid., p. 13.
20. Rieckmann et al., '*Plasmodium vivax* resistance to chloroquine?', pp. 1183–84.
21. Payne, 'Spread of chloroquine resistance in *Plasmodium falciparum*', pp. 241–6.
22. World Health Organization, 'Advances in malaria chemotherapy'.
23. Karwacki et al., 'Two cases of mefloquine resistant malaria in Thailand', pp. 152–3.
24. Wernsdorfer, 'The development of drug–resistant malaria', pp. 297–303.
25. Rieckmann et al., 'Recent military experience with malaria chemoprophylaxis', pp. 446–9.
26. Mendis, 'Malaria vaccine research—a game of chess', in Target (ed.), *Malaria*, pp. 183–96.
27. Farid, 'The malaria programme—from euphoria to anarchy', pp. 8–22.
28. Schreck and Self, 'Bed nets that kill mosquitoes', pp. 342–4.
29. 'Neil Hamilton Fairley', Obituary, pp. 987–8.
30. AAS 65/26/19, personal (handwritten) letter, Sinton to Fairley, 26 June 1945.
31. Shortt and Garnham, 'The pre-erythrocytic development of *Plasmodium cynomolgi* and *Plasmodium vivax*', pp. 785–95.
32. Shortt et al., 'The pre-erythrocytic stage of *Plasmodium falciparum*', pp. 1006–8.
33. Fairley et al., 'Atebrin susceptibility of the Aitape–Wewak strains of *P. falciparum* and *P. vivax*', pp. 229–73.
34. World Health Organization, 'Chemotherapy of malaria'.
35. Cheng et al., 'Measurement of *Plasmodium falciparum* growth rates in vivo', pp. 495–500.
36. Scott et al., 'Synergistic antimalarial activity of dapsone/dihydrofolate reductase inhibitors', pp. 715–72.
37. AAS 65/29/22, Fairley, personal diary, 1951; AAS 65/29/24, Fairley, personal diary, 1952.
38. AAS 65/26/27, letter, Fairley to Major General Norris, 21 July 1954.
39. AAS 65/32/11, RAAF file 132/1/729 A 705, medical meeting at Army Headquarters 28 February 1956.
40. Ford, 'Arthur E. Mills Memorial Oration', pp. 991–6.

Bibliography

Notes on Archival Sources

The major source of archival material for this work is the Basser Library of the Australian Academy of Science, which houses the Fairley papers. Valuable additional documents are in the Australian War Memorial. Australian Army Headquarters were in Melbourne during World War II so there are many relevant documents in the Victorian Accessions of Australian Archives, as well as some material in the Australian Capital Territory holdings of Australian Archives.

Documents relating to American wartime research on malaria are located in the National Academy of Sciences Archives in Washington, DC. These include scientific reports, letters and other papers of the Board for the Co-ordination of Malarial Studies. The minutes of the Board and its panels, as well as some supporting documents, are filed in a chronological series entitled the 'Bulletin on Malaria Research'. This comprises 1400 pages numbered sequentially from the commencement of the program in 1943 until its termination in June 1946. This collection contains many documents relating to the Australian malaria research at Cairns that are not in the Fairley Papers, as well as reports and correspondence concerning British malaria research in World War II.

Books

Bean, C. E. W., *Anzac to Amiens*, Australian War Memorial, Canberra, 1946.
Covell, G., *Anti-mosquito Measures*, Health Bulletin no. 11, Government of India Press, 1943.
Downes, R. M., *The Australian Army Medical Services in the War of 1914–1918*, Vol. 1, Part 2: *The Campaign in Sinai and Palestine*, Australian War Memorial, Melbourne, 1930.
Fairley, N. H., Woodruff, A. W. and Walters, J. H., *Recent Advances in Tropical Medicine*, J. & A. Churchill, London, 1961.
Falls, Cyril, *History of the Great War: Military Operations, Macedonia*, HMSO, London, 1935.
Fry, G. and Fry, C., *Donald Friend: Australian War Artist 1945*, Currey O'Neil, Melbourne, 1982.

Keogh, E. G., *South West Pacific 1941–1945*, Grayflower, Melbourne, 1965.
Lee, D. J. and Woodhill, A. R., *The Anopheline Mosquitoes of the Australasian Region*, Department of Zoology, Monograph no. 2, University of Sydney, 1944.
Long, G., *The Final Campaigns*, Australia in the War of 1939–45, Series 1 (Army), vol. 7, Australian War Memorial, Canberra, 1963.
Macfarlane, Gwyn, *Howard Florey: The Making of a Great Scientist*, Oxford Univesity Press, Oxford, 1979.
Mackie, T. J. and McCartney, J. E., *Handbook of Practical Bacteriology*, E. & S. Livingstone, Edinburgh, 1938.
Macpherson, W. G., Herringham, W. P., Elliott, T. R. and Balfour, J., *History of the Great War: Based on Official Documents; Medical Services, Diseases of the War*, HMSO, London, 1922.
Manchester, William, *American Caesar*, Little, Brown, Boston, 1978.
O'Keefe, Brendan, *Medicine at War: Medical Aspects of Australia's Involvement in Southeast Asian Conflicts 1950–1972*, Allen & Unwin, Sydney, 1994.
Page, Earle, *Truant Surgeon*, Angus & Robertson, Sydney, 1963.
Peters, W., *Chemotherapy and Drug Resistance in Malaria*, Academic Press, London, 1970.
Russell, P. F., West, L. S., Manwell, R. D. and Macdonald, G., *Practical Malariology*, 2nd edn, Oxford University Press, London, 1963.
Selby, David, *Hell and High Fever*, Currawong, Sydney, 1956.
Smyth, John, *The Story of the Victoria Cross*, Frederick Muller, London, 1963.
Trials of War Criminals before the Nuremberg Military Tribunals and Control Council Law no. 10, vol. 2, Nuremberg, October 1946–April 1949, US Government Printing Office, Washington DC, 1949.
Walker, Allan S., *Clinical Problems of War*, Australia in the War of 1939–1945, Series 5 (Medical), vol. 1, Australian War Memorial, Canberra, 1952.
——, *The Island Campaigns*, Australia in the War of 1939–45, Series 5 (Medical), vol. 3, Australian War Memorial, Canberra, 1957.
Wieneke, James, *6th Div. Sketches: Aitape to Wewak*, John Sands, Sydney, 1946.
Wigmore, Lionel, *The Japanese Thrust*, Australia in the War of 1939–1945, Series 1 (Army), vol. IV, Australian War Memorial, Canberra, 1957.
World Health Organization, *Terminology of Malaria and Malaria Eradication*, Geneva, 1963.

Articles, Reports and Theses

Adams, A. R. D. and Sanderson, G., 'Studies on synthetic antimalarial drugs. V. Further investigation of the therapeutic action of 3349 on benign tertian and malignant tertian malaria infections', *Annals of Tropical Medicine and Parasitology*, vol. 39, 1945, pp. 173–9.
Arnold, J., Alving, A. S., Hockwald, R. S., Clayman, C. B., Dern, R. J., Beutler, E. and Jeffrey, G. M., 'The effect of continuous and intermittent primaquine therapy on the relapse rate of Chesson strain vivax malaria', *Journal of Laboratory and Clinical Medicine*, vol. 44, 1954, pp. 429–38.

Australian Anti-Malarial Drug Experimentation Conducted During World War Two, Report of the Repatriation Medical Enquiry, Australian Government, Brisbane, 1999.

Bass, C. C., 'Some observations on the effect of quinine upon growth of malaria plasmodia "in vitro"', *American Journal of Tropical Medicine*, vol. 2, 1922, p. 289.

Berliner, R. W., Taggart, J. V., Zubrod, G., Welch, W. J., Earle, D. P. and Shannon, J. A., 'Pamaquin: 1. Curative antimalarial activity in vivax malaria', *Federal Proceedings*, vol. 5, 1946, p. 165.

Bishop, A. and Birkett, B., 'Acquired resistance to paludrine in *Plasmodium gallinaceum*: Acquired resistance and persistence after passage through the mosquito', *Nature*, vol. 159, 1947, pp. 884–5.

Black, R. H., 'A preliminary note on the cultivation in vitro of New Guinea strains of human malaria parasites', *Medical Journal of Australia*, vol. 2, 1945, pp. 500–1.

——, 'The effect of anti-malarial drugs on *Plasmodium falciparum* (New Guinea strains) developing in vitro', *Transactions of the Royal Society Tropical Medicine and Hygiene*, vol. 40, 1946, 163–70.

——, Studies in Chemotherapy: A Technique for the Cultivation of the Malaria Parasites *Plasmodium falciparum* and *Plasmodium vivax* and the Effects of Various Anti-malarial Drugs on *Plasmodium falciparum* Developing *in vitro*, MD thesis, University of Sydney, 1946.

——, Malaria as a military problem, Paper read at Royal Military College, Duntroon, 14 August 1963, Defence Central Library, Canberra, P616.89362 BLA.

——, 'Report on a visit, on behalf of the Department of Defence, made to Southeast Asia to observe and advise on malaria and other health matters affecting Australian service personnel in January 1966', Dept of Defence file 67/653, CRS A1946, 5 February 1966.

Blackburn, C. R. B., 'Observations on the development of resistance to vivax malaria', *Transactions of the Royal Society of Tropical Medicine and Hygiene*, vol. 42, 1948, pp. 117–62.

——, 'Sir Neil Hamilton Fairley', *Newsletter of the Royal Australasian College of Physicians*, vol. 2, 1969, p. 6.

——, 'Chemoprophylaxis of malaria—an exercise in problem solving', Address given at McMaster University, Hamilton, Ontario, 24 February 1977.

Board for the Co-ordination of Malarial Studies, 'Wartime research in malaria', *Science*, vol. 103, 1946, pp. 8–9.

Boyd, J., 'Neil Hamilton Fairley 1891–1966', *Biographical Memoirs of the Royal Society*, vol. 12, 1966, pp. 123–41.

Carson, P. E., Flanagan, C. L., Ickes, L. E. and Alving, A. L., 'Enzymatic deficiency in primaquine sensitive erythrocytes', *Science*, vol. 124, 1956, pp. 484–5.

Cheng, Q., Lawrence, G., Reed, C., Stowers, A., Ranford-Cartwright, L., Creasey, A., Carter, R. and Saul, A., 'Measurement of *Plasmodium falciparum* growth rates in vivo: A test of malaria vaccines', *American Journal of Tropical Medicine and Hygiene*, vol. 57, 1997, pp. 495–500.

Circular letter no. 153 from the Office of the Surgeon General USARMY, 'The drug treatment of malaria, suppressive and clinical', *Journal of the American Medical Association*, vol. 123, 1943, pp. 205–8.

Ciuca, M., Ballif, L., Chelarescu, M., Isanos, M. and Glaser, L., 'On drug prophylaxis in therapeutic malaria', *Transactions of the Royal Society of Tropical Medicine and Hygiene*, vol. 31, 1937, pp. 241–4.

Clark, W. M., 'History of the co-operative wartime program', in F. Y. Wiselogle (ed.), *A Survey of Antimalarial Drugs, 1941–1945*, Board for the Co-ordination of Malarial Studies, Washington DC, 1946, pp. 1–28.

Coatney, G. R., 'Pitfalls in a discovery: The chronicle of chloroquine', *American Journal of Tropical Medicine and Hygiene*, vol. 12, 1963, pp. 121–8.

Coatney, G. R. and Cooper, W. C., 'The prophylactic effect of sulfadiazine and sulfaguanidine against mosquito-borne *Plasmodium gallinaceum* in the domestic fowl', *Public Health Reports*, vol. 59, 1944, pp. 1455–8.

Coatney, G. R., Cooper, W. C. and Ruhe, D. S., 'Studies in human malaria. VI. The organisation of a program for testing potential antimalarial drugs in prisoner volunteers', *American Journal of Hygiene*, vol. 47, 1948, pp. 113–19.

Coatney, G. R., Cooper, W. C., Young, M. D. and McLendon, S. B., 'Studies in human malaria. I. The protective action of sulfadiazine and sulfapyrazine against sporozoite-induced falciparum malaria', *American Journal of Hygiene*, vol. 46, 1947, pp. 84–104.

Coatney, G. R., Ruhe, D. S., Cooper, W. C., Josephson, E. S. and Young, M. D., 'Studies in human malaria. X. The protective and therapeutic action of chloroquine (SN 7618) against St. Elizabeth strain vivax malaria', *American Journal of Hygiene*, vol. 49, 1949, pp. 49–59.

Coggleshall, L. T., Maier, J. and Best, C. A., 'The effectiveness of two new types of chemotherapeutic agents in malaria', *Journal of the American Medical Association*, vol. 117, 1941, pp. 1077–81.

Council on Pharmacy and Chemistry, 'Chloroquine, non proprietary name for SN-7618', *Journal of the American Medical Association*, vol. 130, 1946, p. 787.

Curd, F. H. S., 'The activity of drugs in the malaria of man, monkeys and birds', *Annals of Tropical Medicine and Parasitology*, vol. 37, 1943, pp. 115–43.

Curd, F. H. S., Davey, D. G. and Rose, F. L., 'Studies on synthetic antimalarial drugs. I. Biological methods', *Annals of Tropical Medical Parasitology*, vol. 39, 1945, pp. 139–56.

Curd, F. H. S., Davey, D. G. and Rose, F. L., 'Studies on synthetic antimalarial drugs. II. General chemical considerations', *Annals of Tropical Medical Parasitology*, vol. 39, 1945, pp. 157–64.

Edeson, J. F. B. and Field, J. W., 'Proguanil-resistant falciparum malaria in Malaya', *British Medical Journal*, vol. 1, 1950, pp. 47–152.

Ehrman, F. C., Ellis, J. M. and Young, M. D., '*Plasmodium vivax* Chesson strain', *Science*, vol. 101, 1945, p. 377.

Fairley, N. H., 'Chemotherapeutic suppression and prophylaxis in malaria: An experimental investigation undertaken by medical research teams in Australia', *Transactions of the Royal Society of Tropical Medicine and Hygiene*, vol. 38, 1945, pp. 311–65.

——, 'The chemotherapeutic control of malaria', *Schweizerische Medizinische Wochenschrift*, vol. 76, 1946, pp. 925–32.

Fairley, N. H., Blackburn, C. R., Andrew, R. R., Mackerras, M. J., Roberts, F. H. S., Allmann, S. L. W., Gregory, T. S., Backhouse, T. C., Tonge, J. I., Black, R. H., Pope,

K. G., Dunn, S. R., Swan, M. S. A., Akhurst, T. A. F. and Roberts, E. M., 'Sidelights on malaria in man obtained by subinoculation experiments', *Transactions of the Royal Society of Tropical Medicine and Hygiene*, vol. 40, 1947, pp. 621–76.

Fairley, N. H., Blackburn, C. R. B., Black, R. H., Gregory, T. S., Tonge, J. I., Pope, K. G., Dunn, S. R., Swan, M. S. A., Akhurst, T. A. F., Mackerras, I. M., Lemerle, T. H. and Ercole, Q. N., 'Researches on paludrine (M.4888) in Australia from the Land Headquarters, Medical Research Unit, Cairns', *Medical Journal of Australia*, vol. 1, 1946, pp. 234–6.

Fairley, N. H., Blackburn, C. R. B., Mackerras, I. M., Gregory, T. S., Black, R. H., Lemerle, T. H., Ercole, Q. N., Pope, K. G., Dunn, S. R., Swan, M. S. A., Akhurst, T. A. F., MacDonald, I. C. and Tonge, J. I., 'Atebrin susceptibility of the Aitape–Wewak strains of *P. falciparum* and *P. vivax*: A field and experimental investigation by L.H.Q. Medical Research Unit', *Transactions of the Royal Society of Tropical Medicine and Hygiene*, vol. 40, 1946, pp. 229–73.

Fairley, N. H., Blackburn, C. R. B., Mackerras, M. J., Gregory, T. S., Black, R. H., Lemerle, T. H., Ercole, Q. N., Pope, K. G., Dunn, S. R., Swan, M. S. A. and Ackhurst, T. A. F., 'Experiments with antimalarial drugs in man. VI. The value of chloroquine diphosphate as a suppressive drug in volunteers exposed to experimental mosquito-transmitted malaria (New Guinea strains)', *Transactions of the Royal Society of Tropical Medicine and Hygiene*, vol. 51, 1957, pp. 493–501.

Fairley, N. H., Blackburn, C. R. B., Mackerras, I. M., Gregory, T. S., Black, R. H., Lemerle, T. H., Ercole, Q. N., Pope, K. G., Dunn, S. R., Swan, M. S. A., Akhurst, T. A. F., MacDonald, I. C. and Tonge, J. I., 'Malaria in the South-West Pacific, with special reference to its chemotherapeutic control', *Medical Journal of Australia*, vol. 2, 1946, pp. 145–62.

Fairley, N. H., Blackburn, C. R. B., Mackerras, I. M., Gregory, T. S., Tonge, J. I., Black, R. H., Lemerle, T. H., Ercole, Q. N., Pope, K. G., Dunn, S. R., Swan, M. S. A., Akhurst, T. A. F., 'Researches on paludrine (M.4888) in malaria', *Transactions of the Royal Society of Tropical Medicine and Hygiene*, vol. 40, 1946, pp. 105–51.

Farid, M. A., 'The malaria programme—from euphoria to anarchy', *World Health Forum*, vol. 1, 1980, pp. 8–22.

Field, J. W., Strahan, J. H., Edeson, J. F. B. and Wilson, T., 'Studies on the chemotherapy of malaria. II. The treatment of acute malaria with proguanil (paludrine)', *Medical Journal of Malaya*, vol. 8, 1954, pp. 303–17.

Findlay, G. M., 'Investigations in the chemotherapy of malaria in West Africa. VI. "Suppressive cure" of malaria', *Annals of Tropical Medicine and Parasitology*, vol. 43, 1948, pp. 1–3.

Ford, E., 'Arthur E. Mills Memorial Oration of the Royal Australian College of Physicians', *Medical Journal of Australia*, vol. 2, 1969, pp. 991–6.

Greenwood, D., 'Conflicts of interest: The genesis of synthetic antimalarial agents in peace and war', *Journal of Antimicrobial Chemotherapy*, vol. 36, 1995, pp. 857–72.

Harinasuta, T., Migasen, S. and Boonnag, D., 'Chloroquine resistance in *Plasmodium falciparum* in Thailand', *UNESCO First Regional Symposium on Scientific Knowledge of Tropical Parasites*, Singapore, 1962, pp. 148–53.

James, S. P., 'Some general results of a study of induced malaria in England', *Transactions of the Royal Society of Tropical Medicine and Hygiene*, vol. 24, 1931, pp. 477–538.

James, S. P. and Tate, P., 'New knowledge on the life cycle of the malaria parasite', *Nature*, vol. 139, 1937, pp. 545–6.

Karwacki, J. J., Webster, H. K., Limsongwong, N. and Shanks, G. D., 'Two cases of mefloquine resistant malaria in Thailand', *Transactions of the Royal Society of Tropical Medicine and Hygiene*, vol. 83, 1989, pp. 152–3.

Keogh, E. V., 'Obituary, Neil Hamilton Fairley', *Medical Journal of Australia*, vol. 2, 1966, pp. 723–6.

Mackerras, I. M., 'Malaria in the South-West Pacific', *Medical Journal of Australia*, vol. 2, 1946, pp. 249–50.

——, 'Australia's contribution to our knowledge of insect-borne disease', *Medical Journal of Australia*, vol. 1, 1948, pp. 157–67.

Mackerras, I. F. M. and Aberdeen, J. E. C., 'A malaria survey at Wewak, New Guinea', *Medical Journal of Australia*, vol. 2, 1946, pp. 763–71.

Mackerras, M. J. and Ercole, Q. N., 'Observations on the life cycle of *Plasmodium malariae*', *Australian Journal of Experimental Medicine and Science*, vol. 26, 1948, pp. 515–19.

Mackerras, M. J. and Ercole, Q. N., 'Observations on the action of paludrine on malarial parasites', *Transactions of the Royal Society of Tropical Medicine and Hygiene*, vol. 41, 1948, pp. 365–76.

Mackerras, M. J. and Ercole, Q. N., 'Observations on the action of quinine, atebrin, and plasmoquin on *Plasmodium vivax*', *Transactions of the Royal Society of Tropical Medicine and Hygiene*, vol. 42, 1949, pp. 443–54.

Mackerras, M. J. and Ercole, Q. N., 'Observations on the action of quinine, atebrin, and plasmoquin on *Plasmodium falciparum*', *Transactions of the Royal Society of Tropical Medicine and Hygiene*, vol. 42, 1949, pp. 455–63.

Malaria Commission, 'Third General Report, Therapeutics of malaria', *Bulletin of the Health Organization of the League of Nations*, vol. 2, 1933, pp. 185–285.

——, 'Fourth General Report, Therapeutics of Malaria', *Bulletin of the Health Organization of the League of Nations*, vol. 6, 1937, pp. 897–1017.

Mendis, K. N., 'Malaria vaccine research—a game of chess', in G. A. T. Targett (ed.), *Malaria: Waiting for the Vaccine*, John Wiley & Sons, Chichester, 1991, pp. 183–96.

Moore, D. V. and Lanier, J. E., 'Observations on two *Plasmodium falciparum* infections with an abnormal response to chloroquine', *American Journal of Tropical Medicine and Hygiene*, vol. 10, 1961, pp. 5–9.

'More about paludrine', *British Medical Journal*, 15 June 1946, Editorial, pp. 919–20.

Most, H., 'Clinical trials of antimalarial drugs', in Medical Department, United States Army, *Internal Medicine in World War II: Vol. II, Infectious Diseases*, Office of the Surgeon General, Department of the Army, Washington DC, 1963, pp. 525–98.

'Neil Hamilton Fairley' Obituary, *Lancet*, vol. 1, 1966, pp. 987–8.

'Paludrine', *Medical Journal of Australia*, vol. 1, 1946, Editorial, p. 229.

Payne, D., 'Spread of chloroquine resistance in *Plasmodium falciparum*', *Parasitology Today*, vol. 3, 1988, pp. 241–6.

Proceedings of conference on certain aspects of prevention of disease in tropical warfare held at Atherton, Queensland on 12–13 June 1944, Australian War Memorial printed records, accession no. 616.936205 C748p.

Rieckmann, K. H., Davis, D. R. and Hutton, D. C., '*Plasmodium vivax* resistance to chloroquine?', *Lancet*, vol. 2, 1989, pp. 1183–4.

Rieckmann, K. H., Yeo, A. E. T., Davis, D. R., Hutton, D. C., Wheatley, P. F. and Simpson, R., 'Recent military experience with malaria chemoprophylaxis', *Medical Journal of Australia*, vol. 158, 1993, pp. 446–9.

Schmid, R., 'History of viral hepatitis: A tale of dogmas and misinterpretations', *Journal of Gastroenterology and Hepatology*, vol. 16, 2001, pp. 718–22.

Schmidt, L. H., Fradkin, R., Genther, C. S. and Hughes, H. B., 'Delineation of the potential of primaquine as a radical curative and prophylactic drug', *American Journal of Tropical Medicine and Hygiene*, vol. 31, 1982, Supplement, pp. 666–80.

Schreck, C. E. and Self, L. S., 'Bed nets that kill mosquitoes', *World Health Forum*, vol. 6, 1995, pp. 342–4.

Schulemann, W., 'Synthetic anti-malarial preparations', *Journal of the Proceedings of the Royal Society of Medicine*, vol. 25, 1932, pp. 897–904.

——, 'Retrospectives and perspectives of chemotherapy of malaria, *World Health Organization Geneva mimeographed document*, 1967, WHO/Mal/67.608.

Scott, H. V., Rieckmann, K. H. and O'Sullivan, W. J., 'Synergistic antimalarial activity of dapsone/dihydrofolate reductase inhibitors and the interaction of antifol, antipyrimidine and antipurine combinations against *Plasmodium falciparum in vitro*', *Transactions of the Royal Society of Tropical Medicine and Hygiene*, vol. 81, 1987, pp. 715–72.

Seaton, D. R. and Lourie, E. M., 'Acquired resistance to proguanil (paludrine) in *Plasmodium vivax*', *Lancet*, vol. 1, 1949, pp. 394–5.

Selby, C. H., 'Malaria in the South-West Pacific: Additional facts about malaria control in the Australian Military Forces', *Medical Journal of Australia*, vol. 2, 1946, pp. 249–50.

Shortt, H. E. and Garnham, P. C. C., 'The pre-erythrocytic development of *Plasmodium cynomolgi* and *Plasmodium vivax*', *Transactions of the Royal Society of Tropical Medicine and Hygiene*, vol. 41, 1948, pp. 785–95.

Shortt, H. E., Fairley, N. H., Covell, G., Shute, P. G. and Garnham, P. C. C., 'The pre-erythrocytic stage of *Plasmodium falciparum*', *British Medical Journal*, 5 November 1949, pp. 1006–8.

Shute, P. G., 'Thirty years of malaria therapy', *Journal of Tropical Medicine and Hygiene*, vol. 61, 1958, pp. 57–61.

Sinton, J. A., Smith, S. and Pottinger, S., 'Studies in malaria, with special reference to treatment. Part XII. Further researches into the treatment of chronic benign tertian malaria with plasmoquine and quinine', *Indian Journal of Medical Research*, vol. 17, 1930, pp. 793–814.

Smith, J., 'The transfusion of whole blood', *Australian and New Zealand Journal of Surgery*, vol. 10, 1941, pp. 384–92.

'This was our longest and dearest campaign', *Salt*, vol. 9, no. 1, Sept. 11 1944, pp. 10–14.

'Triumph against malaria', *British Medical Journal*, 10 November 1945, Editorial, pp. 653–4.

'The war, quinine and the medical profession in Australia', *Medical Journal of Australia*, vol. 2, 1942, Editorial, p. 83.

Wernsdorfer, W. H., 'The development of drug-resistant malaria', *Parasitology Today*, vol. 7, 1991, pp. 297–303.

Williamson, J., Bertram, D. S. and Lourie, E. M., 'Effects of paludrine and other antimalarials', *Nature*, vol. 159, 1947, pp. 885–6.

Wilson, T., Munro, D. S. and Richard, D. R., 'Proguanil resistance in Malayan strains of *P. vivax*', *British Medical Journal*, vol. 1, 1952, pp. 564–8.

World Health Organization, 'Chemotherapy of malaria', WHO Technical Report Series no. 376, Geneva, 1967.

——, 'Advances in malaria chemotherapy', WHO Technical Report Series no. 711, Geneva, 1984.

Yorke, W. and Macfie, J. W. S., 'Observations of malaria made during treatment of general paralysis', *Transactions of the Royal Society of Tropical Medicine and Hygiene*, vol. 18, 1924, pp. 13–44.

Index

Abbott Laboratories 256
Aberdeen, J. E. C., Major 178, 183
Adams, A. R. D., Dr 157, 160–1
Aitape–Wewak campaign: analysis of malaria epidemic 184–90, 269; area of operations 167–8; investigation of malaria cases in 168–83; *see also* Fairley, Brigadier Sir Neil Hamilton
Albert, Adrien, Dr 20, 22, 24, 26, 178
Alving, A. S., Dr 252–3
Anderson, J. H., Colonel 160, 196–200
Andrew, R. R., Lieutenant Colonel 43, 54–6, 64–5, 90–1, 223
Anopheles mosquitoes: *A. amictus* 60; *A. annulipes* 60; *A. farauti* 49, 60, 121; *A. hilli* 60; *A. punctulatus* 60, 121–3, 211; biting habits 27–8, 172; collections for experiments 49–50, 60, 121–3, 211; infecting for Australian experiments 50–2, 203; rearing and handling for experiments 41, 43, 49, 51–2, 232
Anti Malaria Advisory Committee, *see* Tropical Diseases Advisory Committee
antimalarial drugs: 4-amino-quinolines 105, 128, 148; 8-amino-quinolines 105, 150, 251–3; causal prophylactic, search for 38, 102, 149, 156; development by Germans 14, 104–6; post-war development in USA 252–3; screening with bird malaria 14, 38–9, 94, 96, 128, 149, 156–7; shipping difficulties 19, 22, 34; shortages of supplies 18–25; trials by Malaria Commission of the League of Nations 14–15; *see also* Australian experiments
A-S drugs, *see* sulphonamides
A-S I, *see* sulphamerazine
A-S II, *see* sulphamezathine
A-S III, *see* sulphadiazine
atebrin: Australian experiments 55–8, 64–7, 90; blood levels 63–4, 70–2, 79, 119–20; compliance in taking 80, 170, 174, 186, 188, 243; dosages 62–3; effects on blood stages 204; for prophylaxis 23, 36, 44, 58, 62, 79–81, 83–5, 101, 159, 170–2, 186, 239, 241, 243; for treatment 150–1; malaria resistance to 175–6, 179, 182–5, 188, 269; misinformation about 83–5, 110; shortages of supplies 22–5, 33–4; side-effects 22, 62, 73, 75, 80; synthesis by Germans 14; *see also* chloroquine; Japanese forces; sontochin
Australian Army units: Army Malaria Institute 267; Army Malaria Research Unit 267, 270; 11 Australian Army Malaria Control Unit 49; 5 Australian Camp Hospital 42–4, 50, 67–8; 2/2 Australian General Hospital 43, 45, 87–8, 116, 231; 116 Australian General Hospital 68, 226–7; 2 Australian Mobile Entomological Section 49; 6 Australian Mobile Entomological Section 122; 2/22 Battalion 1, 3–4, 6, 85, 245; 2/1 Convalescent Depot 116, 226, 230–3; 1 Malaria Research Laboratory 267
Australian Department of Veterans' Affairs 234, 236
Australian experiments: benefits of results for Allied forces 243–5, 253–4; blood-induced malaria 46, 111; command and control 42, 98; comments in press 83, 196–202, 225–6, 258–63; field-type, *see* long-term experiments; high-altitude simulation 73–4, 79; *in vitro* cultivation of *Plasmodium falciparum* 206–7; long-term experiments 65, 68–70, 78, 124, 139–40, 193, 233–4; on differences between *Plasmodium vivax* and *P. falciparum* tissue phases 90–3; on immunity to *P. vivax* 214–22; on mode of action of antimalarial drugs 204–13; on *Plasmodium malariae* 210–11; on time that sporozoites remain in the blood 88–90;

348

plan at Cairns 45, 47, 50, 61; plan at Rocky Creek 46–7; sporozoite-induced 46–7, 111, 203, 232; subinoculation 87–93, 120, 127, 163, 231, 270; *see also Anopheles* mosquitoes; atebrin, chloroquine; diamodine stilbene; M.4430; malaria; paludrine; plasmoquine; quinine; sontochin; sulphonamides
Australian Repatriation Commission 245–8

Backhouse, T. C., Major 44, 60
Baldwin, A. H., Wing Commander 33, 73
Bancroft, Joseph 48
Bancroft, Thomas 48
Bang, Frederick, First Lieutenant 63–4
Bass, C. C. 206
Bayer Laboratories, Elberfeld 14, 104–5
Bayne-Jones, S., Colonel 71
Bean, C. E. W. 11
Berryman, Frank, Major General 48, 81
Best, C. A., Dr 39
Biggam, A. G., Major General 21, 158
Birch, A. R., Private 212
bird malaria 12, 37; *see also* antimalarial drugs, screening with bird malaria
Bishop, Ann, Dr 38
Bishopp, Fred C., Dr 115–17, 132
Black, R. H., Captain 205–7, 212–13, 265–6
Blackburn, C. R. B., Lieutenant Colonel 34, 65–6, 68, 70–1, 88, 91, 119–20, 125, 133, 139, 153, 162, 174–5, 177, 203, 212–28 *passim*, 234, 242, 247–9
Bladon, D. I., Private 212
Blake, Francis, Dr 116
Blamey, Thomas, General 30–1, 33, 175, 177
Blanchard, Kenneth 104, 129–30, 250
Blesse, F., Brigadier General 106
Board for the Co-ordination of Malarial Studies, USA: Chesson strain, isolation of 141–3, 146; chloroquine, decision for accelerated development of 130–1; conference for a review of the wartime program 101–3; drug screening in birds, problems with 94–6; formation of 39, 59–60; human testing, lack of facilities for 96–100; malaria mission to South West Pacific Area 115–17; problems in liaison with British Medical Research Council 254–6; proposal to import Australian experimental strain to USA 140–1; reorganisation and specialist panels 96; request for Australian trials of sontochin and chloroquine 112–14, 126–7, 132–3; scope and achievements of wartime program 251; selection of drugs for human tests 100–3;

Index 349

staff shortages 97–8; survey numbers for drug designation 104
Boots company 23
Boyd, J. S. K., Colonel 16–17, 40
Boyd, M. F., Dr 138
Bretherton, R. V., Lieutenant Colonel 44
British Medical Research Council 38, 156, 158; problems in liaison with Board for the Co-ordination of Malarial Studies, USA 254–6; request for Australian tests of paludrine 161, 198; *see also* paludrine
British wartime malaria program: formation of 156–7; *see also* Imperial Chemical Industries; human testing, lack of facilities for 158; *see also* paludrine; plasmoquine; sulphonamides
Brockhurst, J. H., Sergeant 210
Brodie, B. B. 63, 183
Bruce, Stanley M. 23
Burbidge, B. E., Captain 44
Burgess, Robert W., Dr 99
Burston, S. R., Major General 32–4, 81–2, 161, 175, 200–1, 241
Bush, Vannevar 98
Butler, T. C., Dr 132

Cameron, D. A., Sergeant 60
Carden, G. A. 96, 98, 103, 109, 255–6
Carr, H. H., Lieutenant Colonel 1, 3
Chesson strain (of vivax malaria) 141–3, 146, 155, 252–3
Chittleborough, A. R., Private 226–7
chloroquine: Australian experiments 135–6, 144–6; efficacy against atebrin-resistant malaria 189; malaria resistance to 265, 267; naming by Americans 250–1; patents 129–30; synthesis by Germans 105, 250; toxicity 105, 129, 131–2, 134–5; US experiments 128, 129, 132, 144–6, 250; *see also* Board for the Co-ordination of Malarial Studies, USA
Christison, Lieutenant General 244
Christophers, Sir (Samuel) Rickard 158
Churchill, Winston 23
Cinchona 12
Ciuca, M. 37
Clark, W., Mansfield, Dr 96, 106–7, 118
Clarke, K. R., Private 212
Coatney, G. Robert, Dr 39, 58, 60, 96, 99, 108, 111, 114, 118, 138, 143, 253–4
Coggleshall, L. C., Dr 39, 133–4, 148–9
Combined Advisory Committee on Tropical Medicine, Hygiene, and Sanitation 33–4, 41, 59, 64, 82

350 Index

Commander-in-Chief's Card 234–5
Conference of Chemotherapy of Malaria, *see* Board for the Co-ordination of Malarial Studies, USA
Cook, C. E., Major 81
Cooper, W. C., Dr 39
Covell, G., Brigadier 243
Crowley, Leo 21–2
Curd, F. H. S., Dr 156–7
Curtin, John 31, 34–5, 66
cycloguanil 270

Dale, Sir Henry 254–5
dapsone 266, 270
Davey, D. G., Dr 156–7, 160–1, 200–1
Davey, T. H., Professor 159
Davies, H. E., Staff Sergeant 212
DDT 109, 178, 268
Decourt, P., Dr 105
diamadino stilbene, Australian experiments 125
Dieuaide, Francis, R., Lieutenant Colonel 101, 121, 143, 151
Dixon, Sir Owen 21
donors: criteria for selection 45; recruitment 43; transport arrangements from New Guinea to Cairns 47–8
Downie, Ewen, Colonel 109, 111–4, 118, 128, 132–3, 140, 256
doxycycline 267
Duncan, Sir Andrew 24
Dunn, S. R., Lieutenant 212
Dupont company 254–5

Earle, D. P., Dr 98
Emerson, G. V., Colonel 142
English, J. C., Lieutenant Colonel 81, 177
erion, *see* atebrin
erythrocytes 13

Fairley, Brigadier Sir Neil Hamilton: as Chairman of Combined Advisory Committee on Tropical Medicine, Hygiene, and Sanitation 33, 64; as mediator between US and British malaria workers 254, 257; early research in Australia, India and England 15; investigation of Aitape–Wewak epidemic 175–8, 182; involvement in recruitment of volunteers 224, 228–9, 243; involvement with Earle Page enquiry on malaria 34–5; personality and leadership 242–3; post-war appointments 248, 259, 270; post-war illness 253, 270; presentations of Cairns results 78–81, 158–9, 177, 183–4, 241; quinine mission to Java 18–19; response to press reports on paludrine 199–201; service in Middle East during World War II 16–17; service in World War I 15; visits (to Cairns) 34, 51, 54–5, 74, 77, 121, 125, 176–7, (to New Guinea) 27–8, 47, 55, 177, 183, (to South East Asia Command) 165, 175, (to Sydney) 34, 42, (to USA and UK) 20–5, 124–6, 147–9, 152, 158–61
Fenner, E. M. B., Captain 87, 123
Fenner, Frank, Major 122, 174
Findlay, G. M., Dr 40
Fisher, H. M., Colonel 170–1
Fitzherbert, Patrick, Corporal 125
Florey, Howard, Dr 255
Ford, E., Lieutenant Colonel 21, 30, 32, 44, 67, 75, 122, 242, 271
Forde, Frank 258
Fraser, J. M., Senator 258
Friend, Donald, Gunner 230–2
Fryberg, A., Major 51

gametocyte carriers, *see* donors
gametocytes 13, 151; infectivity for mosquitoes 203–4; *see also* paludrine; plasmoquine
Garnham, P. C. C., Professor 268
Geiling, E. M. K., Dr 106, 128
German synthesis and development 14, 105, 156–7, 250; *see also* Nuremburg Code
Glover, K. G., Private 233–4
Gore, R. E., Corporal 44, 125
Goulston, S. J. M., Major 160, 192
Gregory, T. S., Major 60, 212

Hairston, Nelson, Second Lieutenant 63
Hakansson, E. G., Captain 58, 131
Harris, T., Father 7
Hastings, Dr 109
Helsinki Declaration 236–8
Hendersen, L. T. E., Private 238
Heyden, George, Dr 41, 49
Heysen, Nora, Captain 232
Holmes, M. J., Colonel 33, 116
Hughes, Gary 261

ICI, *see* Imperial Chemical Industries
Imperial Chemical Industries 23–5, 38, 156–7, 254–6, 259–61; *see also* paludrine

Jaboor, R. F., Lieutenant Colonel 174
Jacobs, W. A., Dr 106
James, S. P., Colonel 37, 86, 92, 150, 152, 158–9, 238

Jamieson, Sir William 24
Japanese forces: atebrin use by 187; malaria problem in 239; Milne Bay landing 29; New Guinea north coast landing 28; Rabaul landing 3
Joekes, M., Flight Lieutenant 162

Keilin, Professor 38
Kellaway, Charles, Dr 15, 111
Keogh, E. V., Colonel 30, 41, 44, 161, 195, 206, 243
Kikuth, Walter 14, 105
King, Harold, Dr 255–6
King, R., Brigadier 183
Kirk, N. T., General 97

Laird, R. L., Dr 141
Landsborough Thomson, A., Dr 198, 200
lariam, *see* mefloquine
Laurabada yacht 8, 9
League of Nations, Malaria Commission 14–15
Ledger, Charles 14
Lee, D. J. 109
Lemerle, T. H., Lieutenant 121–2, 125
Leverholme, Lord 197–8
LHQ Medical Research Unit: establishment 61; conversion to AIF 61; relocation to Jungara 67–8; visit of US Malaria Mission 116
lichen planus 75; *see also* atebrin, side-effects
Lippmann, Henry 262
Lloyd, C. E. M., Major General 78
Loeb, R. F., Dr 96–7, 101, 103, 112, 114, 116, 140–1, 257

M.3349 157, 197, 254; *see also* paludrine
M.4430 158, 162, 197; Australian experiments 194–5
M.4888, *see* paludrine
MacArthur, Douglas, General 33, 35, 41, 75, 83, 116
McCoy, O. R., Major 101
Macdonald, I. C., Major 178
Macfie, J. W. S. 37, 92
McIntyre, Admiral 21
Mackerras, I. M., Lieutenant Colonel 27, 33, 41, 48, 108–13, 125, 129, 138, 175, 177–8, 184–9
Mackerras, M. J., Major 48–9, 52, 121, 123, 177, 203–4, 207–8, 211, 213
McNamara, J. W., Staff Sergeant 210
Maegraith, B., Lieutenant Colonel 159, 196, 198, 200, 202
Maier, John, Dr 39, 105

Maierhofer, Father 5
Maitland, G. B. G., Brigadier 66, 171–2, 177, 189
malaria: blackwater fever 15, 75–6, 230; cerebral 8, 16, 80, 85, 190; characterisation by Hippocrates 11–12; drug resistance 175, 179, 182–3, 184–5, 264–9; during World War I 10–11, 16; during World War II, in South West Pacific Area and South East Asia Command 6–7, 9, 28–31, 77–8, 239, 243–4, *see also* Aitape–Wewak campaign; immunity 63, 214, *see also* Australian experiments; in Australian troops (during Malayan Emergency) 265, (during Vietnam War) 265–6; in birds, *see* bird malaria; in Japanese Army 239; in monkeys 39, 253, *see also Plasmodium cynomolgi*; incidence in returned troops 244; manpower wastage due to 32; personal protection against 27–8, 33, 35, 78, 81, 172, 240–1, 243, *see also* mosquito control; *Plasmodium falciparum* cycle in humans 47, 92–3; *Plasmodium vivax* relapses 47, 92–3, 137–9, 144–6; therapy for treatment of syphilis 37, 96–8, 214, *see also* US experiments; tissue phase 37–8, 86, 102, 268–9; transmission cycle in humans and mosquitoes 12–13; treatment of demobilised troops 245–8; *see also* paludrine
Malaria Commission of the League of Nations 14–15
malaria parasites, *see Plasmodium* parasites
Malaria Experimental Group: decision to establish at Cairns 42; entomology laboratory 50; establishment at 5 Australian Camp Hospital 42–4, 50, 67–8; proposal to establish at University of Sydney 41–2
Marshall, E. K., Dr 94, 96, 101, 105–7, 112–13, 118, 134, 148–9, 252
Martin, J. E. G., Brigadier 176, 183
Marvel, C. S., Dr 131
Mascot launch 8
Maud, Sir John 24
Mauss, H. 14
May & Baker 23–4
mefloquine 267
Mellanby, Sir Edward 161, 254–5, 257
mepacrine, *see* atebrin
Merck & Co. 255
merozoites 13
methaemalbumin 15
Mietzsch, F. 14
Morgan, Hugh, Brigadier General 131, 141–2
Morris, B. M., Major General 28

Morshead, Leslie, Lieutenant General   77
mosquito control   32–3, 35, 36, 78, 81, 178; nets   3, 20, 27, 31, 35, 81, 172, 240, 243, 268; netting   20, 25; repellents   20, 35, 109, 172, 240, 243
mosquitoes *see Anopheles* mosquitoes
Mote, Dr   23–4
Moten, M. J., Brigadier   183

National Research Council, USA   39
neostam   125
Nickerson, W. H. S., Major General   10
Nicole, W. D.   150
National Institutes of Health: NIH 204   100; NIH 700   100
Noad, K. B., Lieutenant Colonel   66
Nuremburg Code   236–8

Office of Research and Development   98
oocysts   13, 207, 209–10
ookinetes   13
O'Sullivan, P., Staff Sergeant   49
Owen, W. T., Major   6–7

Packer, Henry, Dr   97
Page, Sir Earle   34, 41, 66
Palmer, E. C. Major   3–9 *passim*
paludrine: Australian experimental plan   160–3; Australian experiments   163–6, 191–4, 211–13; blood levels   195–6; British experiments   161–2, 198–9; effect on gametocytes   204–5; effects on blood stages   204; effects on mosquito infections   207–10; efficacy against atebrin-resistant malaria   188; for treatment of demobilised troops   246–8; malaria resistance to   264–5; name confusion with M.3349   197, 259; press reports   196–202, 259; synthesis and development by ICI   159, 160; toxicity data   192
pamaquine, *see* plasmoquine
Paris green   33
penicillin   81, 255
pentaquine   252
Peruvian bark   12
Pinchoffs, Maurice, G., Colonel   59, 63–4, 82, 116
Plasmodium parasites: *P. cathemerium*   94, 128, 157–8; *P. cynomolgi*   253, 269; *P. falciparum*, 12, 92, *see also* Australian experiments, and malaria, cycle in humans; *P. gallinaceum*   39, 95, 128, 157–8; *P. knowlesi*   39; *P. lophurae*   94, 106, 128, 158, 252; *P. malariae*   12, 210–11, *see also* Australian experiments; *P. ovale*   12; *P. relictum*   14, 38, 156, 158; *P. vivax*   12, 214–22, *see also* Australian experiments; malaria, *Plasmodium vivax* relapses
plasmoquin E, *see* atebrin
plasmoquine: activity against gametocytes of *Plasmodium falciparum*   14, 151; as causal prophylactic   150, 154–5; Australian experiments   152–5; development by Germans   14; experimental plan for Cairns experiments   153–4; experiments in USA   152, 155; for treatment of demobilised troops   246–8; Indian and British tests   14, 150, 152, 155; shortages of supplies   19; toxicity   14, 150, 153, 165, 237, 247
Pope, K. G., Lieutenant   71, 212
press reports   83, 196–202, 225–6, 258–63
primaquine   253, 265–6
Priority NEILL   48, 224
pyrethrum   25
pyrimethamine   266

QAP therapy   47, 66, 151, 185–6, 215, 231–2, 247–8
quinacrine, *see* atebrin
quinine: Australian experiments   74, 78, 144; early use of   12, 14; effects on blood stages   204; experiments in USA   108, 144; for prophylaxis   28, 73–4, 190; for treatment   3–9, 15, 34, 74–6, 247–8; shortages of supplies   18–25

Ratcliffe, Francis, Major   60, 133
Read, G., Major   168–70
red blood cells   13
Reid, J., Major   162
Repatriation Medical Authority   263
resochin, *see* chloroquine
Rhône-Poulenc company   105
Richards, A. N., Dr   116, 254
Rivers, Captain   110
Roberts, F. H. S., Captain   49
Roehl, Wilhelm   14, 156–7
Roosevelt, Franklin   21, 98
Rose, F. L., Dr   156
Ross, Ronald, Captain   12
Russell, P. F., Lieutenant Colonel   58
Ryle, Gerald   261

Salter, D. M., Colonel   177
SB, *see* sontochin
Scanlan, J. J., Colonel   2–3

Schaudinn, Fritz 37, 86
schizonts 13
Schmidt, Leon, Dr 129, 252
Schneider, J., Dr 106–7, 113
Schonhofer, F. 14, 105
Schuleman, W. 14
Scott, Bruce 263
Scott, C. M., Dr 161, 198, 257
Sebrell, W. H., Dr 96, 99, 131
Selby, C. H., Lieutenant Colonel 174–5, 185–6
Selby, D. M., Lieutenant 7–8
Shannon, James A. Dr 58, 60, 96, 101–3, 107–9, 111–12, 114, 118, 129, 132, 134, 137–8, 148–9, 151, 155, 253–4, 257
Shortt, H. E., Colonel 268
Shute, P. G. 150, 162
Simmons, J. S., Brigadier 63, 97, 251
Sinton, J. A., Brigadier 14, 150, 158, 160, 165, 175–7, 244, 268
Sioli, F. 14, 105, 250
Small, L. F., Dr 39
Smart, Edward K., Lieutenant General 25
Smibert, R. S., Lieutenant Colonel 171, 174–5
Smith, Julian, Dr 87
SN-13,276 *see* pentaquine
SN-183 *see* sontochin
SN-6911 *see* sontochin
SN-7618 *see* chloroquine
sontochin: Australian experiments 120, 123–7, 144–6; efficacy against atebrin-resistant malaria 189; experiments in USA 106–8, 112, 144–6; plans for Australian experiments 115, 118–20; provision to Australians of toxicological data 117–18; synthesis and development by Germans 105–6; toxicity 105, 129, 131; Tunisian field trials by Vichy French 105–7, 131; *see also* Board for the Co-ordination of Malarial Studies, USA
sontoquine, *see* sontochin
Southworth, Hamilton, Dr 151, 254
sporozoites 13; *see also* Australian experiments
SS *Dunera* 260, 262
SS *Klang* 18–19
SS *Orcades* 18
Steigrad, J., Brigadier 75
Stevens, J. E., Major General 167, 169, 177, 189
Sturdee, V. A. H., Lieutenant General 77, 82, 241
sulphadiazine 42, 44, 100, 108
sulphaguanidine 16, 40, 60, 81

sulphamerazine 40, 42
sulphamezathine 38, 40, 42, 231
sulphapyrazine 40, 60
sulphonamides: Australian experiments 46, 53–8, 64–5, 90; development of plans for tests in Australia 40–2; experiments in USA and Britain 38–40, 58–60, 100, 108
Survey of Antimarial Drugs 104–5
Suter, C. M., Dr 256
Sutton, Harvey, Professor 41
Swan, M. S. A., Lieutenant 44, 70–1, 73
Sydenham, T. 12

Taggart, J. V., Dr 98
Taliaferro, W. H., Dr 95
Tate, P. 37, 86
Thomas, Henry M., Colonel 116
Tonge, J. I., Major 178, 212
Torti, F. 12
Trager, William, First Lieutenant 63, 70
Tropical Diseases Advisory Committee 33, 53–5

Udenfriend, S. J. 63, 183
US experiments: blood-induced 96, 99, 129; in prisoner volunteers 99, 111, 252; on 8-amino-quinolines 251–3; sporozoite-induced 96–7, 99, 144–6; using malaria therapy patients 96–9, 111, 129, 141; *see also* Board for the Co-ordination of Malarial Studies, USA; chloroquine; Fairley, Brigadier Sir Neil Hamilton; LHQ Medical Research Unit; National Research Council, USA; plasmoquine; quinine; sontochin; sulphonamides; Winthrop Chemical Company, New York

Viant, E. E., Corporal 232–3, 235, 238
volunteers: contribution to solving the malaria problem 238; criteria for selection 44–5, 228–9; ethical considerations 236–8; extra leave 223, 226; memorial at Rocky Creek 238; personal experiences 230–4; recruitment 43, 51, 223–9; repatriation benefits, ineligibility for 234–6; shortages of 164, 212, 224, 227–8, 243; sickness with malaria 223–4, 233–4, 238; supervision at drug parades 72–3, 224
Von Jauregg, Wagner, Professor 36

Warburton, Mr 21–2
Ward, H. K., Professor 20, 41–2
Waterhouse, D. F., Captain 109

Watson, Robert B., Dr 97, 115–17, 132, 139, 141–3
Wavell, Archibald, Commander-in-Chief 16–17
Weed, L. H. 97
Weir, Sir Cecil 24–5
West, R. F. K., Lieutenant Colonel 172, 177
Westmoreland, William, General 266
Whiteley, R. W., Corporal 233–4
Wilson, Sir Charles 23
Windeyer, W. J. V., Brigadier 81
Wingler, A. 14
Winterbottom, W. J., Warrant Officer Class 2 69, 124, 212, 224, 233
Winthrop Chemical Company, New York 105–7, 113, 129–30, 133, 256–7, 260
Wiselogle, Frederick, Dr 104
Wood, I. J., Lieutenant Colonel 42, 46
Woodhill, A. R., Captain 49, 109

Yorke, Warrington, Professor 21, 37, 92, 156
Young, Martin D., Dr 99, 142